**A Clinical Guide to
Urologic Emergencies**

A Clinical Guide to Urologic Emergencies

Edited by

Hunter Wessells, MD, FACS
Professor and Nelson Chair of Urology
Department of Urology
University of Washington School of Medicine
Seattle, WA, USA

Shigeo Horie, MD, PhD
Professor and Chairman
Department of Urology
Juntendo University Graduate School of Medicine
Tokyo, Japan

Reynaldo G. Gómez, MD, FACS
Chief of Urology
Hospital del Trabajador
Santiago, Chile

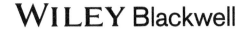

Registered Offices
John Wiley & Sons, Inc., 111 River Street, Hoboken, NJ 07030, USA
John Wiley & Sons Ltd, The Atrium, Southern Gate, Chichester, West Sussex, PO19 8SQ, UK

Editorial Office
9600 Garsington Road, Oxford, OX4 2DQ, UK

For details of our global editorial offices, customer services, and more information about Wiley products visit us at www.wiley.com.

Wiley also publishes its books in a variety of electronic formats and by print-on-demand. Some content that appears in standard print versions of this book may not be available in other formats.

Library of Congress Cataloging-in-Publication Data
Names: Wessells, Hunter, editor. | Horie, Shigeo, 1960– editor. | Gómez,
    Reynaldo Guillermo, editor.
Title: A clinical guide to urologic emergencies / edited by Hunter
    Wessells, Shigeo Horie, Reynaldo Guillermo Gómez.
Description: Hoboken, NJ : Wiley-Blackwell, [2021] | Includes
    bibliographical references and index.
Identifiers: LCCN 2020040342 (print) | LCCN 2020040343 (ebook) | ISBN
    9781119021476 (cloth) | ISBN 9781119021483 (Adobe PDF) | ISBN
    9781119021490 (epub)
Subjects: MESH: Male Urogenital Diseases | Urogenital System–injuries |
    Emergencies
Classification: LCC RC874.8 (print) | LCC RC874.8 (ebook) | NLM WJ 140 |
    DDC 616.6/025–dc23
LC record available at https://lccn.loc.gov/2020040342
LC ebook record available at https://lccn.loc.gov/2020040343

Cover Design: Wiley
Cover Images: X-ray and ultrasound images © Hunter Wessells, Image of the kidneys and their association with adjacent organs © Daniel Burke, University of Washington

Set in 9.5/12.5pt STIXTwoText by SPi Global, Pondicherry, India

10 9 8 7 6 5 4 3 2 1

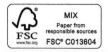

Dedication

To all those who served in the COVID-19 pandemic and to those we lost.

To the patients, students, residents, fellows and colleagues at UW Medicine and Harborview who contributed to the knowledge in this volume, as well as my family for their unwavering support. H.W.

To my patients, colleagues, and students past, present and future. To my family for their support. To my mentors of emergency medicine, Drs. Mii, Toyooka and Morita for enlightening and inspiring me. S.H.

To my parents for the effort they put into my education, my masters for guiding my curiosity, my patients for their trust, my hospital's staff support along over 35 years and my family for their patience and for inspiring my work. R.G.G.

Contents

List of Contributors   *ix*
Preface   *xii*
List of Abbreviations   *xiv*
About the Companion Website   *xviii*

Section I   Upper Urinary Tract   *1*

1   Blunt Renal Injuries   *3*
Lindsay A. Hampson and Nnenaya Mmonu

2   Penetrating Renal Trauma: A Civilian and Military Perspective   *25*
Jonathan Wingate

3   Renal Infections   *40*
Brusabhanu Nayak, Nitin Srivastava, and Rajeev Kumar

4   Acute Kidney Stone Management   *64*
Justin S. Ahn and Jonathan D. Harper

5   Traumatic Adrenal Hemorrhage   *83*
Hong Truong and Bradley D. Figler

6   External Ureteral Trauma   *91*
Humberto G. Villarreal and Steven J. Hudak

7   Iatrogenic Ureteral Injury   *105*
Haruaki Kato, Kazuyoshi Iijima, Tomohiko Oguchi, and Seiji Yano

Section II   Lower Urinary Tract   *117*

8   Bladder Injuries   *119*
Yosuke Nakajima

9 Traumatic Urethral Injuries *126*
Laura G. Velarde and Reynaldo G. Gómez

10 Acute Management of Urethral Stricture *144*
Akio Horiguchi

11 Prostatitis and Prostatic Abscess *158*
Hunter Wessells

Section III External Genitalia *165*

12 Fournier's Gangrene *167*
Kosuke Kitamura and Shigeo Horie

13 Traumatic Penile Injuries *179*
Ariel Fredrick and Alex J. Vanni

14 Priapism *189*
Akash A. Kapadia, Kevin Ostrowski, and Thomas J. Walsh

15 Traumatic Scrotal and Testicular Injuries *202*
Marios Hadjipavlou and Davendra Sharma

16 Testicular Torsion *216*
Alexander J. Skokan and Dana A. Weiss

17 Epididymitis and Orchitis *232*
Norman Zambrano and Juan Fullá

Section IV Pediatric *245*

18 Urologic Neonatal Emergencies *247*
Nicolas Fernandez and Nayib Fakih

Section V COVID-19 *271*

19 Urologic Emergency Care in the COVID-19 Pandemic Era *273*
Rishi R. Sekar, Sarah K. Holt, Joseph Meno, Rachel McKenzie, and Hunter Wessells

Index *280*

List of Contributors

Justin S. Ahn
Department of Urology, UCSF School of
Medicine, San Francisco, CA, USA

Nayib Fakih
Division of Urology, Hospital Universitario
San Ignacio, Pontificia Universidad
Javeriana, Bogota, Colombia

Nicolas Fernandez
Division of Pediatric Urology, Seattle
Children's Hospital, University of
Washington, Seattle, WA, USA

Bradley D. Figler
Department of Urology, University of
North Carolina-Chapel Hill, Chapel
Hill, NC, USA

Ariel Fredrick
Lahey Hospital and Medical Center,
Lahey Institute of Urology at Portsmouth
and Rochester, Portsmouth and
Rochester, NH, USA

Dr. Juan Fullá
Clinica Las Condes, Las Condes, Chile

Reynaldo G. Gómez
Urology Service, Hospital del Trabajador,
Santiago, Chile

Marios Hadjipavlou
Guy's Hospital, London, UK

Lindsay A. Hampson
Department of Urology, UCSF School
of Medicine, San Francisco, CA, USA

Jonathan D. Harper
Department of Urology, University
of Washington School of Medicine,
Seattle, WA, USA

Sarah K. Holt
Department of Urology, University
of Washington School of Medicine,
Seattle, WA, USA

Shigeo Horie
Department of Urology, Juntendo
University Graduate School of Medicine,
Tokyo, Japan

Akio Horiguchi
Department of Urology, National Defense
Medical College, Tokorozawa, Japan

Steven J. Hudak
UT Southwestern Medical Center,
Dallas, TX, USA

Kazuyoshi Iijima
Department of Urology, Nagano Municipal
Hospital, Nagano, Japan

Akash A. Kapadia
Department of Urology, University
of Washington School of Medicine,
Seattle, WA, USA

Haruaki Kato
Department of Urology, Nagano Municipal
Hospital, Nagano, Japan

Kosuke Kitamura
Department of Urology, Juntendo
University Graduate School of Medicine,
Tokyo, Japan

Rajeev Kumar
All India Institute of Medical Sciences,
New Delhi, India

Rachel McKenzie
Department of Urology, University
of Washington School of Medicine,
Seattle, WA, USA

Joseph Meno
Department of Urology, University
of Washington School of Medicine,
Seattle, WA, USA

Nnenaya Mmonu
Department of Urology, UCSF School of
Medicine, San Francisco, CA, USA

Yosuke Nakajima
Kawasaki Municipal Ida Hospital,
Kawasaki, Japan

Brusabhanu Nayak
All India Institute of Medical Sciences,
New Delhi, India

Tomohiko Oguchi
Department of Urology, Nagano Municipal
Hospital, Nagano, Japan

Kevin Ostrowski
Department of Urology, University
of Washington School of Medicine,
Seattle, WA, USA

Rishi R. Sekar
Department of Urology, University
of Washington School of Medicine,
Seattle, WA, USA

Davendra Sharma
St George's Hospital, London, UK

Alexander J. Skokan
Harborview Medical Center, University
of Washington School of Medicine,
Seattle, WA, USA

Nitin Srivastava
All India Institute of Medical Sciences,
New Delhi, India

Hong Truong
Department of Urology, Thomas
Jefferson University Hospital,
Philadelphia, PA, USA

Alex J. Vanni
Center for Reconstructive
Urologic Surgery, Lahey Hospital
and Medical Center, Burlington,
MA, USA

Laura G. Velarde
Urology Service, Hospital del Trabajador,
Santiago, Chile

Humberto G. Villarreal
Loma Linda University Medical Center,
Loma Linda, CA, USA

Thomas J. Walsh
Department of Urology, University
of Washington School of Medicine,
Seattle, WA, USA

Dana A. Weiss
The Children's Hospital of Philadelphia,
Philadelphia, PA, USA

Hunter Wessells
Department of Urology, University
of Washington School of Medicine,
Seattle, WA, USA

Jonathan Wingate
Madigan Army Medical Center,
Tacoma, WA, USA

Seiji Yano
Department of Urology, Nagano Municipal
Hospital, Nagano, Japan

Norman Zambrano
Clinica Las Condes, Las Condes, Chile

Preface

A Clinical Guide to Urologic Emergencies

The burden of urological disease worldwide is driven by a range of common conditions, some of which impair health acutely and others through chronic pathophysiological processes. Urological emergencies, when untreated, can lead to death, permanent disability, and lifelong reductions in quality of life. History is replete with examples including urinary stone disease in ancient Egypt and descriptions of combat wounds by Ambrose Pare in the Renaissance; this book will highlight common indications for acute urological intervention as well the emergence of unforeseen mechanisms of injury such as necrotizing genital skin infections associated with the introduction of novel sodium-glucose cotransporter 2 (SGLT2) inhibitors for diabetes and the contemporary battlefield injuries of such immense complexity as to require the re-engineering of military care.

Variation in population demographics, access to care, workforce capacity, and technology have a profound effect on how a given segment of the population will experience illness. The Global Burden of Disease, a tool to quantify health loss from hundreds of diseases, injuries, and risk factors, demonstrates that the determinants of health vary greatly by geography, whether continent-, country-, or county-level. These disparities have been brought into sharper focus by the pandemic of COVID-19, which exerts a disproportionate impact on individuals from minority populations in the United States and worldwide. These same at-risk populations also shoulder an excess burden of disease due to war, cyclic violence, road traffic injuries, and diseases for which access to emergency care is essential.

Population growth worldwide, changing epidemiology of disease, and human migration and displacement will exacerbate emergency urological needs across the lifespan and across the spectrum of global wealth. For healthcare providers in high income countries (HIC), motor vehicle collisions, obstructing urinary calculi, urinary tract infections (UTI), and the cumulative burden of urological diseases associated with aging and comorbid chronic disease such as diabetes and cardiovascular disease will drive urgent and emergent healthcare utilization. Urological surgery to improve health in low and middle-income countries (LMIC) has a critical focus on the broader impact of road traffic accidents, urethral stricture, advanced benign prostatic obstruction and genitourinary infections. The Lancet Commission on Global Surgery achieved consensus that HIC actors should work in equal partnership with LMIC actors and should situate efforts to improve the delivery of surgical care within the broader health systems strengthening agenda.

The editors have collaborated to present a global perspective, encompassing a diversity of healthcare environments, patient populations, and authors to ensure that the content of this book will be relevant to the widest range of healthcare providers. Acknowledging that not all urological care can or should be delivered by urologists, we provide detailed information for first-line providers in urgent care, emergency, and office-based settings. Where indicated we call out alternative laboratory testing, imaging, and treatments for situations in which resources preclude the use of technology intensive and costly choices. Similarly, the publisher has aimed to provide a low-cost textbook with digital imprint to ensure wide accessibility.

We organized the content by organ systems, allowing the reader to go from "top to bottom" of the genitourinary system, or cut to the chase and find a specific chapter as a point of reference. An important feature incorporates perspectives on traumatic injuries from the civilian and military environments. Unfortunately, war and road traffic will place increasing burdens on civilian populations and healthcare systems. Thus, the inclusion of military and civilian perspectives allows for innovation, cross pollination, and preparedness. The burden of congenital anomalies cannot be eradicated and will require surgical and non-surgical interventions across decades of a person's life; early treatment can have enormous benefit and thus we include a chapter on neonatal emergencies.

Completing this book in the midst of a global pandemic, it is important to recognize that diagnosis and treatment of many urological conditions will be deferred because of limited access to routine care, surgery, and even emergency services. The frequency of extreme weather events, resource scarcity, and other factors will likely lead to other severe disease outbreaks that will further limit access to care and drive greater pressure on emergency urological services. Thus, it is instructive to estimate the burden of the COVID-19 toll of deferred urological problems, which will come to the fore as pressure eases on ICU and Emergency Departments worldwide. We have added a special chapter on the topic.

References

http://www.healthdata.org/gbd/about

Ng-Kamstra JS, Greenberg SLM, Abdullah F, et al. Global Surgery 2030: a roadmap for high income country actors. BMJ Glob Health. 2016; 1(1): e000011.

https://www.brookings.edu/research/the-climate-crisis-migration-and-refugees/

List of Abbreviations

Abbreviation	Expansion
AAST	American Association for the Surgery of Trauma
ACCI	Age Adjusted Charlson Comorbidity Index
ACTH	adrenocorticotropic hormone
AFB	acid fast bacilli
ATLS	Advance Trauma and Life Support
AUA	American Urological Association
AUA-SI	American Urological Association Symptom Index
AVF	arteriovenous fistula
BCG	bacillus Calmette Guérin (vaccine)
BI	blast injury
BRI	blunt renal injury
Ca	calcium
CAH	congenital adrenal hyperplasia
CBC	complete blood count
CDC	Centers for Disease Control and Prevention
CDUS	color Doppler ultrasound
CKD	chronic kidney disease
Cl	chloride
CMV	cytomegalovirus
CNS	central nervous system
COPUM	congenital obstructing posterior urethral membranes
CT	computed tomography
DHT	dihydrotestosterone

DMSA	dimercaptosuccinic acid
DSD	disorders of sex development
DVIU	direct vision internal urethrotomy
EAU	European Association of Urology
ED	erectile dysfunction
EP	extraperitoneal
EPA	excision and primary anastomosis
EPN	emphysematous pyelonephritis
ESRD	end-stage renal disease
ERMS	embryonal rhabdomyosarcoma
FG	Fournier's gangrene
FGSI	Fournier's Gangrene Severity Index
FSH	follicle stimulating hormone
GSW	gunshot wound
GU	genitourinary
GUTB	genitourinary tuberculosis
HbS	hemoglobin S
HCT	hematocrit
HIC	high income countries
HIV	Human Immunodeficiency Virus
ICU	intensive care unit
IDSA	Infectious Disease Society of America
IED	improvised explosive devices
IgA	Immunoglobulin A
IIEF	International Index of Erectile Function
IM	intramuscular
INR	international normalized ratio
IP	intraperitoneal
IR	interventional radiology
IRSG	Intergroup Rhabdomyosarcoma Study Group
ISS	Injury Severity Score
IVC	inferior vena cava
IVU	intravenous urogram/urography

LH	luteinizing hormone
LMIC	low- and middle-income countries
LS	lichen sclerosus
MEDC	more economically developed countries
MET	medical expulsive therapy
MiGUTS	Multi-institutional Genito-Urinary Trauma Study
MRI	magnetic resonance imaging
Na	sodium
NIE	noninfectious epididymitis
NOM	non-operative, management
NPWT	negative-pressure wound therapy
NSAID	nonsteroidal anti-inflammatories
NSTI	necrotizing soft tissue infection
NTDB	National Trauma Data Bank
NTT	neonatal testicular torsion
OEIS	omphalocele, exstrophy of the bladder, imperforate anus, and spinal abnormalities complex
OIS	Organ Injury Scaling
ORIF	open reduction internal fixation
Osm	osmolarity
PCD	percutaneous drainage
PCN	percutaneous nephrostomy
PCO_2	partial pressure of carbon dioxide
PCR	polymerase chain reaction
PDDU	penile duplex doppler ultrasonography
PDE-5	phosphodiesterase-5
PDS	polydioxanone suture
PFUI	pelvic fracture urethral injury
PO_2	partial pressure of oxygen
PRI	penetrating renal injury
PROM	patient reported outcome measurement
PSV	peak systolic velocity
PT	prothrombin time
PTT	partial thromboplastin time

PUV	posterior rethral valves
PVR	post void residual
ROC	receiver operator characteristic
RUG	retrograde urethrogram
SCD	sickle cell disease
SD	standard deviation
SIU	Societe Internationale d'Urologie
STI	sexually transmitted infections
T1	T1 weighted image
T2	T2 weighted image
TUR	transurethral resection
TWIST score	Testicular Workup for Ischemia and Suspected Torsion
UA	urinalysis
UFGSI	Uludag Fournier's Gangrene Severity Index
UPEC	uropathogenic *E. coli*
UPJ	ureteropelvic junction
US	ultrasound
USG	ultrasonography
US-PVR	ultrasonographic post void residual
UTI	urinary tract infection
VAC	vacuum-assisted closure
VCUG	voiding cystourethrography
VUR	vesicoureteral reflux
WHO	World Health Organization
XGP	xanthogranulomatous pyelonephritis
XR	x-ray

About the Companion Website

This title is accompanied by a website:

www.wiley.com/go/wessells/urologic

The website contains key videos related to the following chapters in the book:

Chapter 2.   CT scan of penetrating renal injury
Chapter 4.   Ureteroscopic stone treatment (laser lithotripsy and basket extraction)
Chapter 6.   Robotic ureteral reconstruction with buccal mucosa graft
Chapter 9.   Urethral elongation after pelvic fracture urethral injury
Chapter 9.   Urethral disruption after pelvic fracture urethral injury
Chapter 9.   Endoscopic urethral realignment after pelvic fracture urethral injury
Chapter 10.   Excision and primary anastomosis of bulbar urethral stricture
Chapter 11.   Transurethral drainage of prostatic abscess

Section I

Upper Urinary Tract

1

Blunt Renal Injuries

Lindsay A. Hampson and Nnenaya Mmonu

Department of Urology, UCSF School of Medicine, San Francisco, CA, USA

Epidemiology, Etiology, Pathophysiology

Epidemiology and Etiology

Kidneys are the most injured genitourinary organ in external trauma, and it is estimated that 1–5% of all traumas and 10% of abdominal traumas sustain a renal injury [1–4]. In a series consisting purely of blunt abdominal trauma mechanism, 15% of patients were found to have an injury to the kidneys [5]. Of all patients who sustain genitourinary trauma, over half of them involve the kidney [6]. A population-based study found the incidence of renal trauma to be 4.9 per 100 000 population ≥16 years of age in the United States [4]. The majority of these patients were young and male, with 72% between the ages of 16 and 44 and 75% male. In an analysis of pediatric genitourinary injuries, renal injuries were found to make up 3.5% of the cohort, but the incidence has not been defined [7].

There is variation in the etiology of renal trauma based on geographical location; series from Low and Middle-Income Countries (LMIC) suggest that the rates of penetrating trauma are high, with the majority of blunt trauma caused by road traffic accidents, assault, and falls [8–11]. In the More Economically Developed Countries (MEDC), the vast majority (90–95%) of renal injury is sustained by blunt trauma, which is caused by motor vehicle collisions (63%), falls (14%), sports injuries (11%), pedestrian accidents (4%), motorcycle crashes (2%), assault (2%), and the remaining from other causes [6, 12, 13]. In a recent blunt renal trauma series, 80% of injuries were found to be grade I–II renal injuries, 9.5% grade III, 8.1% grade IV, and 2.7% grade IV [5]. Thus, imaging all renal injuries is unnecessary, and criteria have been developed (see below). Table 1.1 summarizes the large (n > 100) series with emphasis on blunt injuries.

Pathophysiology

Blunt trauma injury to the kidney is thought to occur as a result of kinetic energy transmission, often as a consequence of rapid deceleration forces or direct interaction of structures in the environment with the soft tissues and bones of the flank and then the

A Clinical Guide to Urologic Emergencies, First Edition. Edited by Hunter Wessells, Shigeo Horie, and Reynaldo G. Gómez.
© 2021 John Wiley & Sons Ltd. Published 2021 by John Wiley & Sons Ltd.
Companion website: www.wiley.com/go/wessells/urologic

Table 1.1 Demographics of renal trauma.

SERIES[a]	[6]	[14]	[15]	[1][b]	[4]	[16]	[5][b]	[17]	[18]	[19]
Year published	1984	1986	1995	2001	2003	2012	2012	2013	2013	2014
Renal injury (N)	154	132	2254	227	6231	1505	221	338	9002	105
Renal injury (%)	2.9	3.25	n/a	1.4	1.2	n/a	n/a	n/a	n/a	n/a
Blunt (%)	93.5	95.4	89.8	93.4	81.6	95.0	100	96.2	82.0	96.1
Penetrating (%)	6.5	4.6	10.2	6.6	18.4	5.0	0	3.9	17.8	3.9
Grade IV–V (%)	n/a			14.6			10.9	29.3	21.1	23.5
Initial non-operative management among *all* trauma (%)		92.6	92.6	n/a	88.6	94.5	n/a	92.6	86.8	98.0
Initial non-operative management among *blunt* trauma (%)			98.3	89.5/92.9?	96.3		92.3	92.6	94.4	
Nephrectomy (%) among *all* trauma	3.8	3.2			7.9	3.1	n/a	7.1	8.6	1.9
Nephrectomy (%) among *blunt* trauma			0	7.2	3.3		5.4	7.4	4.7	

Blank cells indicate missing data.

[a] Series with N <100 not included.

[b] Data showing grade and management of blunt renal injuries only.

kidney. Studies using animal models have shown that the kidney has viscoelastic proper-ties and that damage occurs as a result of stresses that cause tissue deformations exceeding an impact energy threshold of 4 J [20, 21]. A three-dimensional animal model also demon-strated that the primary site of load-bearing, where injuries result from, is the junction between the renal pelvis and the renal cortex [21]. Research has also demonstrated that the kidney with a fluid-filled structure (i.e. ureteropelvic junction obstruction, hydrone-phrosis, or renal cyst) may be more prone to rupture due to the hydrostatic pressure and resulting distribution of forces within the kidney [20, 22].

Children may have a higher risk of significant renal injury from blunt trauma and this is thought to be related to the proportionately larger kidney for their body size as compared to that of adults, the possibility of children retaining fetal lobulations that may predispose to parenchymal disruption, and the pediatric kidney having less protection due to lower perirenal fat content, weaker abdominal muscles, and less ossification of the rib cage [23, 24].

The proportion of patients with renal trauma found to have congenital anomalies varies, depending on different series, ranging from 1 to 23% [23]. One series that reviewed 193 pediatric renal trauma patients found that just over 8% of patients had a congenital anomaly [25]. Data regarding renal trauma and congenital anomalies is somewhat mixed, with most studies suggesting that congenital anomalies increase the risk of significant renal injury and decrease the possibility of renal salvage, while other series suggest that there is no effect on morbidity or mortality [25-30]. Overall consensus is that pre-existing renal anomalies likely increase the vulnerability of kidneys in blunt renal trauma [4, 30]. They may also complicate the management of a renal laceration involving the collecting system or parenchyma (e.g. horseshoe kidney with complex arterial vasculature, UPJ (ureteropelvic junction) obstruction, etc.).

Diagnosis

Workup

A complete history, including the crash mechanics and velocity of impact as well as known pre-existing renal disease or abnormality, should be obtained if possible. For example, renal injury frontal and side impact collisions may be impacted by direct contact from seatbelt and steering column [31]. Seatbelt use and airbag deployment are also important character-istics to note; absence of a seatbelt is associated with higher probability of thoracoabdomi-nal injury [32]. Compared to individuals who did not have airbag deployment with vehicle collision, those with frontal and side airbags have a 46 and 53% decrease in renal injury, respectively [33]. Vehicle characteristics are important given the association of increased crash test rating (i.e. safer car) with lower likelihood of thoracoabdominal injury [32].

Blunt trauma caused by a blow to the flank, rib fracture, or rapid deceleration injury should make clinicians suspicious for possible renal injury. Such mechanisms include inju-ries related to sports (in particular ice hockey, soccer, and football), ski and snowboarding, and motor vehicle versus pedestrian. Signs of renal injury from blunt trauma that may be noted on physical examination include gross hematuria, flank hematoma, and abdominal or flank tenderness. Vital signs are important to obtain and monitor both in the field and upon arrival at the hospital, as hemodynamic stability drives evaluation and management of renal trauma. Laboratory examinations, including a creatinine, hematocrit, and urinalysis with microscopic analysis to evaluate for hematuria, should be obtained.

Radiographic Evaluation

The American Urological Association (AUA) has released guidelines to provide indications for imaging of suspected renal trauma [34]. Patients sustaining blunt injury that require diagnostic imaging are those who have gross hematuria, or those who have a systolic blood pressure of less than 90 mmHg with microscopic hematuria. Additionally, any patients who are stable but have a mechanism of injury (e.g. fall from a great height) or physical examination (see above) findings concerning renal injury should also be imaged, as trauma patients may have renal injury, even in the absence of hematuria or shock [14, 35]. Based on the AUA Urotrauma Guidelines, children should be imaged with the same modality and criteria as adults.

If imaging is obtained, a contrast enhanced CT (computed tomography) abdomen pelvis with immediate and delayed images is recommended, in order to visualize the kidney parenchyma and collecting system and to look for evidence of bleeding or urinary extravasation. The immediate phase is typically an arterial or early venous phase, which highlights the renal parenchyma and can be useful for evaluating for parenchymal laceration, intravascular contrast extravasation, and hematoma. The delayed phase, typically obtained at 10–15 minutes after contrast administration, is useful to evaluate the collecting system of the kidney and the ureter. In addition, subtle findings on initial venous imaging such as perinephric stranding, hematoma, and low-density retroperitoneal fluid may prompt imaging with delayed phase to evaluate for a ureteropelvic or ureteral injury; a large medial urinoma or contrast extravasation on delayed images without distal ureteral contrast visualized is concerning for a renal pelvis or ureteral avulsion injury [36, 37].

Evaluating the size of a perinephric hematoma, the presence of intravascular contrast extravasation, and a medial laceration on CT can be useful, as these factors can predict bleeding complications and help guide management, as discussed in the management section (below).

Renal injuries are classified by the Organ Injury Scaling of the American Association for Surgery of Trauma (AAST) [38] (Table 1.2, Figures 1.1 and 1.2). Grade I injuries are renal contusions or subcapsular hematomas without parenchymal laceration. Grade II injuries involve perirenal hematomas of the renal retroperitoneum or parenchymal renal lacerations that extend for less than 1 cm. Once the laceration extends for greater than 1 cm into the renal parenchyma, this becomes a grade III injury, with an elevation to grade IV if there is collecting system involvement (i.e. urinary contrast extravasation from the renal collecting system). Grade IV injuries also include contained hilar vascular injuries, such as injury to the main renal artery or vein. Grade V injuries are so-called "shattered" kidneys and renal hilar avulsion injuries that cause devascularization of the kidney. Revisions have been proposed to this classification in order to include previously undescribed injuries and reclassify other injuries to facilitate more appropriate alignment of classification and management/outcomes, particularly in order to better classify vascular (such as segmental vessel injury) and collecting system injuries, though these revisions have not been formally accepted [40–43].

Table 1.2 2018 American Association for the Surgery of Trauma (AAST) organ injury scale [38].

Grade	Description of Injury
I	Subcapsular hematoma and/or parenchymal contusion without laceration
II	Perirenal hematoma confined to Gerota fascia
	Renal parenchymal laceration ≤1 cm depth without urinary extravasation
III	Renal parenchymal laceration >1.0 cm parenchymal depth without collecting system rupture or urinary extravasation
	Any injury in the presence of a kidney vascular injury or active bleeding contained within Gerota fascia
IV	Parenchymal laceration extending into urinary/collecting system with urinary extravasation
	Renal pelvic laceration and/or complete ureteropelvic disruption
	Segmental renal vein or artery injury
	Active bleeding beyond Gerota fascia into retroperitoneum or peritoneum
	Segmental or complete kidney infarction(s) due to vessel thrombosis without active bleeding
V	Main renal artery or vein laceration or avulsion of hilum
	Devascularized kidney with active bleeding
	Shattered kidney with loss of identifiable parenchymal renal anatomy

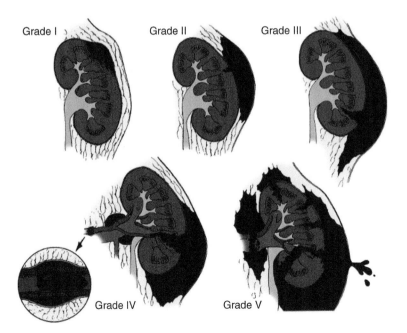

Figure 1.1 American Association for the Surgery of Trauma (AAST) Organ Injury Severity Score for the Kidney. *Source:* from Campbell-Walsh, 10th Edition with permission [39].

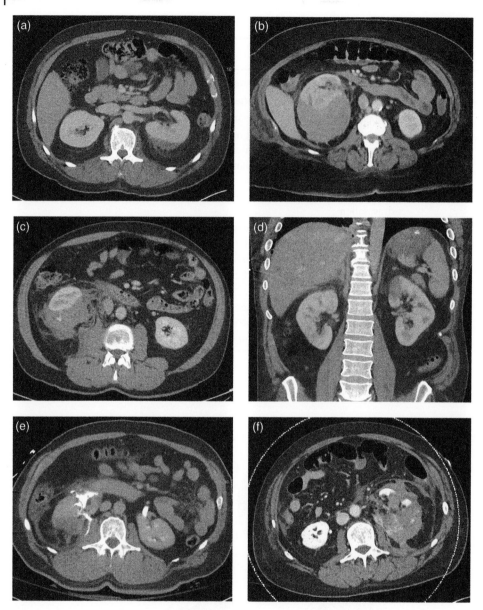

Figure 1.2 CT images of renal injuries including: (a) axial view of a left subcapsular hematoma (AAST Grade I); (b) a large right perinephric hematoma and a 2-cm parenchymal laceration (Grade III); (c) intravascular contrast extravasation into a right perinephric hematoma (Grade III); (d) coronal view of a left upper pole perfusion defect consistent with a segmental vascular injury (Grade IV); (e) a right medial parenchymal laceration with urinary contrast extravasation (Grade IV); and (f) a shattered left kidney with hematoma, contrast extravasation and multiple parenchymal fragments (Grade V). *Source:* courtesy of Alex Skokan, MD.

If CT is not available, or if the patient is brought directly to the operating room for exploration without first obtaining imaging, and renal injury is suspected due to hematuria or a perinephric hematoma, a one-shot intravenous pyelogram (IVP) can be useful, primarily to confirm the presence of a contralateral kidney, and secondarily to identify injury of the kidney of interest, although it is much less sensitive to detect injuries than CT (see image) [44]. A one-shot IVP is obtained by administering 2 ml/kg IV bolus of contrast with a single x-ray of the abdomen obtained 10–15 minutes later. The radiographic image quality can be limited by under-resuscitation, hypotension, significant edema, or renal dysfunction. One study evaluated the quality and usefulness of one-shot IVP in the operative setting, finding that the average quality score was 3.84/5 with only 1/50 studies found to be unintelligible, and the majority (66%) were good or of excellent quality. The average usefulness score was 3.96/5, with only 1 imaging study considered worthless and the majority (72%) considered important or critical for determining urological management.

Other imaging modalities such as ultrasound, radionucleotide scintigraphy, and angiography are not recommended for initial evaluation of renal injuries but may be useful during subsequent management.

Management

Non-operative Management

Patients with high-grade renal injuries who are hemodynamically stable can be managed non-operatively, involving hospital admission, intensive care monitoring, bed-rest, hydration, and serial hematocrit checks [34]. Over time, data have shown that the majority of renal injuries can be safely managed in a non-operative manner, with the potential benefits of preserving renal function and limiting morbidity [45].

Most stable patients with urinary extravasation can be managed non-operatively initially, as long as they do not have concern for a renal pelvis or ureteropelvic junction injury. Management may involve bladder drainage in order to facilitate collecting system drainage and/or antibiotics, although evidence is lacking to support these. Urinary extravasation can resolve spontaneously without intervention, with rates of spontaneous resolution near to 90% [46–48]. Guidelines support initial non-operative management of patients with urinary extravasation, given the possibility of spontaneous resolution and avoiding risks of injury during stent placement, risks of anesthesia, and the possibility of retained stents due to patients being lost to follow-up [34]. If there is any concern for complications with non-operative management (such as fever, enlarging urinoma, ileus, infection) or the urinary extravasation is found to be persistent on repeat imaging, ureteral stent placement is indicated. Some of these patients will require additional drainage with a nephrostomy tube and/or perinephric drain [47-48].

The AUA Urotrauma Guidelines suggest that patients who sustain high-grade injury (AAST IV-V) that are managed non-operatively should undergo repeat imaging after 48 hours or earlier, if needed, given the higher risk of complications and possibility of requiring future intervention [34]. In addition, conservatively managed patients who have clinical signs of complications – such as fevers, persistent severe pain, dropping hematocrit, hemodynamic instability, worsening flank or abdominal pain – should also undergo repeat imaging [34].

Repeat imaging may be tailored, based on an individuals' specific injury [49]. A recent analysis of repeat imaging in patients with grade IV and V renal trauma at three Level 1 trauma centers over 19 years (1999–2017) demonstrated that in asymptomatic patients, one in eight patients would need to undergo repeat imaging to identify a patient who needs surgical intervention. The primary goal of repeat imaging is to evaluate for complications and to evaluate clinical deterioration. Hence, it may be more worthwhile to obtain repeat imaging in patients who have signs of bleeding or history of collecting system injury as in this study. Stable patients with grade I–III injuries generally do not require repeat imaging. Repeat imaging with ultrasound instead of CT has also been advocated, based on studies showing that imaging of asymptomatic patients would not have altered clinical decision-making and concerns that standardized repeat imaging with CT exposes patients to unnecessary radiation exposure, and drives up healthcare costs, and ultrasound has been shown to be an effective alternative for detecting clinically relevant complications [20, 50, 51].

Indications for Intervention

As per AUA guidelines, "the surgical team must perform immediate intervention (surgery or angioembolization in selected situations) in hemodynamically unstable patients with no or transient response to resuscitation" [34]. Intervention is also required in the face of an enlarging or pulsatile perinephric hematoma seen on exploratory laparotomy, suspected renal pedicle avulsion, or a ureteropelvic junction disruption [52]. Depending on the clinical circumstances, these patients may require surgery or angioembolization. Several studies have evaluated high-risk criteria for bleeding associated with renal trauma, finding that intravascular contrast extravasation, perinephric hematoma of more than 3.5 cm in distance from the parenchymal edge to the hematoma edge, and medial renal laceration are risk factors associated with surgery for hemodynamic instability and the presence of two or more of these risk factors predicts the need for intervention [41–43, 53]. Studies have also evaluated these predictors for angiographic embolization, finding that perirenal hematoma size and intravascular contrast extravasation are indicators for embolization [54]. One study showed that patients without intravascular contrast extravasation and who have a perirenal hematoma rim distance of less than 25 mm are unlikely to benefit from angioembolization, and that combining CT scan-specific criteria such as intravascular contrast extravasation, perirenal hematoma size, and discontinuity of Gerota's fascia, can be predictive of the need for renal embolization [55]. Intravascular contrast extravasation alone is not an indication for angioembolization or other interventions. It is important to consider the hemodynamic status of the patient and blood transfusion requirements.

Building on these single institution series, the Multi-institutional Genito-Urinary Trauma Study Group created a nomogram to predict bleeding interventions after high-grade renal injury [56]. The variables in the nomogram (Figure 1.3) include mechanism of injury, hemodynamic status, associated injuries, and the following radiographic features: intravascular contrast extravasation; para-renal hematoma; and hematoma size.

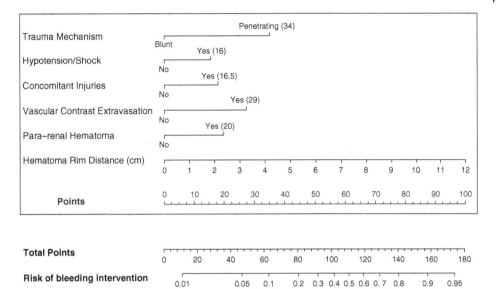

Figure 1.3 Nomogram predicting bleeding interventions after high-grade renal injury. Points are awarded for "Yes" responses for the first 5 parameters; the Hematoma Rim Distance is scored by tracing a line down to the Points scale in red. Total Points is based on the sum of the first 5 scores and the points from the scale in red. Source: from the MiGUTS Study, with permission [56].

With an area under the ROC (receiver operator characteristic) curve of 0.83, the nomogram performed better than AAST grade alone (which was not included in the nomogram). The nomogram, once externally validated, could provide a means to incorporate imaging data into decision-making on renal trauma management. Future work will be necessary to determine how to apply the nomogram in clinical care settings. Potential applications include its use to triage patients to ICU (intensive care unit) versus floor care for isolated grade III and IV injuries; ensure appropriateness of transfer from a lower to higher trauma designation hospital; to select treatment of bleeding with embolization versus transfusion alone; and support decisions for operative management [57].

Non-operative Versus Operative Management

Published series of blunt trauma patients suggest that when patients are matched by grade and mechanism injury in an operative cohort compared to a more conservatively managed cohort, the rate of nephrectomy is lower, complication rates are similar, and length of hospital stay is shorter with non-operative management [45–47]. Further supporting these data, hospitals that have changed their policy toward renal trauma management to adopt a non-operative approach have shown significant (two- to six-fold) decreases in renal exploration and nephrectomy without seeing an increase in complications [46, 58, 59].

In comparing series of grade IV blunt injuries that were managed non-operatively versus those who underwent exploration, higher rates of exploration are associated with higher rates of nephrectomy [45]. Finally, there are published series of patients who have sustained blunt grade V injuries, usually complex parenchymal lacerations (e.g. shattered kidney), who have been managed non-operatively. One such series showed a decreased rate of transfusions, shorter ICU length of stay, and fewer complications for the conservatively managed patients [60]. A recent series showed that just over 50% of grade V injuries were able to be managed non-operatively [61].

Predictors of Failure of Non-Operative Management in Blunt Renal Trauma

Of patients with blunt trauma that are managed non-operatively, some will ultimately require intervention. One series evaluated 154 patients (74.8%) with grade IV and V blunt renal trauma, who were initially managed non-operatively, with a non-operative management failure rate of 7.8% [62]. The vast majority of the patients who failed non-operative management did so because of their kidney injury and none of these patients had complications as a result of delayed operative management. The mean time to failure was just over 24 hours and the majority (83.3%) failed due to hemodynamic instability. Independent predictors based on multivariate analysis found that those who were older than 55 years of age or who were injured as a result of a motor vehicle collision were more likely to fail non-operative management.

Patients with a devitalized parenchymal segment were more likely to require delayed surgical intervention in a series of grade IV and V blunt renal injuries [46]. Of 40 patients with grade III–V blunt renal injury initially managed non-operatively, the risk of delayed nephrectomy in three was associated with grade IV injuries and secondary hemorrhage which necessitated intervention [8].

Management of Renal Trauma in Children

Many studies have evaluated management of renal trauma in children, with the consensus being that most cases of pediatric renal trauma can be safely managed non-operatively [63–67]. Rates of delayed intervention vary from very low to as high as 30–40% [64, 68–70]. In one series of 16 patients managed non-operatively, 44% required intervention with a mean time to intervention of 11 days; collecting system clot and larger urinoma were significant predictors of failure of non-operative management [70]. Consistent with findings in adults, another group found that medial contrast extravasation among grade IV renal injuries was a significant predictor of failure of non-operative management [71].

Given the lack of age specific guidelines, pediatric blunt renal trauma guidelines were established recently by the Eastern Association for Surgery of Trauma and Pediatric Trauma society [72]. These guidelines advocate for nonoperative management in high-grade trauma sustained by hemodynamically stable patients based on synthesis of evidence. For those undergoing intervention, angioembolization is highly recommended. Finally, routine blood pressure monitoring is recommended after injury.

Operative Technique

Absolute criteria for renal exploration include life-threatening hemorrhage with hemodynamic instability, renal pedicle avulsion, and expanding, pulsatile, or uncontained retroperitoneal hematoma [25]. Renal exploration and repair in the acute injury setting is accomplished through a midline abdominal incision. While prior literature supported early

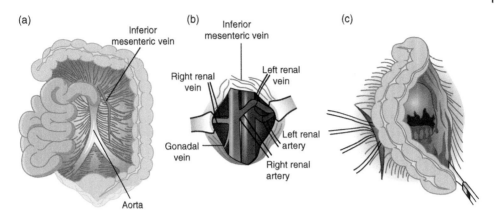

Figure 1.4 Surgical approach to renal vessels and hilum. (a) Relationship between the aorta, posterior peritoneum, and inferior mesenteric vein. (b) Window in posterior peritoneum made between aorta and inferior mesenteric vein demonstrating each renal artery and vein. (c) After vascular exposure and isolation, exploration of Gerota fascia obtained by incising the peritoneum lateral to the descending colon (for a left-sided injury). *Source:* from Campbell-Walsh, 10th Edition, with permission [39].

vascular control, more recent literature is inconclusive on this approach [73-77]. Surgical exploration often results in nephrectomy [4]. The renal vessels can be isolated before Gerota's fascia is opened in order be able to rapidly occlude hilar vessels if significant bleeding is encountered; some advocate that this technique may lead to a lower rate of nephrectomy, whereas other data have shown no difference in nephrectomy rate, transfusion requirements, or blood loss with potential for increased operative time [76, 77]. If early vascular control is desired, an incision can be made in the mesentery medial to the inferior mesenteric vein and extended to the ligament of Treitz in order to expose the aorta [78] (Figure 1.4). The left renal vein will be visualized first as it passes anterior to the aorta and the renal arteries can then be identified posterior to the left renal vein, and the right renal vein will be identified anterior to the right renal artery. Once the hilar vessels have been isolated, the colon can then be reflected medially by incising the peritoneum lateral to the colon and exposing Gerota's fascia. The kidney can then be fully exposed in order to identify any injuries. The other approach to the renal hilum involves initial reflection of the colon and its mesentery, keeping out of Gerota's fascia, followed by isolation of the renal hilum for early vascular control, and renorrhaphy, partial nephrectomy, or nephrectomy.

Repair of the kidney depends on the injuries present, and should involve debridement of nonviable tissue, suture ligation of individual bleeding vessels to obtain hemostasis, watertight closure of any collecting system defects, and closure or re-approximation of the parenchymal defect when possible. If parenchymal closure is difficult, techniques such as thrombin-soaked Gelfoam bolsters or omental interposition or pedicle flap may be helpful.

In terms of renovascular injuries, segmental arterial and venous injuries can be managed with suture ligation, realizing that ligation of segmental arteries will result in ischemia to the corresponding renal parenchyma. Repair of the main renal artery and vein should be attempted when safe with 4-0 or 5-0 prolene suture; however, many injuries of the main hilar vessels will result in nephrectomy (Figure 1.5).

(a)   (b)   (c)

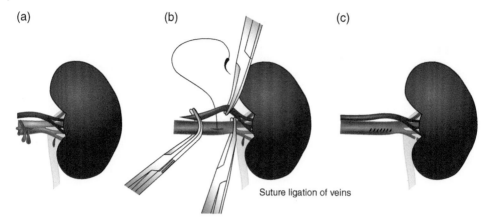

Suture ligation of veins

Figure 1.5 Surgical management of vascular injuries. (a) Schematic showing injury to different portions of the renal vein. Injuries are repaired (b) or divided (c), depending on location and size. *Source:* from Campbell-Walsh, 10th Edition, with permission [39].

Issues in Operative Technique for Blunt Trauma

Renal trauma may be incompletely staged and this can be an important determinant for renal exploration. If exploration occurs before complete staging has been accomplished, a one-shot IVP or retrograde pyelograms can be performed in the operating room (see above), or the kidney and/or ureters can be directly inspected during an abdominal exploration [79].

In cases of renal trauma, it is important to have familiarity with damage control maneuvers. It is particularly important in patients who do not have life-threatening renal injury. In cases of uncontrolled bleeding, vascular control is paramount. Renal pedicle access by blunt dissection over psoas fascia allows for application of a large vascular clamp. Once this is done, then the kidney can be evaluated and nephron sparing techniques can be applied. Another consideration is in cases where the patient is unstable for kidney exploration and repair in the setting of active bleeding. In this case, packing the renal fossa with delated intervention is an alternative to nephrectomy. This would allow for appropriate staging in patients who were initially unstable for imaging. This staging may allow for the patient to have non-operative management and/or angioembolization.

Complications and Follow-Up

Complications after renal trauma are reported to be rare, occurring in about 5% of cases in modern series, although true rates of long-term complications are difficult to define given the lack of long-term follow-up in the trauma population [25]. One retrospective series of grade IV and V blunt renal trauma evaluated the incidence of complications among patients who underwent immediate intervention versus those who were conservatively managed, subdividing the conservatively managed patients into successes and failures of conservative management [62]. Most were successfully managed conservatively. Of those who underwent successful conservative management (n = 142), 10.6% developed urinoma

Table 1.3 Long-term follow-up recommendations.

AUA [34]	EAU [81, 82]	SIU/WHO [30]
Periodic monitoring of blood pressure up to a year after injury. Do not recommend routine DMSA (dimercaptosuccinic acid) or other functional nuclear scans.	Physical exam, urinalysis, "individualized radiological investigation," serial blood pressure monitoring, and determination of renal function. Follow-up should continue until healing is complete and lab findings have stabilized. Monitoring may need to be continued for years to evaluate for latent renovascular hypertension.	No specific recommendations, but consensus statement does cite a study that recommends that all grade IV/V injuries follow-up with documentation of renal function by quantitative assessment

(n = 15) and 16.9% had hematuria (n = 24). Of those who failed conservative management (n = 12), 8.3% developed urinoma (n = 1) and 8.3% had persistent hematuria (n = 1).

Short-term monitoring and follow-up of trauma patients as previously specified is intended to detect complications and offer appropriate additional interventions. In terms of long-term follow-up, there is no consensus and most trauma series do not have the luxury of long-term follow-up, given the difficulty in following up the acutely injured population [80]. Follow-up recommendations are outlined in Table 1.3.

Secondary Hemorrhage

Delayed hemorrhage can be a life-threatening complication of renal trauma that can arise as a result of the parenchymal injury itself, segmental arterial bleeding, or ruptured arterio-venous fistulas (AVFs) or pseudoaneurysm. One series of grade III–IV blunt injuries managed conservatively showed a 13–25% rate of delayed bleeds, with the caveats that this number varies significantly by series and the majority of the literature on delayed bleeds is derived from cases of penetrating trauma [83-85]. Delayed bleeds occur most commonly in the first 2–3 weeks after trauma, although case reports have described trauma-associated bleeds occurring as late as 15 or 20 years after the initial insult [83-84]. Renal trauma from stab wounds demonstrate the onset of secondary hemorrhage in the 2–36 day time-frame [30, 85].

Most often, delayed hemorrhage is caused by AVF or pseudo-aneurysm [30]. The occurrence of pseudoaneurysm after blunt renal trauma has been described in several case reports but is a rare event [83, 86–88]. Pseudoaneurysms are believed to form within the surrounding tissue after an arterial injury, likely due to shear stress in blunt renal trauma, where the space around the vascular injury is temporarily tamponaded by coagulation. Eventually, the intravascular and extravascular space may recannulate after degradation of the clot and necrosis of the surrounding tissue, leading to the formation of a pseudoaneurysm which can then grow and rupture [88, 89].

AVF after blunt trauma is also a rare event and has been reported in several case reports [89–92]. The fistula is thought to form as a result of injury to an arterial and venous vessel in close proximity to one another, usually within the renal parenchyma. Initially the bleeding may be tamponaded by a clot; as the hematoma resorbs the arterial bleeding can resume, draining into the nearby lacerated vein [30].

New-onset or worsening hematuria, flank pain or mass, a hematocrit drop, or even new-onset hypertension, should raise suspicion of a delayed bleed. CT angiogram or conventional angiography is the preferred imaging modality, although diagnosis can be made with ultrasound in some cases. Depending on the etiology, either surgical management or super-selective embolization is employed, with the goal of controlling the bleeding while preserving as much renal function as possible [93, 94]. Complications of embolization can include abscess, infarction, renal insufficiency, and pulmonary embolization of coils [25, 84, 94, 95].

Urinary Extravasation and Perinephric Abscess

AUA guidelines recommend that clinicians perform urinary drainage in the presence of complications such as enlarging urinoma, fever, increasing pain, ileus, fistula, or infection [34].

Renal injuries with urinary extravasation at initial presentation can for the most part be managed conservatively given the high rates (90%) of spontaneous resolution, although repeat imaging is intended to evaluate for persistent leaks, urinomas, or perinephric abscesses that require additional intervention such as stenting or percutaneous drainage [30, 46–48, 98]. Patients with devitalized renal parenchyma in conjunction with urinary extravasation tend to have increased morbidity and may require more aggressive management [80, 96–98]. Furthermore, patients with concomitant injuries, such as pancreatic or colonic injuries, may also have a higher likelihood of developing complications [25, 99–101].

In practice, approximately 29% of patients with high-grade renal trauma undergo ureteral stent placement [102]. To date, there are no standard guidelines on duration of stent and Foley placement for high-grade renal trauma. In a single center series, an indwelling stent for six to eight weeks was associated with favorable outcomes [103]. Generally, maintaining a Foley catheter while a stent is in place helps with healing by preventing antegrade reflux of urine to the kidney, minimizing pressure in the collecting system, and enhancing urinoma drainage. Percutaneous drains may be necessary in cases of increasing urinoma size, complexity, and/or infection [34].

Renal Insufficiency

The lack of long-term follow-up after renal trauma makes it difficult to determine the true rates of renal insufficiency after trauma. One study evaluating pediatric blunt renal trauma patients managed conservatively found that the decline in percentage of renal function of the injured renal unit correlated to the severity of renal injury, with $44.7 \pm 8.4\%$ residual function for grade II–III injuries, $41.8 \pm 9.2\%$ residual function for grade IV injury, and $29.5 \pm 7.9\%$ residual function for grade V injuries [104]. Notably, all patients had normal serum creatinine at follow-up. This group re-assessed renal function for a subset of these patients at one year post-injury, finding that renal function remained stable over this time period [105]. These results are supported by another study of 67 renal injuries (36% blunt trauma) that underwent post-injury dimercapto-succinic acid renal scan and found that the mean decrease in renal function corresponded to injury grade (p < 0.005 in multivariate analysis), with a mean decrease in renal function of 15% for grade III, 30% for grade IV, and 65% for grade V injuries [106]. In multivariate analysis, there was no difference in the decrease in renal function between blunt and penetrating renal injury or in those injuries that were managed operatively versus conservatively.

A study evaluating 52 patients who underwent renal reconstruction after renal trauma found that renal function on the reconstructed side had a mean 39.3% preservation of function, with 81% of patients having more than one-third function of the injured kidney based on radionucleotide scintigraphy [107].

Two studies evaluated the rates of chronic kidney disease after renal trauma. One compared trauma patients with and without renal injuries, finding that 230 patients without renal injury had an incidence of acute kidney injury of 17.4% compared to 11.4% in the patients with renal injury [108]. Another multi-institutional study evaluating grade IV and V renal injuries (49% blunt trauma) found that 6/89 patients developed chronic kidney disease (CKD) (serum creatinine range 2.0–15.6 mg/dl), and of these 6 patients, 3/5 with long-term follow-up developed progressive and permanent renal failure requiring dialysis [80].

Hypertension

Patients who sustain renal injuries have an increased risk of renovascular hypertension, with the incidence of renal trauma-related hypertension estimated between less than 1 and 5% [80, 109–113]. As a result, the European Association of Urology (EAU) Guidelines on Urologic Trauma, the AUA Urotrauma Guidelines, and the Societé Internationale d'Urologie (SIU)/World Health Organization (WHO) consensus statement on renal trauma all recommend periodic monitoring of blood pressure for the first year after injury, at least for a subset patients who have sustained high-grade injuries [30, 37, 82].

Renovascular hypertension after trauma may develop through several mechanisms: renal arterial stenosis or occlusion, parenchymal compression caused by perinephric hematoma (Page kidney), or chronic scar formation [109, 111, 112]. All of these result in a reduction in renal blood flow, which can then cause a unilateral hypersecretion of renin and resultant hypertension [25]. Diagnosis can be made with selective angiography and renal vein renin levels. Older studies of renal trauma patients show rates of new-onset hypertension of 4–5%, with onset between two weeks and eight months of injury [80, 112]. A more recent study contradicts these data, showing that patients who develop hypertension after renal trauma typically manifest it during their initial hospitalization and do not develop delayed hypertension during long-term follow-up [114].

Management with medications, renal artery bypass surgery, or partial or total nephrectomy has been shown to be effective [109, 111]. In studies evaluating conservative treatment, treatment rates range from 28 to 50% [111, 112, 114, 115]. In terms of surgical management, elevated renin levels from the affected kidney have been shown to predict a good response to surgical treatment [111, 116]. Similarly, one study showed that in cases of arterial stenosis or occlusion, early nephrectomy within the first year after injury had better response rates compared to delayed nephrectomy [108].

Other Complications

Other rare complications may include chronic pyelonephritis, post-trauma hydronephrosis, stone formation, fistulae, or flank pain [82].

Mortality

Mortality following renal trauma is nearly always related to associated injuries, with estimates of renal trauma driven mortality at less than 0.1% of all deaths [25].

Conclusions

The majority of renal trauma is caused by blunt mechanisms, making it vital for emergency providers and surgeons to have an understanding of renal trauma. Evaluation and management of blunt renal trauma has evolved significantly over the past decade. Guidelines from urologic societies have helped to disseminate indications for imaging and managing high-grade kidney injuries. Over time, there has been an evolution toward non-operative management, as data have shown good success with conservative approaches. The goal of diagnosing and managing renal trauma should be to preserve renal function, and this includes appropriate treatment of complications and failed conservative management. Long-term follow-up and assessment of renal function in these patients is lacking and requires updating.

References

1 Baverstock, R., Simons, R., and McLoughlin, M. (2001). Severe blunt renal trauma: a 7-year retrospective review from a provincial trauma centre. *Can. J. Urol.* 8 (5): 1372–1376.

2 McAninch, J.W., Carroll, P.R., Klosterman, P.W. et al. (1991). Renal reconstruction after injury. *J. Urol.* 145 (5): 932–937.

3 McAninch, J.W. (1999). Genitourinary trauma. *World J. Urol.* 17 (2): 65.

4 Wessells, H., Suh, D., Porter, J.R. et al. (2003). Renal injury and operative management in the United States: results of a population-based study. *J. Trauma* 54 (3): 423–430.

5 Aragona, F., Pepe, P., Patanè, D. et al. (2012). Management of severe blunt renal trauma in adult patients: a 10-year retrospective review from an emergency hospital. *BJU Int.* 110 (5): 744–748.

6 Krieger, J.N., Algood, C.B., Mason, J.T. et al. (1984). Urological trauma in the Pacific Northwest: etiology, distribution, management and outcome. *J. Urol.* 132 (1): 70–73.

7 Tasian, G.E., Bagga, H.S., Fisher, P.B. et al. (2013). Pediatric genitourinary injuries in the United States from 2002 to 2010. *J. Urol.* 189 (1): 288–293.

8 Prasad, N.H., Devraj, R., Chandriah, G.R. et al. (2014). Predictors of nephrectomy in high grade blunt renal trauma patients treated primarily with conservative intent. *Indian J. Urol.* 30 (2): 158–160.

9 Madiba, T.E., Haffejee, A.A., and John, J. (2002). Renal trauma secondary to stab, blunt and firearm injuries – a 5-year study. *S. Afr. J. Surg.* 40 (1): 5–9; discussion 9–10.

10 Gray, N. (1985). Renal trauma in a South African hospital: a two year study. *J. R. Army Med. Corps* 131 (1): 19–20.

11 Ersay, A. and Akgün, Y. (1999). Experience with renal gunshot injuries in a rural setting. *Urology* 54 (6): 972–975.

12 Bretan, P.N., McAninch, J.W., Federle, M.P., and Jeffrey, R.B. (1986). Computerized tomographic staging of renal trauma: 85 consecutive cases. *J. Urol.* 136 (3): 561–565.

13 Voelzke, B.B. and Leddy, L. (2014). The epidemiology of renal trauma. *Transl. Androl. Urol.* 3 (2): 143–149.

14 Cass, A.S., Luxenberg, M., Gleich, P., and Smith, C.S. (1986). Clinical indications for radiographic evaluation of blunt renal trauma. *J. Urol.* 136 (2): 370–371.

15 Miller, K.S. and McAninch, J.W. (1995). Radiographic assessment of renal trauma: our 15-year experience. *J. Urol.* 154 (2 Pt 1): 352–355.

16 Sugihara, T., Yasunaga, H., Horiguchi, H. et al. (2012). Management trends, angioembolization performance and multiorgan injury indicators of renal trauma from Japanese administrative claims database. *Int. J. Urol.* 19 (6): 559–563; author reply 564.

17 Shoobridge, J.J., Bultitude, M.F., Koukounaras, J. et al. (2013). A 9-year experience of renal injury at an Australian level 1 trauma centre. *BJU Int.* 112 (Suppl. 2): 53–60.

18 McClung, C.D., Hotaling, J.M., Wang, J. et al. (2013). Contemporary trends in the immediate surgical management of renal trauma using a national database. *J. Trauma Acute Care Surg.* 75 (4): 602–606.

19 Breen, K.J., Sweeney, P., Nicholson, P.J. et al. (2014). Adult blunt renal trauma: routine follow-up imaging is excessive. *Urology* 84 (1): 62–67.

20 Schmidlin, F.R., Schmid, P., Kurtyka, T. et al. (1996). Force transmission and stress distribution in a computer-simulated model of the kidney: an analysis of the injury mechanisms in renal trauma. *J. Trauma* 40 (5): 791–796.

21 Bschleipfer, T., Kallieris, D., Hauck, E.W. et al. (2002). Blunt renal trauma: biomechanics and origination of renal lesions. *Eur. Urol.* 42 (6): 614–621.

22 Esho, J.O., Ireland, G.W., and Cass, A.S. (1973). Renal trauma and preexisting lesions of kidney. *Urology* 1 (2): 134–135.

23 Kuzmarov, I.W., Morehouse, D.D., and Gibson, S. (1981). Blunt renal trauma in the pediatric population: a retrospective study. *J. Urol.* 126 (5): 648–649.

24 Brown, S.L., Elder, J.S., and Spirnak, J.P. (1998). Are pediatric patients more susceptible to major renal injury from blunt trauma? A comparative study. *J. Urol.* 160 (1): 138–140.

25 Al-Qudah, H.S. and Santucci, R.A. (2006). Complications of renal trauma. *Urol. Clin. North Am.* 33 (1): 41–53-vi.

26 McAleer, I.M., Kaplan, G.W., and LoSasso, B.E. (2002). Congenital urinary tract anomalies in pediatric renal trauma patients. *J. Urol.* 168 (4 Pt 2): 1808–1810; discussion 1810.

27 Cass, A.S. (1983). Blunt renal pelvic and ureteral injury in multiple-injured patients. *Urology* 22 (3): 268–270.

28 Morse, T.S., Smith, J.P., Howard, W.H., and Rowe, M.I. (1967). Kidney injuries in children. *J. Urol.* 98 (5): 539–547.

29 Onen, A., Kaya, M., Cigdem, M.K. et al. (2002). Blunt renal trauma in children with previously undiagnosed pre-existing renal lesions and guidelines for effective initial management of kidney injury. *BJU Int.* 89 (9): 936–941.

30 Santucci, R.A., Wessells, H., Bartsch, G. et al. (2004). Evaluation and management of renal injuries: consensus statement of the renal trauma subcommittee. *BJU Int.* 93 (7): 937–954.

31 Kuan, J.K., Kaufman, R., Wright, J.L. et al. (2007). Renal injury mechanisms of motor vehicle collisions: analysis of the crash injury research and engineering network data set. *J. Urol.* 178 (3 Pt 1): 935–940; discussion 940. Epub 2007 Jul 16.

32 Figler, B.D., Mack, C.D., Kaufman, R. et al. (2014). Crash test rating and likelihood of major thoracoabdominal injury in motor vehicle crashes: the new car assessment program side-impact crash test, 1998–2010. *J. Trauma Acute Care Surg.* 76 (3): 750–754. https://doi.org/10.1097/TA.0b013e3182aafd5b.

33 Smith, T.G. 3rd, Wessells, H.B., Mack, C.D. et al. (2010). Examination of the impact of airbags on renal injury using a national database. *J. Am. Coll. Surg.* 211 (3): 355–360. https://doi.org/10.1016/j.jamcollsurg.2010.05.009. Epub 2010 Jul 14.

34 Morey, A.F., Brandes, S., Dugi, D.D. et al. (2014). Urotrauma: AUA guideline. *J. Urol.* 192 (2): 327–335.

35 Brandes, S.B. and McAninch, J.W. (1999). Urban free falls and patterns of renal injury: a 20-year experience with 396 cases. *J. Trauma* 47 (4): 643–649; discussion 649–50.

36 Ortega, S.J., Netto, F.S., Hamilton, P. et al. (2008). CT scanning for diagnosing blunt ureteral and ureteropelvic junction injuries. *BMC Urol.* 8: 3.

37 Kawashima, A., Sandler, C.M., Corriere, J.N. et al. (1997). Ureteropelvic junction injuries secondary to blunt abdominal trauma. *Radiology* 205 (2): 487–492.

38 Moore, E.E., Shackford, S.R., Pachter, H.L. et al. (1989). Organ injury scaling: spleen, liver, and kidney. *J. Trauma* 29 (12): 1664–1666.

39 Wein, A.J., Kavoussi, L.R., Novick, A.C. et al. (2011). *Campbell-Walsh Urology*. Elsevier Health Sciences 1 p.

40 Buckley, J.C. and McAninch, J.W. (2011). Revision of current American Association for the Surgery of Trauma Renal Injury grading system. *J. Trauma* 70 (1): 35–37.

41 Dugi, D.D., Morey, A.F., Gupta, A. et al. (2010). American Association for the Surgery of Trauma grade 4 renal injury substratification into grades 4a (low risk) and 4b (high risk). *J. Urol.* 183 (2): 592–597.

42 Chiron, P., Hornez, E., Boddaert, G. et al. (2015). Grade IV renal trauma management. A revision of the AAST renal injury grading scale is mandatory. *Eur. J. Trauma Emerg. Surg.* 42 (2): 237–241.

43 Figler, B.D., Malaeb, B.S., Voelzke, B. et al. (2013). External validation of a substratification of the American Association for the Surgery of Trauma renal injury scale for grade 4 injuries. *J. Am. Coll. Surg.* 217 (5): 924–928.

44 Morey, A.F., McAninch, J.W., Tiller, B.K. et al. (1999). Single shot intraoperative excretory urography for the immediate evaluation of renal trauma. *J. Urol.* 161 (4): 1088–1092.

45 Santucci, R.A. and Fisher, M.B. (2005). The literature increasingly supports expectant (conservative) management of renal trauma – a systematic review. *J. Trauma* 59 (2): 493–503.

46 Moudouni, S.M., Hadj Slimen, M. et al. (2001). Management of major blunt renal lacerations: is a nonoperative approach indicated? *Eur. Urol.* 40 (4): 409–414.

47 Matthews, L.A., Smith, E.M., and Spirnak, J.P. (1997). Nonoperative treatment of major blunt renal lacerations with urinary extravasation. *J. Urol.* 157 (6): 2056–2058.

48 Alsikafi, N.F., McAninch, J.W., Elliott, S.P., and Garcia, M. (2006). Nonoperative management outcomes of isolated urinary extravasation following renal lacerations due to external trauma. *J. Urol.* 176 (6 Pt 1): 2494–2497.

49 Bayne, D.B., Tresh, A., Baradaran, N. et al. (2019). Does routine repeat imaging change management in hihg-grade renal trauma? Results from three level 1 trauma centers. *World J. Urol.* 37 (7): 1455–1459. https://doi.org/10.1007/s00345-018-2513-2. Epub 2018 Oct 1.

50 Shirazi, M., Sefidbakht, S., Jahanabadi, Z. et al. (2010). Is early reimaging CT scan necessary in patients with grades III and IV renal trauma under conservative treatment? *J. Trauma* 68 (1): 9–12.

51 Eeg, K.R., Khoury, A.E., Halachmi, S. et al. (2009). Single center experience with application of the ALARA concept to serial imaging studies after blunt renal trauma in children – is ultrasound enough? *J. Urol.* 181 (4): 1834–1840; discussion 1840.

52 Voelzke, B.B. and McAninch, J.W. (2008). The current management of renal injuries. *Am. Surg.* 74 (8): 667–678.

53 Hardee, M.J., Lowrance, W., Brant, W.O. et al. (2013). High grade renal injuries: application of Parkland Hospital predictors of intervention for renal hemorrhage. *J. Urol.* 189 (5): 1771–1776.

54 Nuss, G.R., Morey, A.F., Jenkins, A.C. et al. (2009). Radiographic predictors of need for angiographic embolization after traumatic renal injury. *J. Trauma* 67 (3): 578–582; discussion 582.

55 Charbit, J., Manzanera, J., Millet, I. et al. (2011). What are the specific computed tomography scan criteria that can predict or exclude the need for renal angioembolization after high-grade renal trauma in a conservative management strategy? *J. Trauma* 70 (5): 1219–1227; discussion 1227-8.

56 Keihani, S., Rogers, D.M., Putbrese, B.E. et al. (2019). A nomogram predicting the need for bleeding interventions after high-grade renal trauma: results from the American Association for the Surgery of Trauma Multi-institutional Genito-Urinary Trauma Study (MiGUTS). *J. Trauma Acute Care Surg.* 86 (5): 774–782.

57 Hagedorn, J.C., Quistberg, D.A., Arbabi, S. et al. (2019). Factors associated with secondary overtriage in renal trauma. *Urology* 130: 175–180.

58 Danuser, H., Wille, S., Zöscher, G., and Studer, U. (2001). How to treat blunt kidney ruptures: primary open surgery or conservative treatment with deferred surgery when necessary? *Eur. Urol.* 39 (1): 9–14.

59 Schmidlin, F.R., Rohner, S., Hadaya, K. et al. (1997). The conservative treatment of major kidney injuries. *Ann. Urol. (Paris)* 31 (5): 246–252.

60 Altman, A.L., Haas, C., Dinchman, K.H., and Spirnak, J.P. (2000). Selective nonoperative management of blunt grade 5 renal injury. *J. Urol.* 164 (1): 27–30; discussion 30-1.

61 Lanchon, C., Fiard, G., Arnoux, V. et al. (2015). High grade blunt renal trauma: predictors of surgery and long-term outcomes of conservative management. A prospective single center study. *J. Urol.* 195 (1): 106–111.

62 van der Wilden, G.M., Velmahos, G.C., Joseph, D.K. et al. (2013). Successful nonoperative management of the most severe blunt renal injuries: a multicenter study of the research consortium of New England Centers for Trauma. *JAMA Surg.* 148 (10): 924–931.

63 Haller, J.A., Papa, P., Drugas, G., and Colombani, P. (1994). Non-operative management of solid organ injuries in children. Is it safe? *Ann. Surg.* 219 (6): 625–628; discussion 628-31.

64 Levy, J.B., Baskin, L.S., Ewalt, D.H. et al. (1993). Nonoperative management of blunt pediatric major renal trauma. *Urology* 42 (4): 418–424.

65 Gill, B., Palmer, L.S., Reda, E. et al. (1994). Optimal renal preservation with timely percutaneous intervention: a changing concept in the management of blunt renal trauma in children in the 1990s. *Br. J. Urol.* 74 (3): 370–374.

66 Henderson, C.G., Sedberry-Ross, S., Pickard, R. et al. (2007). Management of high grade renal trauma: 20-year experience at a pediatric level I trauma center. *J. Urol.* 178 (1): 246–250; discussion 250.

67 Baumann, L., Greenfield, S.P., Aker, J. et al. (1992). Nonoperative management of major blunt renal trauma in children: in-hospital morbidity and long-term followup. *J. Urol.* 148 (2 Pt 2): 691–693.

68 Smith, E.M., Elder, J.S., and Spirnak, J.P. (1993). Major blunt renal trauma in the pediatric population: is a nonoperative approach indicated? *J. Urol.* 149 (3): 546–548.

69 Lee, J.N., Lim, J.K., Woo, M.J. et al. (2015). Predictive factors for conservative treatment failure in grade IV pediatric blunt renal trauma. *J. Pediatr. Urol.* 12 (2): 93.e1–93.e7.

70 Reese, J.N., Fox, J.A., Cannon, G.M., and Ost, M.C. (2014). Timing and predictors for urinary drainage in children with expectantly managed grade IV renal trauma. *J. Urol.* 192 (2): 512–517.

71 Bartley, J.M. and Santucci, R.A. (2012). Computed tomography findings in patients with pediatric blunt renal trauma in whom expectant (nonoperative) management failed. *Urology* 80 (6): 1338–1343.

72 Hagedorn, J.C., Fox, N., Ellison, J.S. et al. (2019). Pediatric blunt renal trauma practice management guidelines: collaboration between the Eastern Association for the Surgery of Trauma and the Pediatric Trauma Society. *J. Trauma Acute Care Surg.* 86 (5): 916–925. https://doi.org/10.1097/TA.0000000000002209.

73 Carlton CE Jr, Scott R Jr, Goldman M. The management of penetrating injuries of the kidney. J Trauma. 1968 Nov;8(6):1071-83.

74 Holcroft JW, Trunkey DD, Minagi H, Korobkin MT, Lim RC. Renal trauma and retroperitoneal hematomas-indications for exploration. J Trauma. 1975 Dec;15(12):1045-52.

75 Atala A, Miller FB, Richardson JD, Bauer B, Harty J, Amin M. Preliminary vascular control for renal trauma. Surg Gynecol Obstet. 1991 May;172(5):386-90.

76 McAninch, J.W. and Carroll, P.R. (1982). Renal trauma: kidney preservation through improved vascular control – a refined approach. *J. Trauma* 22 (4): 285–290.

77 Gonzalez, R.P., Falimirski, M., Holevar, M.R., and Evankovich, C. (1999). Surgical management of renal trauma: is vascular control necessary? *J. Trauma* 47 (6): 1039–1042; discussion 1042-4.

78 Meng, M.V., Brandes, S.B., and McAninch, J.W. (1999). Renal trauma: indications and techniques for surgical exploration. *World J. Urol.* 17 (2): 71–77.

79 Smith, T.G. 3rd and Coburn, M. (2013). Damage control maneuvers for urologic trauma. *Urol. Clin. North Am.* 40 (3): 343–350. https://doi.org/10.1016/j.ucl.2013.04.003. Epub 2013 Jun 29.

80 Knudson, M.M., Harrison, P.B., Hoyt, D.B. et al. (2000). Outcome after major renovascular injuries: a Western trauma association multicenter report. *J. Trauma* 49 (6): 1116–1122.

81 Serafetinides, E., Kitrey, N.D., Djakovic, N. et al. (2015). Review of the current management of upper urinary tract injuries by the EAU Trauma Guidelines Panel. *Eur. Urol.* 67 (5): 930–936.

82 Lynch, T.H., Martínez-Piñeiro, L., Plas, E. et al. (2005). EAU guidelines on urological trauma. *Eur. Urol.* 47 (1): 1–15.

83 Jebara, V.A., El Rassi, I., Achouh, P.E. et al. (1998). Renal artery pseudoaneurysm after blunt abdominal trauma. *J. Vasc. Surg.* 27 (2): 362–365.

84 Chazen, M.D. and Miller, K.S. (1997). Intrarenal pseudoaneurysm presenting 15 years after penetrating renal injury. *Urology* 49 (5): 774–776.

85 Heyns, C.F., de Klerk, D.P., and de Kock, M.L. (1983). Stab wounds associated with hematuria – a review of 67 cases. *J. Urol.* 130 (2): 228–231.

86 Swana, H.S., Cohn, S.M., Burns, G.A., and Egglin, T.K. (1996). Renal artery pseudoaneurysm after blunt abdominal trauma: case report and literature review. *J. Trauma* 40 (3): 459–461.

87 Lee, R.S. and Porter, J.R. (2003). Traumatic renal artery pseudoaneurysm: diagnosis and management techniques. *J. Trauma* 55 (5): 972–978.

88 Farrell, T.M., Sutton, J.E., and Burchard, K.W. (1996). Renal artery pseudoaneurysm: a cause of delayed hematuria in blunt trauma. *J. Trauma* 41 (6): 1067–1068.

89 Tomita, K., Iwaki, H., Kageyama, S. et al. (2010). Renal arteriovenous fistula induced by blunt renal trauma: a case report. *Hinyokika Kiyo* 56 (1): 25–28.

90 Aulakh, T.S., Hayne, D., and Hinwood, D. (2007). Delayed presentation of arteriovenous fistula 20 years after blunt renal trauma. *Int. Urol. Nephrol.* 39 (3): 713–715.

91 Armstrong, A.L., Birch, B.R., and Jenkins, J.D. (1994). Renal arteriovenous fistula following blunt trauma. *Br. J. Urol.* 73 (3): 321–322.

92 Benson, D.A., Stockinger, Z.T., and Mcswain, N.E. (2005). Embolization of an acute renal arteriovenous fistula following a stab wound: case report and review of the literature. *Am. Surg.* 71 (1): 62–65.

93 Uflacker, R., Paolini, R.M., and Lima, S. (1984). Management of traumatic hematuria by selective renal artery embolization. *J. Urol.* 132 (4): 662–667.

94 Reilly, K.J., Shapiro, M.B., and Haskal, Z.J. (1996). Angiographic embolization of a penetrating traumatic renal arteriovenous fistula. *J. Trauma* 41 (4): 763.

95 Tucci, P., Doctor, D., and Diagonale, A. (1979). Embolization of post-traumatic renal arteriovenous fistula. *Urology* 13 (2): 192–194.

96 Reigle, M.D., Selzman, A.A., Elder, J.S., and Spirnak, J.P. (1998). Use of ureteral stents in the management of major renal trauma with urinary extravasation: is there a role? *J. Endourol.* 12 (6): 545–549.

97 Buckley, J.C. and McAninch, J.W. (2006). Selective management of isolated and nonisolated grade IV renal injuries. *J. Urol.* 176 (6 Pt 1): 2498–2502; discussion 2502.

98 Heyns, C.F. (2004). Renal trauma: indications for imaging and surgical exploration. *BJU Int.* 93 (8): 1165–1170.

99 Moudouni, S.M., Patard, J.J., Manunta, A. et al. (2001). A conservative approach to major blunt renal lacerations with urinary extravasation and devitalized renal segments. *BJU Int.* 87 (4): 290–294.

100 Husmann, D.A. and Morris, J.S. (1990). Attempted nonoperative management of blunt renal lacerations extending through the corticomedullary junction: the short-term and long-term sequelae. *J. Urol.* 143 (4): 682–684.

101 Keihani, S., Anderson, R.E., Fiander, M. et al. (2018). Incidence of urinary extravasation and rate of urethral stenting after high-grade renal trauma in adults: a meta-analysis. *Transl. Androl. Urol.* 7 (Suppl. 2): S169–S178. https://doi.org/10.21037/tau.2018.04.13.

102 Prakash, S.V., Mohan, C.G., Reddy, V.B. et al. (2015). Salvageability of kidney in Grade IV renal trauma by minimally invasive treatment methods. *J. Emerg. Trauma Shock* 8 (1): 16–20. https://doi.org/10.4103/0974-2700.145418.

103 Keller, M.S., Eric Coln, C., Garza, J.J. et al. (2004). Functional outcome of nonoperatively managed renal injuries in children. *J. Trauma* 57 (1): 108–110; discussion 110.

104 Keller, M.S. and Green, M.C. (2009). Comparison of short- and long-term functional outcome of nonoperatively managed renal injuries in children. *J. Pediatr. Surg.* 44 (1): 144–147; discussion 147.

105 Tasian, G.E., Aaronson, D.S., and McAninch, J.W. (2010). Evaluation of renal function after major renal injury: correlation with the American Association for the Surgery of Trauma Injury Scale. *J. Urol.* 183 (1): 196–200.

106 Wessells, H., Deirmenjian, J., and McAninch, J.W. (1997). Preservation of renal function after reconstruction for trauma: quantitative assessment with radionuclide scintigraphy. *J. Urol.* 157 (5): 1583–1586.

107 McGonigal, M.D., Lucas, C.E., and Ledgerwood, A.M. (1987). The effects of treatment of renal trauma on renal function. *J. Trauma* 27 (5): 471–476.

108 Watts, R.A. and Hoffbrand, B.I. (1987). Hypertension following renal trauma. *J. Hum. Hypertens.* 1 (2): 65–71.

109 Lebech, A. and Strange-Vognsen, H.H. (1990). Hypertension following blunt kidney injury. *Ugeskr. Laeger* 152 (14): 994–997.

110 Meyrier, A., Rainfray, M., and Lacombe, M. (1988). Delayed hypertension after blunt renal trauma. *Am. J. Nephrol.* 8 (2): 108–111.

111 Chedid, A., Le Coz, S., Rossignol, P. et al. (2006). Blunt renal trauma-induced hypertension: prevalence, presentation, and outcome. *Am. J. Hypertens.* 19 (5): 500–504.

112 Montgomery, R.C., Richardson, J.D., and Harty, J.I. (1998). Posttraumatic renovascular hypertension after occult renal injury. *J. Trauma* 45 (1): 106–110.

113 Goldblatt, H., Lynch, J., Hanzal, R.F., and Summerville, W.W. (1934). Studies on experimental hypertension: I. The production of persistent elevation of systolic blood pressure by means of renal ischemia. *J. Exp. Med.* 59 (3): 347–379.

114 Fuchs, M.E., Anderson, R.E., Myers, J.B., and Wallis, M.C. (2015). The incidence of long-term hypertension in children after high-grade renal trauma. *J. Pediatr. Surg.* 50 (11): 1919–1921.

115 von Knorring, J., Fyhrquist, F., and Ahonen, J. (1981). Varying course of hypertension following renal trauma. *J. Urol.* 126 (6): 798–801.

116 Working Group on Renovascular Hypertension (1987). Detection, evaluation, and treatment of renovascular hypertension. Final report. *Arch. Intern. Med.* 147 (5): 820–829.

2

Penetrating Renal Trauma

A Civilian and Military Perspective

Jonathan Wingate

Madigan Army Medical Center, Tacoma, WA, USA

Introduction

The World Health Organization (WHO) defines traumatic injuries as either intentional (interpersonal violence related, war-related, or self-inflicted injuries) or unintentional injuries (motor vehicle collisions, falls, etc.). Traumatic injuries are the leading cause of death in the United States for people aged 1–44 years [1]. Worldwide, traumatic injuries are the ninth leading cause of death and disproportionately affects males and those in low and middle-income countries (LMIC) [2]. By 2030, the WHO projects a 28% increase in global deaths due to trauma and injury [3].

Civilian Versus Military Trauma

In civilian trauma, the kidneys are the most commonly injured genitourinary (GU) organ. The kidneys are injured in 1–5% of trauma patients and comprise up to 24% of traumatic solid abdominal organ injuries [4–6]. Stratifying by mechanism, there is wide geographical variation for penetrating renal injury (PRI) versus blunt renal injury (BRI) and the reported range for PRI is between 10.9 and 43.9% of all renal injuries [7–9].

Historically, in wartime trauma, the kidneys were the predominant GU organ injured during conflicts in the early and mid-twentieth century. Hugh Hampton Young described the GU injury patterns for Allied Forces in World War I and noted a 7.3% incidence of renal trauma at time of laparotomy with a 50% mortality rate [10]. These were almost all penetrating injuries, with 93.9% of soldiers having a concomitant hollow viscous injury. Surprisingly, the nephrectomy rate was only 18.1% [10]. There has been a paradigm shift in GU injuries due to advancements in technology – specifically the use of Kevlar body armor – resulting in a significant decline of PRIs and an increase in complex lower tract blast injuries, the signature GU injury of the recent conflicts in the Middle East [11–14].

Although penetrating trauma is seen in both civilian and military trauma, mechanistically they vastly differ. Civilian penetrating trauma has an equal distribution between stab

A Clinical Guide to Urologic Emergencies, First Edition. Edited by Hunter Wessells, Shigeo Horie, and Reynaldo G. Gómez.
© 2021 John Wiley & Sons Ltd. Published 2021 by John Wiley & Sons Ltd.
Companion website: www.wiley.com/go/wessells/urologic

and gunshot wounds (GSW) and the majority of GSW are low-velocity handguns [15]. Military penetrating trauma is usually due to high kinetic weapons such as rifles or due to blast injury (BI). However, due to the global increase of terror attacks and mass shootings, managing patients with injuries from these high kinetic weapons among civilian surgeons is increasing, so understanding how to manage these injuries is paramount.

Pathophysiology of Penetrating Trauma

Low-velocity weapons, such as knives, lead to local tissue damage and effects along the tract of penetration. High-velocity projectiles, such as bullets and shrapnel, result in wider tissue injury. This is governed by the formula $KE = \frac{1}{2} MV^2$, where KE is kinetic energy, M is the bullet mass, and V is the velocity. On average, a rifle (such as the AK-47 or M-16A1) has a bullet velocity 2–3 times greater than a standard handgun. This translates into 4–9 times greater kinetic energy (holding mass constant), thus causing greater damage. There are two areas of projectile-tissue interaction in missile wounds – the permanent and temporary cavity. The permanent cavity is due to local tissue damage and necrosis due to the projectile, whereas the temporary cavity is caused by the transient lateral displacement of tissue [16]. Due to varying bullet characteristics, such as fragmentation, weight, and yaw patterns, bullets can cause variable and significant damage in the temporary cavity that may seem out of proportion to the entry or exit wound.

Injury from explosions are classified into: (i) primary BI due to the interaction of the blast wave with gas-filled structures; (ii) secondary BI due to ballistic trauma resulting from fragmentation wounds from the explosive device or the environment; (iii) tertiary BI due to displacement of the victim or environmental structures, which are largely blunt injuries; and (iv) quaternary BI or burns, toxins, and radiation contamination [17]. Most primary BI do not result in surviving causalities because these patients would have been so close to the blast epicenter that they likely sustained lethal injuries. The pressure wave caused by blasts cause damage primarily to gas-containing organs, such as the lung; the kidneys are remarkably resilient to the pressure effects of blasts, although renal pelvis injuries have been documented [18]. The kidneys are mainly injured by the secondary and tertiary mechanisms. The PRI from blasts have pathophysiology similar to more common injury patterns, such as GSW. Although these fragments are often much smaller than bullets, they may cause more tissue damage due to the sheer number of fragments and because the velocity of these fragments can be over twice that of a rifle.

Anatomy

It is imperative to have a sound understanding of renal anatomy, as it is foundational for understanding associated injury patterns, surgical approach/reconstruction, and comprises the basis of non-operative management (NOM). The kidneys are paired retroperitoneal organs extending from vertebral levels T12 to L3. From deep to superficial, the layers surrounding the kidney are as follows: renal capsule, peri-renal fat, renal fascia (Gerota's fascia), and para-renal fat. Both Gerota's fascia and the renal capsule are responsible for tamponade of renal hematomas and they are both critical layers for renorrhaphy. The vascular supply consists of one main renal artery and vein, although about 25% of

Table 2.1 AAST Renal injury classification, revised in 2018.

Grade I	• Contusion or nonexpanding subcapsular hematoma
Grade II	• Nonexpanding perirenal hematoma
	• <1 cm cortical laceration without urinary extravasation
Grade III	• Cortical laceration >1 cm without urinary extravasation
	• Any injury in the presence of a kidney vascular injury or active bleeding contained within Gerota's fascia
Grade IV	• Laceration into collecting system
	• Segmental renal artery or vein injury
	• Active bleeding beyond Gerota's fascia
	• Segmental or complete kidney infarction due to vessel thrombosis without active bleeding
Grade V	• Main renal artery or vein laceration or hilar avulsion
	• Devascularized kidney with active bleeding
	• Shattered kidney with loss of identifiable parenchymal renal anatomy

Figure 2.1 The kidneys and their association with adjacent organs. *Source:* figure courtesy of Daniel Burke, University of Washington.

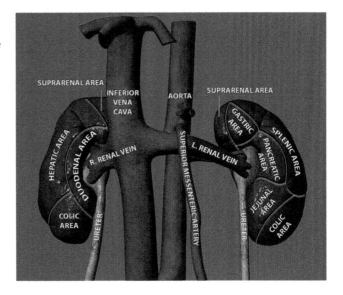

kidneys have accessory vessels. The internal structure can grossly be divided into the renal parenchyma and collecting system. The latter is comprised of minor and major calyces that coalesce into the renal pelvis. This distinction between the parenchyma and collecting system is important in renal injury grading (Table 2.1).

The diaphragm, 11th and 12th ribs, quadratus lumborum, and psoas major surround both kidneys. Anteriorly, the right kidney is associated with the liver, duodenum, and right colic flexure; the left kidney is associated with the spleen, stomach, pancreas, left colic flexure, and jejunum (Figure 2.1). Even with the safeguards of their retroperitoneal location, they are susceptible to penetrating trauma and it is due to their close anatomical relationship with other organs that isolated PRI is rare.

Evaluation

The initial evaluation and management of trauma patients has been standardized according to set protocols with the development of the Advance Trauma Life Support (ATLS) guidelines. Thus, the initial management of the trauma patient has often been completed by the trauma team prior to the involvement of a urologist [19, 20]. Vitals sign monitoring is imperative in patients with PRI, as patient stability dictates management.

For suspected renal trauma, the evaluation should include a thorough history and physical examination to evaluate for penetrating entry and exit wounds, flank ecchymosis, rib fractures, and gross hematuria. In addition to standard laboratory testing, a urinalysis should be obtained to evaluate for microscopic hematuria – defined as three or more red blood cells per high power field. Hematuria is the best indicator of significant renal trauma; however, it is not a sensitive marker, as up to 20.8% of patients with renal trauma lack hematuria [21, 22].

Imaging

The goals of imaging are to grade the renal injury, identify injuries to other organs, and demonstrate the presence of a functioning contralateral kidney should operative management be necessary. The stability of the patient determines the initial imaging; unstable patients cannot obtain computed tomography (CT) scans if they require immediate intervention and the kidneys and retroperitoneum can be assessed in the operating room at time of laparotomy. In military trauma, due to forward deployment of combat support hospitals and the technological progression of expeditionary medicine, CT capabilities are available in war zones and the imaging principles remain congruent with civilian trauma [23].

All stable patients with penetrating abdominal trauma should get diagnostic imaging with IV contrast enhanced CT. To fully evaluate and stage renal trauma (Table 2.1), the American Urological Association (AUA) and European Association of Urology (EAU) recommend a three-phase CT [24, 25]:

1) *Arterial phase*: to assess for vascular injury and active contrast extravasation
2) *Nephrographic phase*: to demonstrate parenchymal contusions and lacerations
3) *Delayed phase*: to identify collecting system injury.

In clinical practice, however, whole-body trauma imaging is often obtained prior to the involvement of the urologist and delayed phase imaging is not routinely performed. As the optimal timing for delayed phase imaging is 9–10 minutes after contrast injection, another CT can be performed without repeat IV contrast injection if performed within this time window [26]. If there is a PRI on initial imaging and delayed phase imaging was not obtained, a repeat CT with delayed phase imaging is still recommended and can be performed with low risk of contrast-induced nephropathy [27].

The American Association for the Surgery of Trauma (AAST) organ injury scale is the most commonly-used tool to grade traumatic solid organ injuries. The AAST staging for renal trauma is shown in Table 2.1. Although it was not originally designed to be a prognostic tool, studies have shown good correlation between higher-grade renal injuries and need for surgical intervention, such as nephrectomy [28, 29].

Findings on CT that are risk factors for hemorrhage and need for urgent invasive intervention are hematoma with a diameter greater than 3.5 cm, medial renal laceration, and intravascular contrast extravasation. In patients with two or more of these risk factors, the risk of intervention to control bleeding was 66.7% [30].

For higher-grade renal lacerations (Grade IV–V), penetrating trauma, or patients experiencing complications (fever, ileus, etc.), both the AUA and EAU recommend repeat CT imaging two to four days after the initial trauma, because these are prone to developing complications from their initial injury, such as urinoma or persistent bleeding [24, 25].

Management

Non-Operative

Traditionally, penetrating trauma has been managed with surgical exploration. However, there has been a shift toward more conservative management of trauma patients due to the improvements in imaging, interventional radiology, and resuscitation techniques. For hemodynamically stable patients, NOM with close patient observation should be offered as first-line therapy [25].

Although there is no consensus algorithm for NOM and there is significant institutional variance, NOM generally comprise of bedrest, strict hemodynamic monitoring in a critical care unit, and serial hematocrit (HCT) checks. If patients are hemodynamically stable with down-trending HCTs, they should be resuscitated with blood products. The presence of active bleeding on imaging, combined with transfusion requirement or hemodynamic instability, indicate that interventional radiology should be consulted for selective embolization. For patients with urinary extravasation, ureteral stenting should be considered, although optimal timing for stenting (early vs. late) is not currently known. We propose one management strategy in Figure 2.2. NOM, however, should not be equated to non-interventional management. Rather, NOM should be viewed as an algorithmic approach with stepwise escalation of intervention based on patient dynamics (see Figure 2.3).

For renal injuries, the site of the wound, hemodynamic stability, and diagnostic imaging (grade of injury) are the main determinants for intervention. Although higher-grade injuries (Grade IV and V) are more likely to require surgical exploration, with careful selection and staging, patients with PRI may be offered a trial of expectant management.

In one series, 54% of stab wounds were successfully managed non-operatively, with only 3% of patients requiring exploration for delayed bleeding [31]. Another series found that stab wounds were more likely to be successfully managed with NOM if the site of abdominal wound penetration is posterior to the anterior axillary line [32].

PRI from low-velocity GSWs can be managed with NOM. In one large series, approximately 30% of gunshot PRIs were successfully managed with observation [33]. As there is also a shift toward selective NOM for gunshot abdominal trauma wounds, there may be a larger impetus for NOM in patients with PRI who would not otherwise undergo surgical exploration [34].

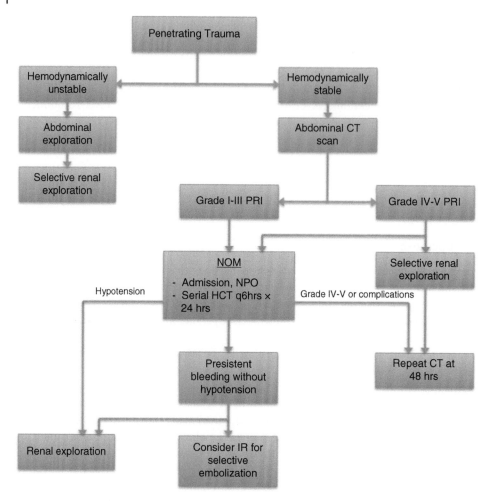

Figure 2.2 Proposed Proposed treatment algorithm. CT, computed tomography; HCT, hematocrit; IR, interventional radiology; NOM, non-operative management; NPO nothing by mouth; PRI, penetrating renal injury.

One quandary has been the management of suspected renal trauma in patients without pre-operative CT imaging. Data suggests that even if patients are undergoing surgical exploration for associated non-urologic injuries, renal exploration is not always necessary. The only absolute indication for renal exploration is a pulsatile or expanding retroperitoneal hematoma. Stable retroperitoneal hematomas should not be explored [24]. Obvious urinary leakage from a penetrating mechanism requires evaluation to exclude a renal pelvis or ureteral injury (see Figure 2.4). In one large series of patients undergoing exploratory laparotomy for renal GSWs, 56% of patients did not need renal exploration and renal exploration was associated with a 50% nephrectomy rate [35]. If patients undergo emergent laparotomy without imaging and a stable zone II (retroperitoneal flank) hematoma is not explored, they should receive appropriate renal imaging once stable, in order to evaluate the extent of the injury.

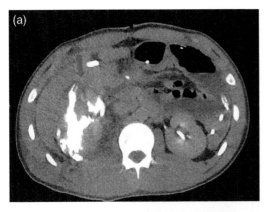
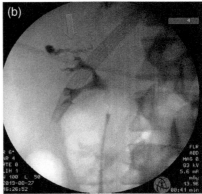
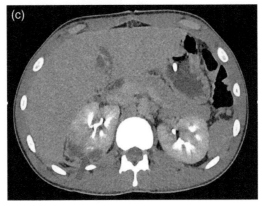

Figure 2.3 Twenty-one-year-old male who sustained a GSW to the abdomen. He had a grade IV right PRI, with injuries to the liver and duodenum. (a) CT demonstrates a significant urine leak on initial delayed phase imaging. (b) He was taken to the operating room for retrograde pyelogram and ureteral stenting. Pyelogram demonstrates contrast extravasation from the middle calyx. Arrow depicts area of contrast extravasation. (c) Repeat CT scan with delayed phase imaging at two weeks demonstrates improved, but persistent contrast extravasation. He was taken to the operating room six weeks after ureteral stenting where retrograde pyelogram demonstrated complete healing of his collecting system and his stent was removed. *Source:* courtesy of Jonathan Wingate, MD.

Operative

Operative management of PRI is not as nuanced as NOM – an unstable patient, unresponsive to resuscitation, requires immediate surgical exploration. Surgical exploration is traditionally performed via a midline transabdominal approach. These cases are often performed in conjunction with trauma surgeons, as the rates of concomitant non-GU organ injuries are very high [8, 36].

Prior to exploring a zone II hematoma, the surgeon should ensure there is a contralateral kidney if no pre-operative imaging was obtained. This can be performed by manual palpation of the contralateral kidney or a single shot urogram (2 ml/kg of IV contrast followed by a KUB at 10 minutes).

(a)

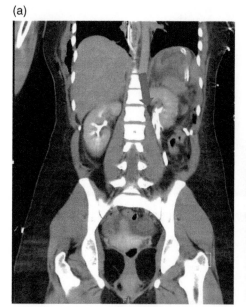

(b)

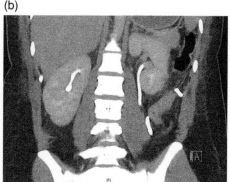

Figure 2.4 Twenty-five-year-old female who sustained multiple stab wounds with a machete. (a) CT scan demonstrates contrast extravasation from the left collecting system. Intra-operatively, she was noted to have a 1.5 cm renal laceration in the inferior pole. There was active urine extravasation from the wound. A renorrhaphy was performed. She also had injuries to the small bowel and right chest. (b) CT performed 48 hours after renorrhaphy demonstrates resolution of the urine leak. *Source:* courtesy of Jonathan Wingate, MD.

Principles of damage control surgery are abbreviated operation, intensive care resuscitation, and definitive surgery. For penetrating trauma, if there is concern for active bleeding at time of laparotomy, source control should be obtained. If there is an expanding zone II hematoma consistent with active renal bleeding, this should be explored. However, for non-expanding hematomas, if the patient is unstable, four-quadrant packing with temporary abdominal closure may be performed in order to allow for resuscitation.

There are two surgical approaches to the kidney – medial or lateral. In the medial approach, the renal vessels are isolated prior to renal exploration as early vascular control may decrease nephrectomy rates and blood loss during surgery [37]. The retroperitoneum is incised over the aorta superior to the inferior mesenteric artery and medial to the inferior mesenteric vein. The anterior surface of the aorta is explored until the left renal vein is encountered crossing anteriorly over the aorta. Vessel loops are then placed around the renal hilum and early vascular control is obtained. The kidney is then exposed by incising the peritoneum lateral to the colon and mobilizing the peritoneum off Gerota's fascia. This approach takes longer and may be difficult in the setting of large hematomas.

In cases of active hemorrhage or an unstable patient, one may not have time to get proximal renal vascular access. For rapid exposure, the kidney can be approached laterally – the retroperitoneum lateral to the kidney is opened and the kidney is delivered into the operative field. Manual compression of the renal parenchyma can help tamponade the bleeding.

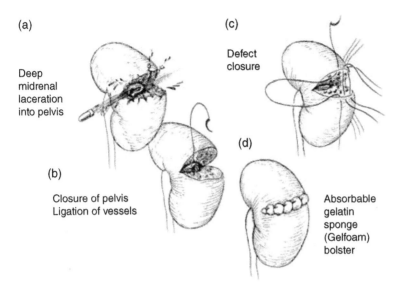

Figure 2.5 Renorrhaphy. (a) Deep midrenal laceration into pelvis. Basic reconstructive principles of renorrhaphy include (b) closure of pelvis and ligation of vessels, (c) defect closure, and (d) placement of Gelfoam® bolsters. *Source:* from Buckley and McAninch [48], with permission.

The hilum can also be manually compressed then a vascular clamp is applied. For significant bleeding, more proximal control can be temporarily obtained through digital compression of the aorta at the diaphragmatic hiatus or with the use of a padded Richardson retractor [38].

Regardless of approach, after vascular control, the renal fascia is opened and the kidney is dissected from the surrounding hematoma. Renal reconstruction is then performed. The principles include complete renal exposure, debridement of nonviable parenchyma, suture ligation of bleeding vessels, closure of any collecting system injuries, and re-approximation of the parenchyma (see Figure 2,5). For injuries to the renal pelvis, a ureteral stent should be placed. This can be placed antegrade via the collecting system defect. Then the renal pelvis should be repaired with a fine, absorbable suture (i.e. 5–0 PDS: polydioxanone suture). Collecting system defects with overlying renal parenchyma, even large ones, do not require routine stenting. Omental flaps may be used for coverage of the repair.

All sutures during the renorrhaphy should be absorbable. The renorrhaphy is performed using an absorbable suture (i.e. 2–0 polysorb) in interrupted horizontal mattress fashion. Pledgets made out of Surgicel can be used to prevent tearing of the sutures from the renal parenchyma. Some urologists place a bolster dressing in the renorrhaphy bed with a hemostatic agent such as Gelfoam or Surgicel (see Figure 2.6). A closed suction drain should be placed in the retroperitoneum but not directly on the renorrhaphy site.

Thrombosis of the renal artery and vein should be managed conservatively. Although surgical revascularization has a high technical success rate, most patients have irreversible ischemic damage or delayed thrombosis [39, 40]. These repairs should only be attempted on patients with solitary kidneys or if they have bilateral occlusion.

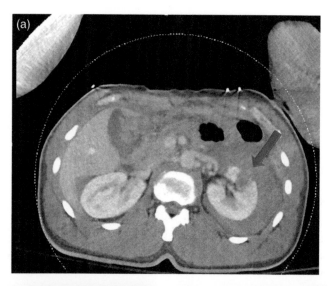

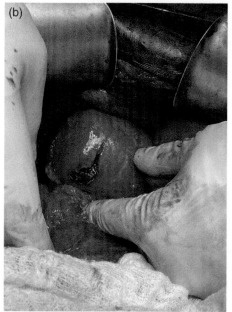
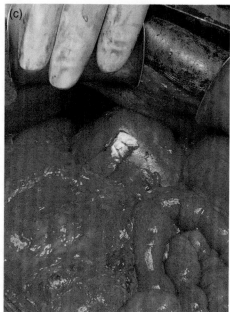

Figure 2.6 Forty-four-year-old male who sustained a GSW with a grade III left renal laceration. While undergoing exploratory laparotomy for multiple abdominal organ injuries, the urology service was consulted for management of his renal injury. (a) Pre-operative CT scan demonstrated a left grade III renal injury without collecting system injury (delayed imaging not shown). (b) Intra-operative photo showing the anterior-medial renal laceration. (c) This was repaired by renorrhaphy. Final appearance shows interrupted 4-0Vicryl sutures over a Gelfoam® bolster. *Source:* photo courtesy of Alexander Skokan, MD, University of Washington.

Indications for nephrectomy include an unreconstructable kidney, significant vascular injury, or an unstable patient who cannot tolerate an attempted repair. In the civilian trauma literature, the nephrectomy rate for PRI ranges from 19 to 31% [8, 41, 42].

For the recent military conflicts in the Middle East, renal trauma comprised 29.6% of the GU injuries, with a 65.5% nephrectomy rate [13, 43]. These rates are much higher than civilian penetrating trauma and seem dissonant with the protective effects of body armor. These high nephrectomy rates are driven by two variables unique to expeditionary medicine: (i) high kinetic energy weapons, such as assault rifles and improvised explosive devices which rendered the majority of the kidneys unreconstructable; and (ii) the unique logistical limitations of battlefield to intercontinental evacuation. The combat damage control paradigm involves up to 10 stages to allow for battlefield evacuation, multiple surgeries and resuscitations, and intercontinental transport, which may contribute to higher nephrectomy rates independent of the mechanistic differences of the PRI [44]. Furthermore, expeditionary surgical teams do not have the same access to resources such as blood products and intensivists. These factors contribute to more aggressive measures to gain definitive hemodynamic stability, even in light of damage control principles.

Complications

Persistent urinary extravasation can lead to urinoma and perinephric abscesses. These can be managed using maximal drainage with the placement of an internal ureteral stent and percutaneous drainage of the abscess or urinoma. Stents are usually left for six weeks with at least seven days of Foley catheter drainage to prevent reflux of urine during voiding [45].

Delayed renal bleeding can occur in up to 23.5% of patients who undergo NOM [46]. This usually occurs within the first seven days after injury and the majority of these cases can be managed by angiography with embolization. Renin-mediated hypertension (Page kidney) from chronic ischemia or compressive hematoma is rare.

Conclusion

During his analysis of GU trauma during World War II, Army urologist and veteran James Kimbrough stated that "conservative treatment has proved sufficient in renal damage [47]." Indeed, the management pendulum of penetrating renal trauma seems to be returning to what was discovered during the two World Wars. Urologists must be prepared with a treatment algorithm should patients fail NOM or have complications, including renorrhaphy and nephrectomy.

References

1 Centers for Disease Control and Prevention (2017). "Injury Prevention & Control: Data & Statistics.". https://www.cdc.gov/injury/wisqars/pdf/leading_causes_of_death_by_age_group_2017-508.pdf.

2 World Health Organization (2014). "Injuries and Violence: The Facts." http://www.who.int/violence_injury_prevention/media/news/2015/Injury_violence_facts_2014/en.

3 World Health Organization (2004). "The Global Burden of Disease: 2004 Update." doi:https://doi.org/10.1016/S0140-6736(02)51408-2.

4 Meng, M.V., Brandes, S.B., and McAninch, J.W. (1999). Renal trauma: indications and techniques for surgical exploration. *World Journal of Urology* 17 (2): 71–77. https://doi.org/10.1007/s003450050109.

5 Smith, J., Caldwell, E., D'Amours, S. et al. (2005). Abdominal trauma: a disease in evolution. *ANZ Journal of Surgery* 75 (9): 790–794. https://doi.org/10.1111/j.1445-2197.2005.03524.x.

6 Wessells, H., Suh, D., Porter, J.R. et al. (2003). Renal injury and operative management in the United States: results of a population-based study. *Journal of Trauma* 54 (3): 423–430. https://doi.org/10.1097/01.TA.0000051932.28456.F4.

7 Mann, U., Zemp, L., and Rourke, K.F. (2019). Contemporary management of renal trauma in Canada: a 10-year experience at a level 1 trauma centre. *Canadian Urological Association Journal* 13 (6): E177–E182. https://doi.org/10.5489/cuaj.5581.

8 Salem, M.S., Urry, R.J., Kong, V.Y. et al. Traumatic renal injury: five-year experience at a major trauma centre in South Africa. *Injury* 51 (1): 39–44. https://doi.org/10.1016/j.injury.2019.10.034.

9 Colaco, M., Navarrete, R.A., MacDonald, S.M. et al. (2019). Nationwide procedural trends for renal trauma management. *Annals of Surgery* 269 (2): 367–369. https://doi.org/10.1097/SLA.0000000000002475.

10 Young, H.H. (1942). Wounds of urogenital tract in modern warfare. *Journal of Urology* 47 (2): 59–108. https://doi.org/10.1016/s0022-5347(17)70776-8.

11 Nnamani, N.S., Janak, J.C., Hudak, S.J. et al. Genitourinary injuries and extremity amputation in operations enduring freedom and Iraqi freedom: early findings from the Trauma Outcomes and Urogenital Health (TOUGH) Project. *Journal of Trauma and Acute Care Surgery* 81 (5): S95–S99. https://doi.org/10.1097/TA.0000000000001122.

12 Janak, J.C., Orman, J.A., Soderdahl, D.W., and Hudak, S.J. (2017). Epidemiology of genitourinary injuries among male U.S. Service members deployed to Iraq and Afghanistan: early findings from the Trauma Outcomes and Urogenital Health (TOUGH) project. *Journal of Urology* 197 (2): 414–419. https://doi.org/10.1016/j.juro.2016.08.005.

13 Hudak, S.J. and Hakim, S. (2009). Operative management of Wartime genitourinary injuries at Balad Air Force Theater Hospital, 2005 to 2008. *Journal of Urology* 182 (1): 180–183. https://doi.org/10.1016/j.juro.2009.02.150.

14 Banti, M. and Walter, J. (2018). Genitourinary trauma. In: *Managing Dismounted Complex Blast Injuries in Military and Civilian Settings: Guidelines and Principles* (eds. J. Galante, M. Martin, C. Rodriguez and W. Gordon), 151–158. Springer https://doi.org/10.1002/9780470755082.ch10.

15 Sakran, J.V., Mehta, A., Fransman, R. et al. (2018). Nationwide trends in mortality following penetrating trauma: are we up for the challenge? *Journal of Trauma and Acute Care Surgery* 85: 160–166. https://doi.org/10.1097/TA.0000000000001907.

16 Jenkins, D. and Dougherty, P. (2004). Guns and bullets. In: *Ballistic Trauma: A Practical Guide*, 2e (eds. P.F. Mahoney, J.M. Ryan, A.J. Brooks and C.W. Schwab), 31–44. London: Springer.

17 Baskin, T. and Holcombe, J. (2005). Guns and bullets. In: *Ballistic Trauma: A Practical Guide*, 2e (eds. P.F. Mahoney, J.M. Ryan, A.J. Brooks and C.W. Schwab), 31–44. London: Springer.

18 Argyros, G.J. (1997). Management of primary blast injury. *Toxicology* 121 (1): 105–115. https://doi.org/10.1016/S0300-483X(97)03659-7.

19 Brasel, K.J. (2013). Advanced Trauma Life Support (ATLS®): the ninth edition. *Journal of Trauma and Acute Care Surgery* 74 (5): 1363–1366. https://doi.org/10.1097/TA.0b013e31828b82f5.

20 Huber-Wagner, S., Lefering, R., Qvick, L.M. et al. (2009). Effect of whole-body CT during trauma resuscitation on survival: a retrospective, multicentre study. *The Lancet* 373 (9673): 1455–1461. https://doi.org/10.1016/S0140-6736(09)60232-4.

21 Brandes, S.B. and McAninch, J.W. (1999). Urban free falls and patterns of renal injury: a 20-year experience with 396 cases. *Journal of Trauma – Injury, Infection and Critical Care* 47 (4): 643–650. https://doi.org/10.1097/00005373-199910000-00007.

22 Kansas, B.T., Eddy, M.J., Mydlo, J.H., and Uzzo, R.G. (2004). Incidence and management of penetrating renal trauma in patients with multiorgan injury: extended experience at an inner city trauma center. *The Journal of Urology* 172 (4 Pt 1): 1355–1360. https://doi.org/10.1097/01.ju.0000138532.40285.44.

23 Harcke, H.T., Statler, J.D., and Montilla, J. (2006). Radiology in a hostile environment: experience in Afghanistan. *Military Medicine* 171 (3): 194–199. https://doi.org/10.7205/milmed.171.3.194.

24 Serafetinides, E., Kitrey, N.D., Djakovic, N. et al. (2015). Review of the current management of upper urinary tract injuries by the EAU Trauma Guidelines Panel. *European Urology* 67 (5): 930–936. https://doi.org/10.1016/j.eururo.2014.12.034.

25 Morey, A.F., Brandes, S., Dugi, D.D. et al. (2014). Urotrauma: AUA Guideline. *Journal of Urology* 192 (2): 327–335. https://doi.org/10.1016/j.juro.2014.05.004.

26 Keihani, S., Putbrese, B.E., Rogers, D.M. et al. (2019). Optimal timing of delayed excretory phase computed tomography scan for diagnosis of urinary extravasation after high-grade renal trauma. *Journal of Trauma and Acute Care Surgery* 86: 274–281. https://doi.org/10.1097/TA.0000000000002098.

27 Colling, K.P., Irwin, E.D., Byrnes, M.C. et al. (2014). Computed tomography scans with intravenous contrast: low incidence of contrast-induced nephropathy in blunt trauma patients. *The Journal of Trauma and Acute Care Surgery* 77 (2): 226–230. https://doi.org/10.1097/TA.0000000000000336.

28 Kuan, J.K., Wright, J.L., Nathens, A.B. et al. (2006). American Association for the Surgery of Trauma Organ Injury Scale for kidney injuries predicts nephrectomy, dialysis, and death in patients with blunt injury and nephrectomy for penetrating injuries. *Journal of Trauma – Injury, Infection and Critical Care.* 60 (2): 351–356. https://doi.org/10.1097/01.ta.0000202509.32188.72.

29 Santucci, R.A., McAninch, J.W., Safir, M. et al. (2001). Validation of the American Association for the Surgery of Trauma Organ Injury Severity Scale for the kidney. *Journal of Trauma – Injury, Infection and Critical Care* 50: 195–200. https://doi.org/10.1097/00005373-200102000-00002.

30 Dugi, D.D., Morey, A.F., Gupta, A. et al. (2010). American Association for the Surgery of Trauma grade 4 renal injury substratification into grades 4a (low risk) and 4b (high risk). *Journal of Urology* 183 (2): 592–597. https://doi.org/10.1016/j.juro.2009.10.015.

31 Armenakas, N.A., Duckett, C.P., and McAninch, J.W. (1999). Indications for nonoperative management of renal stab wounds. *The Journal of Urology* 161 (3): 768–771.

32 Bernath, A.S., Schutte, H., Fernandez, R.R., and Addonizio, J.C. (1983). Stab wounds of the kidney: conservative management in flank penetration. *The Journal of Urology* 129 (3): 468–470. https://doi.org/10.1016/s0022-5347(17)52182-5.

33 Voelzke, B.B. and McAninch, J.W. (2009). Renal gunshot wounds: clinical management and outcome. *Journal of Trauma – Injury, Infection and Critical Care* 66 (3): 593–600. https://doi.org/10.1097/TA.0b013e318196d0dd.

34 Jansen, J.O., Inaba, K., Resnick, S. et al. (2013). Selective non-operative management of abdominal gunshot wounds: survey of practise. *Injury* 44 (5): 639–644. https://doi.org/10.1016/j.injury.2012.01.023.

35 Rostas, J., Simmons, J.D., Frotan, M.A. et al. (2016). Intraoperative management of renal gunshot injuries: is mandatory exploration of Gerota's fascia necessary? This study was a poster presentation at the 2013 clinical congress of the American College of Surgeons, October 6–10, 2013, Washington DC. *American Journal of Surgery* 211: 783–786. https://doi.org/10.1016/j.amjsurg.2015.09.023.

36 McAninch, J.W., Carroll, P.R., Armenakas, N.A., and Lee, P. (1993). Renal gunshot wounds: methods of salvage and reconstruction. *The Journal of Trauma* 35 (2): 279–283; discussion 283-4.

37 McAninch, J.W. and Carroll, P.R. (1982). Renal trauma: kidney preservation through improved vascular control-a refined approach. *The Journal of Trauma* 22 (4): 285–290.

38 Thal, E., Eastridge, B., and Milhoan, R. (2003). Operative Exposure of Abdominal Injuries and Closure of the Abdomen. In: *ACS Surgery: Principles and Practice* (eds. D. Wilmore, L. Cheung, A. Harken, et al.). WebMD.

39 Haas, C.A., Dinchman, K.H., Nasrallah, P.F., and Patrick Spirnak, J. (1998). Traumatic renal artery occlusion: a 15-year review. *Journal of Trauma – Injury, Infection and Critical Care* 45: 557–561. https://doi.org/10.1097/00005373-199809000-00024.

40 Carroll, P.R., McAninch, J.W., Klosterman, P., and Greenblatt, M. (1990). Renovascular trauma: risk assessment, surgical management, and outcome. *The Journal of Trauma* 30 (5): 547–552; discussion 553-4.

41 Davis, K.A., Lawrence Reed, R., Santaniello, J. et al. (2006). Predictors of the need for nephrectomy after renal trauma. *Journal of Trauma – Injury, Infection and Critical Care* 60 (1): 164–169. https://doi.org/10.1097/01.ta.0000199924.39736.36.

42 Keihani, S., Xu, Y., Presson, A.P. et al. (2018). Contemporary management of high-grade renal trauma: results from the American Association for the Surgery of Trauma Genitourinary Trauma Study. *Journal of Trauma and Acute Care Surgery* 84: 418–425. https://doi.org/10.1097/TA.0000000000001796.

43 Paquette, E.L. (2007). Genitourinary trauma at a combat support hospital during operation Iraqi freedom: the impact of body armor. *Journal of Urology* 177 (6): 2196–2199. https://doi.org/10.1016/j.juro.2007.01.132.

44 Blackbourne, L.H. (2008). Combat damage control surgery. *Critical Care Medicine* 36 (7 Suppl): S304–S310. https://doi.org/10.1097/ccm.0b013e31817e2854.

45 Alsikafi, N.F., McAninch, J.W., Elliott, S.P., and Garcia, M. (2006). Nonoperative management outcomes of isolated urinary extravasation following renal lacerations due to external trauma. *Journal of Urology* 176 (6): 2494–2497. https://doi.org/10.1016/j.juro.2006.08.015.

46 Wessells, H., McAninch, J.W., Meyer, A., and Bruce, J. (1997). Criteria for nonoperative treatment of significant penetrating renal lacerations. *Journal of Urology* 157 (1): 24–27. https://doi.org/10.1016/S0022-5347(01)65271-6.

47 Kimbrough, J. (1946). War wounds of the urogenital tract. *The Journal of Urology* 55 (2): 179–189. https://doi.org/10.1016/S0022-5347(17)69896-3.

48 Buckley, J.C. and McAninch (2008). Reconstructive surgery after renal trauma. In: *Textbook of Reconstructive Urologic Surgery* (ed. D.K. Montague), 99. UK: Informa.

3

Renal Infections

Brusabhanu Nayak, Nitin Srivastava, and Rajeev Kumar

All India Institute of Medical Sciences, New Delhi, India

Introduction

Urinary tract infections (UTI) are among the most common human infections and add substantial morbidity and financial burden on society. Clinical presentation may vary from asymptomatic bacteriuria to an acute febrile illness with chills and rigors or even frank septicaemia. The upper urinary tract is normally sterile, and pathogens usually ascend the urinary tract from the perineum, although other pathways such as hematogenous and iatrogenic routes also contribute to the pathophysiology of UTI. Gram-negative bacteria are the usual pathogens; gram-positive bacteria, fungi, and rarely parasites have also been isolated. The common pathologies include acute and chronic bacterial pyelonephritis, emphysematous pyelonephritis (EPN), xanthogranulomatous pyelonephritis (XGP), renal abscess, pyonephrosis, and genitourinary tuberculosis (GUTB) involving the kidney.

Advances in the understanding of the microbiology and the pathophysiology of UTI have improved the management of renal infections, with introduction of more effective antibiotics and better and judicious usage of drugs and combinations of endoscopic, percutaneous, or surgical interventions. Radiological investigations have become indispensable for clinical decision-making. We review the common pathologies and their management.

Acute Pyelonephritis

Acute pyelonephritis is an infective process of the renal parenchyma and is most often a clinical diagnosis based on signs and symptoms of flank pain, tenderness, and fever, with accompanying laboratory findings of leukocytosis, pyuria, positive urine culture, and occasionally bacteraemia and hematuria [1].

A Clinical Guide to Urologic Emergencies, First Edition. Edited by Hunter Wessells, Shigeo Horie, and Reynaldo G. Gómez.
© 2021 John Wiley & Sons Ltd. Published 2021 by John Wiley & Sons Ltd.
Companion website: www.wiley.com/go/wessells/urologic

Epidemiology

A population-based study from the United States has shown annual rates of 15–17 cases of acute pyelonephritis per 10 000 females and 3–4 cases per 10 000 males [2]. The incidence in females shows 3 peaks, at 0–4 years, 15–35 years, and a gradual increase from 50 years of age until another peak at 80 years. Males showed a peak incidence at 0–4 years of age and a gradual increase after 35 years, with a peak at 85 years of age [2].

Clinical Presentation

Acute pyelonephritis has a spectrum of clinical presentation from mild symptoms to a critically-ill condition with frank sepsis [3]. The classic presentation is of flank pain, fever with chills, nausea and vomiting, and costovertebral angle tenderness which can be elicited with mild firm palpation. These are similar to those of a renal abscess, described later in this chapter. Symptoms of cystitis may or may not be present and bilateral involvement can be seen in up to 25% of patients [4, 5].

Acute pyelonephritis can be described as either uncomplicated or complicated, depending upon associated features and conditions [6]. Acute pyelonephritis in an otherwise healthy premenopausal female with normal urinary tract is generally considered uncomplicated, while all others are classified as complicated [6]. Table 3.1 summarizes the conditions associated with complicated pyelonephritis [7–9].

Table 3.1 Factors associated with complicated UTI (pyelonephritis).

Male gender
Pregnancy
Diabetes mellitus
Immunosuppression
Foreign bodies
Indwelling urinary catheter
Ureteric stents
Functional genitourinary abnormality
Neurogenic bladder
Voiding dysfunction
Structural genitourinary abnormality
Stones, fistulae, polycystic kidney
Renal insufficiency
Obstruction
Surgery
Reflux
Nosocomial
Febrile >3 days
Gross hematuria

Source: adapted from [4, 5].

Laboratory Findings

Urinalysis: The dipstick is a useful test in diagnosing UTI. A combination of positive nitrite and leukocyte esterase has a sensitivity of 75% and specificity of 82% for diagnosing a UTI [10]. However, all these may not necessarily be pyelonephritis. Microscopic analysis of the urine can confirm the findings on the dipstick and may help to rule out contamination of the specimen. Urine microscopy can potentially identify additional supporting features and provide immediate information about the nature of the infecting organism. For example, gram-negative rods seen on gram stain or presence of yeast on microscopy can guide the physician in starting empirical antimicrobial therapy. Presence of white blood cells, along with a negative urine culture, suggests sterile pyuria, which can be associated with GUTB.

Cultures: Urine cultures provide microbiological evidence of a UTI with quantitative assessment of the isolated pathogen. Up to 90% of acute uncomplicated pyelonephritis is associated with $\geq 10^5$ CFU/ml of the pathogen. A colony count of $\geq 10^4$ CFU/ml defines significant bacteriuria in acute uncomplicated pyelonephritis [11]. Urine culture is not necessary for diagnosing UTI, but its usefulness lies in directing treatment, particularly in complicated and recurrent UTI [8].

Microbiology and Pathophysiology

Microorganisms can reach the urinary tract through ascending route, haematogenous route, or lymphatic route, but the ascending route is the most common pathway, especially for the organisms of enteric origin like *Escherichia coli* and *Enterobacteriaceae* [12]. The most common organism isolated for both uncomplicated and complicated UTI is uropathogenic *E coli* (UPEC). In uncomplicated UTI, UPEC is followed by *Klebsiella pneumonae*, *Staphylococcus saprophyticus*, *Enterococcus faecalis*, *Proteus mirabilis*, *Pseudomonas*, *Staphylococcus aureus*, and *Candida* species [12, 13], whereas in complicated UTI, UPEC is followed by *Enterococcus species*, *K. pneumonae*, *Candida species*, *S. aureus*, *P. mirabilis*, and *Pseudomonas aeruginosa* [14, 15]. Table 3.2 summarizes the common pathogens associated with complicated and uncomplicated UTI in general. Table 3.3 summarizes the pathogens commonly associated with acute pyelonephritis.

Table 3.2 Pathogens associated with complicated and uncomplicated UTI.

Uncomplicated UTI	Complicated UTI
Uropathogenic *E. coli*	UPEC
Klebsiella pneumonae	Enterococcus species
Staphylococcus saprophyticus	*Klebsiella pneumonae*
Enterococcus faecalis	Candida species
Proteus mirabilis	*Staphylococcus aureus*
Pseudomonas	*Proteus mirabilis*
Staphylococcus aureus, candida species	Pseudomonas

Table 3.3 Pathogens causing acute pyelonephritis [2].

E. coli (most common)

Klebsiella species

Proteus species

Enterobacter species

Pseudomonas

Imaging

The diagnosis of acute pyelonephritis is typically based on clinical and laboratory findings. Imaging may not be required in uncomplicated UTI and treatment can be started empirically on the basis of clinical and laboratory findings [16]. Early imaging is recommended in cases of complicated pyelonephritis, severe symptoms including nausea and vomiting, no response to intravenous antibiotics in 72 hours, or suspicion of renal abscess [16, 17]. Prompt imaging is required in a patient presenting with, or is developing, signs of sepsis. Imaging in these patients may reveal conditions which are potentially treatable with interventions, e.g. obstruction (hydronephrosis), stones, presence of gas, urinoma, perinephric collections, or a renal abscess.

(USG) is the recommended initial modality for imaging because of its non-invasiveness, but there are limitations like obesity and inter-observer differences. USG can miss mild pyelonephritis and underestimates the severity, although contrast enhanced USG can better demonstrate the involved area in acute pyelonephritis [18]. The common USG findings of acute pyelonephritis include diffuse renal swelling, a diffuse or focal decrease in parenchymal echogenicity, loss of corticomedullary differentiation, and thickening of the pelvicalyceal system [18].

Contrast enhanced computed tomography (CT) scan is the current modality of choice for acute pyelonephritis [19]. The nephrogram phase is superior in delineating lesions in acute pyelonephritis, classically striations of the nephrogram (Figure 3.1) and wedge-shaped

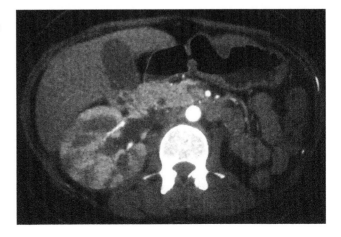

Figure 3.1 Striated nephrogram in right kidney in acute pyelonephritis. *Source:* courtesy of Rajeev Kumar, MD, MCh.

Table 3.4 CT findings in acute pyelonephritis.

Striated nephrogram (Figure 3.1)
Wedge-shaped areas of hypoattenuation, from papilla in medulla to cortical surface
Unifocal or multifocal
Unilateral or bilateral
Focal or global enlargement of kidney
Thickening of Gerota's fascia
Perinephric fat stranding

areas of hypoattenuation. Renal infection CT protocol would include pre-contrast imaging followed by post-contrast and delayed images or urographic phase if obstruction is suspected [20]. Table 3.4 lists the typical CT findings [20].

Magnetic Resonance Imaging (MRI) is being increasingly used in renal infections. Findings of MRI mimic those of a CT scan, typically renal enlargement, areas of poor perfusion, and perinephric fat stranding. Since there is no radiation exposure, MRI becomes an option for evaluation in pregnant women. Furthermore, since iodinated contrast is not used, MRI is useful for patients with impaired renal function. MRI urography may be added for evaluating the pelvicalyceal system, ureter, and bladder. MRI can help in differentiating acute infection from chronic scars, which is difficult on other imaging modalities [21]. However, gas-forming infections and calculi may produce signal voids, interfering with the interpretation [22].

Treatment

The treatment of acute pyelonephritis starts with clinical assessment of the severity and risk factors. Urinalysis and culture should be obtained in every patient. For those with mild symptoms of flank pain and fever without nausea and vomiting, treatment should be started with oral antibiotics, analgesics, and antipyretics along with oral hydration. Imaging, usually USG, is required if any obstruction or stone disease is suspected. Oral ciprofloxacin (500 mg twice daily) for one week, with or without initial intravenous dose of the same, is an appropriate choice of treatment given that the prevalence of resistance of the community uropathogens to fluoroquinolones is not known to exceed 10% [23]. An initial one-time intravenous antimicrobial agent, ceftriaxone or aminoglycoside, can be used in place of intravenous fluoroquinolones [23]. In case the local resistance to fluoroquinolones is known to exceed 10%, an initial one-time intravenous dose of ceftriaxone or aminoglycoside is recommended. [23] Oral trimethoprim-sulfamethoxazole (160/800 mg twice daily for 14 days) is an acceptable choice for therapy if the uropathogen is known to be susceptible [23], and can be used as an alternative if fluoroquinolones cannot be given, for example in cases of known resistance to fluoroquinolones, in elderly patients with increased risk of tendon rupture or in cases of hypersensitivity to fluoroquinolones. If trimethoprim-sulfamethoxazole is given without known susceptibility of the pathogen or an oral beta lactam agent is used to treat pyelonephritis, it is recommended to administer an initial intravenous dose of ceftriaxone/aminoglycoside [23]. If there is no clinical improvement in the first 72 hours, or there are features of deterioration at any time, parenteral antibiotics and hospital admission should be considered. Imaging (see above) is recommended in these patients to assess complicating factors like obstruction or an abscess, which may require drainage along with culture-specific antibiotics.

In cases of severe acute pyelonephritis presenting with systemic symptoms of nausea and vomiting, patients may be unable to take oral medications and should be treated initially with parenteral antibiotics. Infectious Disease Society of America (IDSA) guidelines recommend hospitalization for these patients and treatment with intravenous fluoroquinolones, or an aminoglycoside with or without ampicillin, or an extended-spectrum cephalosporin or an extended-spectrum penicillin with or without an aminoglycoside or a carbapenem [23]. The IDSA guidelines further recommend that the choice between these agents should be based on local resistance data and susceptibility of the pathogen. After clinical improvement, they may be switched to oral antibiotics for 7–10 days [23, 24].

If there is no clinical improvement, parenteral antibiotics are continued and additional urine and blood cultures should be obtained. In the case of severe infection, clinical deterioration, or sepsis, involvement of intensive care unit (ICU) or admission in ICU should be initiated. Additional imaging, preferably with a CT scan, should be performed to look for complicating factors. It can provide the clinician with important information, such as evidence of obstruction (hydronephrosis), gas in the renal parenchyma, or a renal or perinephric abscess. Drainage, in the form of a ureteric stent, percutaneous nephrostomy, or one-time needle aspiration of a renal abscess, can be lifesaving. The choice of drainage procedure largely depends upon the severity of the infection, hemodynamic status of the patient, type and dosage of antiplatelet or anticoagulant agent if any, and the local hospital protocols.

Emphysematous Pyelonephritis

EPN is a life-threatening necrotizing infection of the kidney, characterized by accumulation of gas in the renal parenchyma and surrounding tissue [25]. The disease was first described by Kelly and MacCullem [26], but Schultz and Klorfein [27] first used the term, EPN. There is a spectrum of presentation, with gas seen in renal parenchyma, gas extending to the perinephric space or into the paranephric spaces. When gas is seen only in the collecting system, emphysematous pyelitis, the prognosis is usually good with medical management alone [28]. It should be noted that the gas inside the collecting system can be secondary to instrumentation of the urinary tract, or upper UTI with gas-forming organisms. EPN is notoriously associated with high mortality rates. However, the earlier reported mortality rates of over 70% have now come down to around 20%, due to improved diagnosis and management [29, 30].

There is a female preponderance with a female to male ratio of 3 : 1 [31]. Some studies have described an even higher ratio of 6 : 1 [32, 33]. Up to 95% of cases are associated with diabetes mellitus [29]. Drug abuse, neurogenic bladder, and anatomical anomalies are the other associated factors described in the literature [25, 34]. Almost one-third of patients with EPN may have urinary tract obstruction and this percentage is higher among those who do not have diabetes mellitus as the predisposing cause [35, 36].

Pathogens and Pathogenesis

The most common organisms causing EPN are *E. coli* (70%), followed by *Klebsiella* [36]. Other organisms such as *Acinetobacter, Proteus, Streptococcus*, and *Pseudomonas, Bacteroides* [37], *Clostridium* [38], *Candida* [39] and *Aspergillus* [40] have also been reported. Urine cultures correlating with pus (drained percutaneously) cultures and bacteraemia can be seen in more than 50% of cases [32].

Histopathologic examination of the affected kidney predominantly shows vasculopathy, vascular thrombosis, and widespread micro-abscesses. Other features are interstitial inflammation, glomerulosclerosis, and sloughed papillae [41]. It has been postulated that the high levels of blood glucose in diabetic patients impairs the normal functioning of the leucocytes, thereby reducing the immune response [42].

Gas in renal parenchyma: Huang and Tseng [32] analyzed the gas in renal parenchyma, aspirated radiologically, and found predominantly carbon dioxide and hydrogen. Nitrogen and oxygen were also found with traces of ammonia, methane, and carbon monoxide. It is postulated that microbial infection and increased catabolism causes gas production, which accumulates because ischemic tissue cannot remove it. Presence of gas-forming organisms, high tissue concentration of glucose, and ischemia are the three factors responsible for gas production [32, 43]. Gas in the kidney, and thus severity of the disease, has been classified on the basis of radiological investigations, as shown in Table 3.5. Factors associated with higher mortality are summarized in Table 3.6 [44].

Table 3.5 Classification of emphysematous pyelonephritis.

Classification	Radiological basis	Class	Features
Michael et al. [25]	Plain radiograph and Intravenous pyelogram	Stage 1	Gas present in the renal parenchyma or perinephric tissue
		Stage 2	Gas in the kidney and its surroundings
		Stage 3	Extension of gas through Gerota's fascia and/or bilateral disease
Wan et al. [29]	Computed Tomography	Type 1	Parenchymal destruction with presence of gas but no fluid
		Type 2	Renal or perirenal fluid collection with bubbly or loculated gas or gas in the collecting system
Huang and Tseng [32]	Computed Tomography	Class 1	Gas in the collecting system only
		Class 2	Gas present in the renal parenchyma without extension into extrarenal space
		Class 3A	Extension of gas or abscess into perinephric space
		Class 3B	Extension of gas or abscess into pararenal space
		Class 4	Bilateral EPN or EPN in a solitary kidney

Table 3.6 Factors associated with mortality in emphysematous pyelonephritis.

Significant association with higher mortality
Systolic BP < 90 mmHg
Altered consciousness
Raised serum creatinine levels (>2.5 mg/dl)
Thrombocytopenia
Bilateral EPN
Medical management alone
EPN type 1 based on Wan et al. classification
No significant association with mortality
Diabetes mellitus
Nephrolithiasis
E. coli, Klebsiella pneumonae
Age > 50 years
Female sex
History of UTI
Alcoholism

Clinical Presentation

Women in the fourth and fifth decade of life are the most commonly-affected patients [29]. Patients can present with mild symptoms of fever and flank pain, or may have systemic symptoms of nausea and vomiting, which may be complicated by acute kidney injury, acid base, and electrolyte imbalance, uncontrolled blood glucose, altered consciousness, and sepsis. Rapid progression to septic shock may occur or it may even be the presenting condition [45, 46]. On physical examination, flank tenderness, and sometimes crepitus, can be elicited [46].

Diagnosis

EPN is essentially a radiological diagnosis, and a CT scan is the modality of choice [41]. The usefulness of USG in EPN is limited, because it becomes difficult to differentiate bowel gas from gas in renal parenchyma or abscess. Abdominal distension and obesity can further hamper the assessment [41]. USG misdiagnosed type 1 or type 2 EPN in 50% of patients in the studies carried out by Wan et al. [29]. A CT scan is the modality of choice for diagnosing, staging, and monitoring response to treatment in EPN [41]. A non-contrast CT scan gives excellent information; unless contraindicated, a contrast study should be done to provide details of parenchymal involvement and the extent of disease [29, 41]. Retroperitoneal gas due to other pathologies, like perforation of the second part of duodenum, can mimic EPN, which can be differentiated on the basis of absence of gas in renal parenchyma on the CT scan [47] (Figure 3.2).

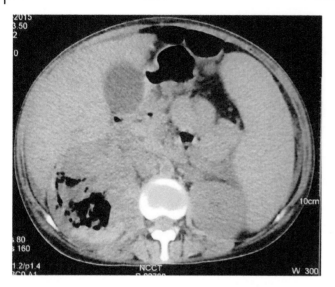

Figure 3.2 Emphysematous pyelonephritis of right kidney. *Source:* courtesy of Rajeev Kumar, MD, MCh.

Treatment

The initial approach to management is resuscitation, parenteral antibiotics, and optimization of glycemic control. The patient may need intensive care admission and multi-organ support. As the condition is known to deteriorate rapidly, aggressive management and prompt surgical intervention, along with intensive care at the earliest sign of deterioration, can improve the outcome. A complete blood count, baseline assessment of renal function, along with urine and blood cultures, should be obtained. Adequate gram-negative coverage is required and should be guided by the local hospital antibiogram. Aminoglycosides, β-lactamase inhibitors, cephalosporins, and quinolones are useful. Aminoglycosides can be used in combination with others [36]. Empirical use of piperacillin and tazobactam is also described [48]. Furthermore, antibiotics should be changed according to the clinical response and culture sensitivity patterns.

The introduction of percutaneous drainage (PCD) techniques has significantly changed the management of EPN. In the 1980s, antibiotics and emergency nephrectomy or open surgical drainage has been described as the management of EPN with a mortality rate of 40–50% [25, 49]. In 1986, Hudson et al. [50] reported favorable outcomes with PCD of affected parts of the kidney using 14Fr tubes under fluoroscopic guidance. Since then, PCD has been used frequently with good results. PCD should be done in patients with localized areas of gas formation and presence of functional renal parenchyma. A large bore (14Fr or higher) catheter should be used for drainage and, in the presence of loculations or multiple areas of gas formation, more than one draining tube can be inserted [51]. Drainage is best performed under CT guidance [41] (Figure 3.3). The PCD tube may have to be retained until the follow-up CT scan shows resolution of gas and subsidence of the infection and inflammation. It can be flushed with an antibiotic solution if required, or changed [51]. Around 13% of patients, treated with medical management and PCD, will still require

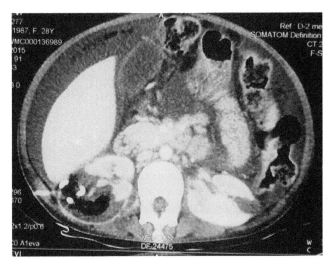

Figure 3.3 Emphysematous pyelonephritis with nephrostomy tube *in situ. Source:* courtesy of Rajeev Kumar, MD, MCh.

nephrectomy, either due to lack of clinical improvement or evidence of a non-functioning kidney on further evaluation, and the reported mortality in this subset is 6.6% [30, 41].

Nephrectomy can be performed by open or laparoscopic approach [52], when there is a non-functioning kidney with no response to conservative management, or Huang class 3A or 3B disease with two or more risk factors. Open nephrectomy is more commonly performed because the laparoscopic approach may be difficult due to extensive inflammation and adhesions as well as risk of intraperitoneal spread of infection.

Xanthogranulomatous Pyelonephritis

XGP, first described by Schlagenhaufer, is an uncommon chronic condition characterized by destruction of renal parenchyma, which is replaced by granulomatous inflammation mainly composed of lipid laden macrophages [52–54]. It is associated with UTI and obstructing renal calculi. Middle-aged women are most often affected and obstructing stones have been reported in 38–83% cases with about half being staghorn calculi [55, 56]. Urine cultures are positive in 50–75% of cases, and the most common organisms are *Proteus* and *E. coli* [57]. *Klebsiella, Pseudomonas,* and *Staphylococcus* are other organisms isolated in urine cultures [58].

There is a higher incidence of XGP in diabetic patients and children [54, 59]. Other factors that may be associated with the development of XGP are abnormal lipid metabolism, altered immunological status, disturbances of leucocytes function like chemotaxis and phagocytosis, malignancy, renal arterial insufficiency, renal venous occlusion and hemorrhage, alcoholism, malnutrition, hyperparathyroidism, renal transplant, prior urological instrumentation or surgery [56, 60]. Bilateral XGP is uncommon [61]. Ninety percent of patients with XGP have diffuse renal involvement, although focal involvement of the kidney can occur [62]. Focal involvement is more common in the pediatric age group and is seen more commonly in children younger than eight years without an associated stone [63, 64].

Clinical Presentation

The onset of the disease is usually subacute or chronic and the duration of symptoms is usually less than six months in the majority of patients [56]. Presenting symptoms may include fever, weight loss/anorexia, and flank pain. Lower urinary tract symptoms and a palpable abdominal mass are less common presenting complaints. Rarely, XGP may present as a nephrocutaneous fistula [60, 62].

Imaging

Diffuse renal enlargement with a central echogenic focus representing a staghorn calculus is the usual finding on USG, but there may be no specific features [65]. CT is the preferred modality for diagnosis and evaluating the extent of the disease [66]. The classical picture is of a staghorn stone, decreased, or absent contrast excretion and a poorly defined mass in an enlarged kidney [67]. The localized or focal XGP can mimic a malignancy, like renal cell carcinoma in adults and Wilms tumor in children, and is sometimes referred to as pseudotumoral or tumefactive form of XGP [67, 68]. On the other hand, the diffuse form has been staged according to the extent of the disease (Table 3.7).

The typical CT findings in a case of diffuse XGP is an enlarged kidney with multiple hypodense egg-shaped areas, likely dilated calices or parenchymal destruction, arranged as in hydronephrosis, with renal calculi [69] (Figure 3.4). XGP has been named as a great imitator, for it resembles other renal diseases both radiologically and pathologically, like acute pyelonephritis, tuberculosis, renal or perinephric abscess, and renal cell carcinoma [70].

Table 3.7 Staging of Xanthogranulomatous pyelonephritis [56, 67].

Stage 1	Involvement is limited to the kidney
Stage 2	Involvement extends to the renal pelvis or the perirenal fat within Gerota's fascia
Stage 3	Involvement extends beyond Gerota's fascia into the retroperitoneum or other organs or both.

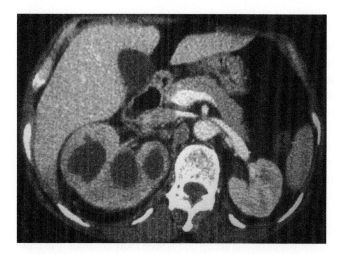

Figure 3.4 Xanthogranulomatous pyelonephritis. *Source:* courtesy of Rajeev Kumar, MD, MCh.

Diagnosis and Treatment

A definitive diagnosis of XGP is made after histopathological analysis of the renal tissue [60]. Grossly, the kidney is enlarged, perinephric tissue may be involved with dense adhesions to surrounding structures, the capsule is thickened with or without necrosis, and there are multiple abscesses in the renal parenchyma, lined by yellowish nodules [58]. On microscopic examination, a mixed inflammatory infiltrate is found with variable numbers of lipid-laden macrophages, neutrophils, giant cells, lymphocytes, and plasma cells [71].

Nephrectomy with antibiotics is the standard treatment of XGP, as most of these kidneys with diffuse involvement are non-functional [72]. A Tc^{99}-DMSA (dimercaptosuccinic acid) scan is used to confirm a non-functioning or poorly-functioning kidney [73]. CT imaging can be helpful in diagnosing XGP in up to 90% cases, but the diagnosis may be difficult as XGP mimics other benign and malignant lesions of the kidney [55]. XGP has been associated with renal cell carcinoma, transitional cell carcinoma of the renal pelvis, and squamous cell carcinoma of the renal pelvis, and therefore a nephrectomy should be performed if malignancy cannot be ruled out [74, 75]. A difficult surgery should be anticipated if a pre-operative CT scan shows pararenal involvement. Separation of the kidney from bowel, diaphragm, or great vessels can be difficult. Segmental resection in an option for stage 1 and stage 2 focal disease [56, 58]. It is very important to relieve any distal obstruction if a nephron sparing surgery is performed. The entire inflammatory mass must be removed to avoid recurrence and fistula formation. Any pre-existing sinus or fistula should also be excised. There are reports of treating focal XGP with antibiotics alone [76]. However, incision and drainage as a single modality can lead to fistulae formation and render nephrectomy more difficult. Open surgery remains the procedure of choice, with the laparoscopic approach restricted to experienced surgeons [77].

Chronic Pyelonephritis

Chronic pyelonephritis is characterized by inflammation, fibrosis, and scarring which is secondary to recurrent or persistent UTI, usually associated with vesicoureteral reflux (VUR) or urinary tract obstruction. It is most commonly seen in children with VUR and patients with anatomic anomalies [78]. In patients with end stage renal disease, 13% have chronic pyelonephritis as the primary cause [79].

Clinical Presentation

A history of recurrent UTI may be elicited in most patients. Some patients, especially children, may present with fever, nausea, vomiting, dysuria, or flank pain. Physical examination may reveal flank tenderness, failure to thrive in young children, or hypertension at a young age. These are typically due to an acute infection, superimposed on chronically diseased kidneys. In fact, there are no specific symptoms of chronic pyelonephritis and the patient can initially present in a state of renal insufficiency.

Radiologic Findings

The typical imaging findings are of renal scarring, atrophy, and cortical thinning. Hypertrophy of normal residual tissue may look like a pseudotumor, and calyceal clubbing may be secondary to retraction of papilla from overlying scar tissue or thickening and dilatation of the calyceal system [80]. Renal asymmetry is often noted, and the kidneys may be smaller in size.

On USG evaluation, kidneys have an irregular outline with areas of atrophic cortex, with dilated underlying calyx. The scar may be hyperechoic as compared to normal surrounding tissue. An intravenous urogram (IVU) will show reduced renal size, irregular outline, caliceal dilatation, and blunting, reaching up to the cortical surface, which is thinned out. Findings on IVU are usually diagnostic. CT scan will demonstrate abnormal renal architecture. Nephrographic and excretory phase will delineate the areas of cortical scars with underlying dilated caliceal system [81]. MRI is comparable to contrast enhanced CT scan for identifying renal scars and abnormal renal architecture [82]. A voiding cystourethrogram will help in diagnosing VUR. A Tc^{99}-DMSA radio isotope scan can also detect renal cortical scars and is more sensitive than IVU [83].

Management

Management includes treating UTI, if present, and preventing further episodes by treating the underlying cause. Recurrent UTIs cause further deterioration of the already compromised renal function and careful monitoring and follow-up is required. Evaluation of the sibling of the patient with VUR is also recommended [84].

Renal Abscess

Renal abscesses present a diagnostic challenge without appropriate radiologic imaging. Renal abscesses caused significant morbidity and mortality in the past due to the lack of early detection; mortality rates in earlier literature varied from 39 to 50% [85]. With improvement in imaging modalities, antibiotics, and PCD, there has been a reduction in morbidity and mortality due to renal abscesses. In recent series, mortality varies from 1.5 to 15% [86, 87].

They can either be intranephric or perinephric in nature. An intranephric abscess is a collection of purulent material within the renal parenchyma, while a perinephric abscess is suppuration within the perirenal fascia. It is usually the result of acute pyelonephritis where inflammation results in liquefactive necrosis and abscess formation. Hematogenous and ascending infections are the two common routes of renal abscess formation. Ascending infection is more common than hematogenous dissemination in renal abscess development. One of the frequent causes is VCR. Perinephric abscess may develop by rupture of an intranephric abscess through the renal capsule into the perinephric space [88, 89].

Epidemiology

The incidence of renal abscesses ranges from <1.3 to 10 cases per 10 000 hospital admissions [90–92]. Hematogenous infection due to gram-positive organisms was commonly responsible for intrarenal abscess development in the pre-antibiotic era. However, most current cases are due to ascending infection from the urinary tract [93, 94]. It affects all age groups without gender predilection, but the incidence increases with age [85, 90, 94]. Predisposing factors (apart from local factors including renal calculi and urinary obstruction) include existing infections at other sites including the skin, teeth, and bones. Additional factors are GUTB, diabetes mellitus, steroid use, and trauma [95, 96]. GUTB remains common in developing countries and causes strictures with obstruction and deformity of the renal parenchyma, thus predisposing to abscess formation. Traumatic hematomas within and around the kidney may get secondarily infected to form an abscess [85]. Renal abscesses are twice as common in diabetic than non-diabetic patients and intravenous drug users contract hematogenous infections through contaminated needles [97–99].

Clinical Presentation

Renal parenchymal abscesses are divided into cortical and medullary abscesses, but this division has little clinical significance [100–102]. Presentation varies from mild symptoms to frank sepsis. Typically, the patient presents with fever, chills, nausea/vomiting, flank pain, and dysuria [103–105]. There is tenderness in the costovertebral angle.

Microbiology

Gram-positive organisms like *Staphylococci* used to be the most commonly responsible for development of renal abscess before the antibiotic era [105, 106]. With widespread use of antibiotics, gram-negative organisms like *E. coli* and *Klebsiella pneumoniae* are most commonly implicated in the development of renal abscess [89, 104, 105, 107, 108].

Laboratory Diagnosis

Urine examination shows presence of white blood cells and bacteriuria. Urine culture often demonstrates the same organism if the abscess is due to a gram-negative organism. If the abscess is due to hematogenous infection by gram-positive organisms, urine culture may not demonstrate any growth. There is marked leukocytosis. Blood culture is usually positive.

Imaging

The most common imaging modalities for diagnosis of renal abscesses are USG and CT. Other modalities that have been used for renal abscesses in the past are excretory urography, angiography, and radioisotope scan. With the increased use of CT, these modalities are no longer used for diagnosis.

USG is the most commonly-used imaging modality for the diagnosis and localization of renal infections [93, 109]. An echo-free or low echodensity space-occupying lesion with increased transmission is seen on the ultrasonogram. USG is also used for percutaneous aspiration of renal abscesses for diagnosis and therapy [109–111]. Contrast enhanced CT is the modality of choice for detecting renal abscesses. The findings depend on the

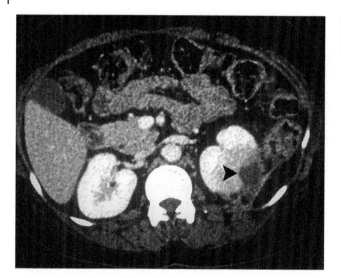

Figure 3.5 Left renal abscess (arrowhead). *Source:* courtesy of Rajeev Kumar, MD, MCh.

duration of the abscess. Initial findings are renal enlargement and areas of decreased attenuation, while chronic abscesses may show a spherical parenchymal mass of low attenuation, surrounded by a higher attenuation inflammatory wall forming a "ring sign" (Figure 3.5).

Radioisotope scans that have been used for evaluating renal abscesses include Galium and Indium scans. The Gallium-67 scan is not very specific for an abscess and has false positive and false negative rates of 15 and 13% respectively [112]. Abnormal accumulation may occur in tumors, vasculitis, and the colon [113]. The radioisotope scan using Indium 111 has the advantage of specific accumulation at the infection site without nonspecific accumulation in the bowel [113]. However, data on the use of this radioisotope in renal abscess detection is limited and its accuracy is not well established.

Management

The standard management of renal abscesses includes drainage and antibiotics followed by management of predisposing causes, if any. The size of the abscess and clinical condition of the patient are important determinants of management. For abscesses less than 3 cm in size, parenteral antibiotics alone may be adequate therapy [114]. For those greater than 5 cm, drainage of the abscess is recommended. Drainage may be achieved by percutaneous or open surgical methods, depending upon feasibility. PCD is possible with minimal morbidity either by USG or CT guidance [88]. For an abscess with intermediate size (3–5 cm), an individualized approach is adopted [115].

The duration of the antibiotic therapy depends upon the patient's clinical condition and response to therapy. The current recommendation is to continue intravenous antibiotics for 48 hours after clinical improvement before switching to oral antimicrobial therapy for 2 weeks thereafter [116]. The choice of antimicrobial therapy depends on the culture and sensitivity of the organisms grown in the aspirate from the abscess. In the absence of an aspirate, antibiotics on the basis of the urine culture are recommended. In the absence of any culture report, empirical antimicrobial therapy with broad-spectrum antibiotics (combination of a third-generation cephalosporin or fluroquinolones and aminoglycoside) is recommended. Nephrectomy is rarely required, usually for patients with diffuse involvement of the kidney with significant parenchymal damage and poor response to therapy. The underlying cause predisposing to abscess formation must be addressed after treating the infection.

Tuberculosis of the Kidney

The genitourinary system is one of the most common sites of extra pulmonary tuberculosis and the kidney is secondarily involved through the hematogenous route. The kidney is the most commonly involved organ in the genitourinary tract. Diagnosis of GUTB is often delayed due to its insidious onset and nonspecific symptoms.

Clinical Presentation

Tuberculosis of the kidney has an insidious onset. Presentation varies from constitutional symptoms like low grade fever, night sweats, and weight loss, to flank pain, dysuria, pyuria, hematuria, discharging sinus in the flank and uremia [117–120]. Bilateral kidney involvement is seen in up to 24% cases [121]. Tuberculosis of the kidney generally affects adults between the second and sixth decades of life [122]. A mean age of 40 years has been reported in the literature [123]. The long latent period ranging from 5 to 40 years between primary pulmonary tuberculosis and its reactivation means that this is rare in children [124].

The most commonly involved organism is *Mycobacterium tuberculosis*. Other mycobacteria like *Mycobacterium bovis* and atypical mycobacterium are rarely involved. Mycobacteria reach the kidney through the hematogenous route from a tubercular focus in the lung [125]. BCG, a live vaccine strain used intravesically for the treatment of bladder cancer, can cause renal lesions by reflux [126, 127]. In the kidney, the mycobacteria form microgranulomas within the periglomerular capillaries and grow further to form macrogranulomas [128].

The upper and lower poles of the kidney are commonly involved [122]. Bacilli from cortical granulomas spill down the nephrons to the loop of Henle to form a new focus of infection within the renal pyramid. The lesions within the renal papilla caseate, cavitate, and form ulcerative lesions. The papillary lesions form extensive papillary necrosis and destruction of adjacent renal parenchyma. The parenchymal lesions extend into the collecting system through erosion. Tubercular lesions cause strictures and obstruction of the pelvicalyceal system. The common sites of strictures within the pelvicalyceal system are the infundibular neck, pelviureteric junction, and vesicoureteric junction. Pelvicalyceal system obstruction along with parenchymal caseation leads to destruction of part or all of the kidney. Rupture of bacilli into the interstitium may cause isolated tubercular interstitial nephritis without any pyuria or hematuria, leading to delayed diagnosis.

Tuberculosis of the kidney can cause chronic kidney disease (CKD) when both the kidneys are involved. The incidence of CKD due to tuberculosis varies from 15 to 24% [121]. Obliterative endarteritis with dystrophic calcification, post-obstructive atrophy due to extensive stricture in the pelvicalyceal system, and tubercular interstitial nephritis are the likely mechanisms. [129, 130]

Laboratory Findings

Examination of early morning urine on 3–5 days for acid fast bacilli (AFB) may identify the disease in around one-third of patients. Polymerase chain reaction (PCR) of urine for mycobacterial antigens is a sensitive test but has doubtful specificity [131]. Newer technology such as the GeneXpert tests may provide results within a few hours [132].

Imaging

Imaging contributes significantly to the diagnosis of GUTB, due to the difficulties associated with obtaining bacteriological proof. USG may identify parenchymal masses, abscesses, cavities, urothelial thickening, and calcifications and hydronephrosis, but has lower sensitivity than IVU or contrast CT due to their ability to detect urothelial changes and deterioration in renal function [133, 134]. IVU is one of the most commonly-used imaging modalities for evaluation of renal tuberculosis. It provides information regarding both structural changes and functional status of the kidneys [135]. The findings of IVU are diverse, depending upon the severity of the infection. Urographic findings will be evident only when the pelvicalyceal system is involved. Approximately 10–15% of patients with active renal tuberculosis will have isolated parenchymal involvement with normal urographic findings [133]. The urographic changes include isolated caliceal dilatation due to infundibular stenosis, gross hydronephrosis, and stricture of the ureteropelvic junction (UPJ). Contrast enhanced CT with delayed images (e.g. CT-IVU) is the most commonly-used imaging modality for renal tuberculosis evaluation in many centers. It helps in diagnosing renal tuberculosis and assessing the severity of loss of function [136]. All the features of the IVU can be delineated with the CT with greater sensitivity.

Treatment

The treatment of renal tuberculosis includes both medical and surgical strategies. Medical management includes antitubercular drugs, as in WHO category I therapy, which includes two months intensive phase of four drugs (Isoniazid, Rifampicin, Pyrizinamide, and Ethambutol) followed by four months continuation phase of Isoniazid and Rifampicin [137]. Surgical therapy may involve draining the kidney, reconstruction of the ureter, bladder, and kidney, or nephrectomy in non-functioning kidneys [137].

Conclusions

Renal infections have a spectrum of presentations, varying from minimal symptoms or asymptomatic to frank sepsis and septic shock. High index of suspicion for renal infection and prompt investigations, as indicated, is required to avoid delay in diagnosis. Knowledge of local resistance patterns of the pathogens could be helpful in formulating antimicrobial therapy. Patients with severe renal infections leading to sepsis may be better managed with ICU involvement or admission. These patients benefit from prompt imaging and interventions for any suspected cause of the infection. A multidisciplinary approach is usually required for patients requiring ICU admission, which may include a urological surgeon, nephrologist, intensive care specialist, and interventional radiologist.

References

1 Talner, L.B., Davidson, A.J., Lebowitz, R.L. et al. (1994). Acute pyelonephritis: can we agree on terminology? *Radiology* 192: 297–305.
2 Czaja, C.A., Scholes, D., Hooton, T.M., and Stamm, W.E. (2007). Population-based epidemiologic analysis of acute pyelonephritis. *Clin. Infect. Dis.* 45: 273–280.
3 Stamm, W. and Hooton, T. (1993). Management of urinary tract infections in adults. *N. Engl. J. Med.* 329: 1328–1334.
4 Scholes, D., Hooton, T.M., Roberts, P.L. et al. (2005). Risk factors associated with acute pyelonephritis in healthy women. *Ann. Intern. Med.* 142: 20–27.
5 Sheffield, J.S. and Cunningham, F.G. (2005). Urinary tract infection in women. *Obstet. Gynecol.* 106: 1085–1092.
6 Hooton, T.M. (2012). Uncomplicated urinary tract infection. *N. Engl. J. Med.* 366: 1028–1037.
7 Neal, D.E. (2008). Jr Complicated urinary tract infections. *Urol. Clin. North Am.* 35: 13–22.
8 Lane, D.R. and Takhar, S.S. (2011). Diagnosis and management of urinary tract infection and pyelonephritis. *Emerg. Med. Clin. North Am.* 29: 539–552.
9 Rubenstein, J.N. and Schaeffer, A.J. (2003). Managing complicated urinary tract infections: the urologic view. *Infect. Dis. Clin. North Am.* 17: 333–351.
10 Hurlbut, T.A. 3rd and Littenberg, B. (1991). The diagnostic accuracy of rapid dipstick tests to predict urinary tract infection. *Am. J. Clin. Pathol.* 96: 582–588.
11 Rubin, R.H., Shapiro, E.D., Andriole, V.T. et al. (1992). Evaluation of new anti-infective drugs for the treatment of urinary tract infection. Infectious Diseases Society of America and the Food and Drug Administration. *Clin. Infect. Dis.* 15 (Suppl 1): S216–S227.
12 Foxman, B. (2014). Urinary tract infection syndromes: occurrence, recurrence, bacteriology, risk factors, and disease burden. *Infect. Dis. Clin. North Am.* 28: 1–13.
13 Ronald, A. (2002). The etiology of urinary tract infection: traditional and emerging pathogens. *Am. J. Med.* 113 (Suppl. 1A): 14S–19S.
14 Levison, M.E. and Kaye, D. (2013). Treatment of complicated urinary tract infections with an emphasis on drug resistant Gram-negative uropathogens. *Curr. Infect. Dis. Rep.* 15: 109–115.
15 Chen, Y.H., Ko, W.C., and Hsueh, P.R. (2013). Emerging resistance problems and future perspectives in pharmacotherapy for complicated urinary tract infections. *Expert Opin. Pharmacother.* 14: 587–596.
16 Kawashima, A., Sandler, C.M., and Goldman, S.M. (1998). Current roles and controversies in the imaging evaluation of acute renal infection. *World J. Urol.* 16: 9–17.
17 Johnson, G.L. and Fishman, E.K. (1997). Using CT to evaluate the acute abdomen: spectrum of urinary pathology. *AJR Am. J. Roentgenol.* 168: 273–276.

18 Kim, B., Lim, H.K., Choi, M.H. et al. (2001). *Ultrasound Med.* 20: 5–14.

19 Goldman, S.M. and Fishman, E.K. (1991). Upper urinary tract infection: the current role of CT, ultrasound and MRI. *Semin. Ultrasound CT MR* 12: 335–360.

20 Gold, R.P., McClennan, B.L., and Rottenberg, R.R. (1983). CT appearance of acute inflammatory disease of the renal interstitium. *AJR Am. J. Roentgenol.* 141: 343–349.

21 Lonergan, G.J., Pennington, D.J., Morrison, J.C. et al. (1998). Childhood pyelonephritis: comparison of gadolinium-enhanced MR imaging and renal cortical scintigraphy for diagnosis. *Radiology* 207: 377–384.

22 Poustchi-Amin, M., Leonidas, J.C., Palestro, C. et al. (1998). Magnetic resonance imaging in acute pyelonephritis. *Pediatr. Nephrol.* 12: 579–580.

23 Gupta, K., Hooton, T.M., Naber, K.G. et al. (2011). International clinical practice guidelines for the treatment of acute uncomplicated cystitis and pyelonephritis in women: a 2010 update by the Infectious Diseases Society of America and the European Society for Microbiology and Infectious Diseases. *Clin. Infect. Dis.* 52 (5): e103–e120. https://doi.org/10.1093/cid/ciq257.

24 Bonkat, G., Pickard, R., Bartoletti, R. et al. (2018). Urological infections. In: *EAU Guidelines*, 16–20. Arnhem: EAU Guidelines Office.

25 Michael, J., Mogle, P., Perlberg, S. et al. (1984). Emphysematous pyelonephritis. *J. Urol.* 131: 203–208.

26 Kelly, H.A. and MacCullem, W.G. (1898). Pneumaturia. *JAMA* 31: 375.

27 Schultz, E.H. Jr., Klorfein, E.H. et al. (1962). *J. Urol.* 87: 762–766.

28 Roy, C., Pfleger, D.D., Lang, H. et al. (2001). Emphysematous pyelitis: findings in five patients. *Radiology* 218: 647–650.

29 Wan, Y.L., Lee, T.Y., Bullard, M.J., and Tsai, C.C. (1996). Acute gas-producing bacterial renal infection: correlation between imaging findings and clinical outcome. *Radiology* 198: 433–438.

30 Somani, B.K., Nabi, G., Thorpe, P. et al. (2008). Is percutaneous drainage the new gold standard in the management of emphysematous pyelonephritis? Evidence from a systematic review. *J. Urol.* 179: 1844–1849.

31 Aboumarzouk, O.M., Hughes, O., Narahari, K. et al. (2014). Emphysematous pyelonephritis: time for a management plan with an evidence-based approach. *Arab. J. Urol.* 12: 106–115.

32 Huang, J.J. and Tseng, C.C. (2000). Emphysematous pyelonephritis: clinical radiological classification, management, prognosis and pathogenesis. *Arch. Intern. Med.* 60: 797–805.

33 Abdul-Halim, H., Kehinde, E.O., Abdeen, S. et al. (2005). Severe emphysematous pyelonephritis in diabetic patients: diagnosis and aspects of surgical management. *Urol. Int.* 75: 123–128.

34 Godec, C.J., Cass, A.S., and Berkseth, R. (1980). Emphysematous pyelonephritis in a solitary kidney. *J. Urol.* 124: 119–121.

35 Stein, J.P., Spitz, A., Elmajian, D.A. et al. (1996). Bilateral emphysematous pyelonephritis: a case report and review of the literature. *Urology* 47: 129–134.

36 Shokeir, A.A., EL-Azab, M., Mohsen, T., and El Diosly, T. (1997). Emphysematous pyelonephritis. A 15 year experience with 20 cases. *Urology* 49: 343–346.

37 Liao, H.W., Chen, T.H., Lin, K.H. et al. (2005). Emphysematous pyelonephritis caused by Bacteroides fragilis. *Nephrol. Dial. Transplant.* 20: 2575–2577.

38 Christensen, J. and Bistrup, C. (1993). Emphysematous pyelonephritis caused by Clostridium septicum and complicated by a mycotic aneurysm. *Br. J. Radiol.* 66: 842–843.

39 Kamalian, M.D., Bhajan, M.A., and Dzarr, G.A. (2005). Emphysematous pyelonephritis caused by candida infection. *Southeast Asian J. Trop. Med. Public Health* 36: 725–727.

40 Ahmad, M. and Dakshinamurty, K.V. (2004). Emphysematous renal tract disease due to Aspergillis fumigatis. *J. Assoc. Physicians India* 52: 495–497.

41 Pontin, A.R. and Barnes, R.D. (2009). Current management of emphysematous pyelonephritis. *Nat. Rev. Urol.* 6: 272–279.

42 Stapleton, A. (2002). Urinary tract infections in patients with diabetes. *Am. J. Med.* 113: 80–84.

43 Yang, W.-H. and Shen, N.C. (1990). Gas forming infection of the urinary tract. An investigation of fermentation as a mechanism. *J. Urol.* 143: 960–964.

44 Falagas, M.E., Alexiou, V.G., Giannopoulou, K.P., and Siempos, I.I. (2007). Risk factors for mortality in patients with emphysematous pyelonephritis: A meta-analysis. *J. Urol.* 178: 880–885.

45 Tang, H.J., Li, C., Yen, M.Y. et al. (2001). Clinical characteristics of emphysematous pyelonephritis. *J. Microbiol. Immunol. Infect.* 34: 125–130.

46 Khaira, A., Gupta, A., Rana, D.S. et al. (2009). Retrospective analysis of clinical profile, prognostic factors and outcomes of 19 patients of emphysematous pyelonephritis. *Int. Urol. Nephrol.* 41: 959–966.

47 Liu, K.-L., Lee, W.-J., Huang, K.-H., and Chen, S.-J. (2007). Right perirenal air: emphysematous pyelonephritis or duodenal perforation? *Kidney Int.* 72: 773–774.

48 Park, B.S., Lee, S.J., Kim, Y.W. et al. (2006). Outcome of nephrectomy and kidney preserving procedures for the treatment of emphysematous pyelonephritis. *Scand. J. Urol. Nephrol.* 40: 332–338.

49 Ahlering, T.E., Boyd, S.D., Hamilton, C.L. et al. (1985). Emphysematous pyelonephritis: a 5-year experience with 13 patients. *J. Urol.* 134: 1086–1088.

50 Hudson, M., Weyman, P.J., van der Vliet, A.H., and Catalona, W.J. (1986). Emphysematous pyelonephritis: successful management by percutaneous drainage. *J. Urol.* 136: 884–886.

51 Ubee, S.S., McGlynn, L., and Fordham, M. (2011). Emphysematous pyelonephritis. *BJU Int.* 107: 1474–1478.

52 Bauman, N., Sabbagh, R., Hanmiah, R., and Kapoor, A. (2005). Laparoscopic nephrectomy for emphysematous pyelonephritis. *Can. J. Urol.* 12: 2764–2768.

53 Schlagenhaufer, F. (1916). Uber eigentumliche Staphylmykosen der Nieven und der pararenalen Bindegewebes. *Frankf. Z Pathol.*: 139–148.

54 Tilkoff-Rubin, N.E., Cotran, R.S., and Rubin, R.H. (2004). Urinary tract infection, pyelonephritis, and reflux nephropathy. In: *Brenner & Rector's The Kidney*, 7e (ed. B.M. Brenner), 1554–1555. Philadelphia: Saunders.

55 Eastham, J., Ahlering, I., and Skinner, E. (1994). Xantogranulomatous pyelnehritis: clinical findings and surgical considerations. *Urology* 43: 295–299.

56 Malek, R.S. and Elder, J.S. (1978). Xanthogranulomatous pyelonephritis: a critical analysis of 26 cases and of the literature. *J. Urol.* 119: 589–593.

57 Chuang, C.K., Lai, M.K., Chang, P.L. et al. (1992). Xanthogranulomatous pyelonephritis: experience in 36 cases. *J. Urol.* 147: 333–336.

58 Levy, M., Baumal, R., and Eddy, A.A. (1994). Xanthogranulomatous pyelonephritis in children. Etiology, pathogenesis, clinical and radiologic features, and management. *Clin. Pediatr. (Phila)* 33: 360–366.

59 Matthews, G.J., McLorie, G.A., Churchill, B.A. et al. (1995). Xanthogranulomatous pyelonephritis in pedriatric patients. *J. Urol.* 153: 1958–1959.

60 Brown, P.S., Dodson, M., and Weintrub, P.S. (1996). Xanthogranulomatous pyelonephritis: Report of nonsurgical management of a case and review of the literature. *Clin. Infect. Dis.* 22: 308–314.

61 Ozcan, H., Akyar, S., and Atasoy, C. (1995). An unusual manifestation of xanthogranulomatous pyelonephritis: bilateral focal solid renal masses. *AJR Am. J. Roentgenol.* 165: 1552–1553.

62 Loffroy, R., Guiu, B., Watfa, J. et al. (2007). Xanthogranulomatous pyelonephritis in adults: clinical and radiological findings in diffuse and focal forms. *Clin. Radiol.* 62: 884–890.

63 Hughes, P.M., Gupta, S.C., and Thomas, N.B. (1990). Case report: xanthogranulomatous pyelonephritis in childhood. *Clin. Radiol.* 41: 360–362.

64 Youngson, G.G. and Gray, E.S. (1990). Neonatal xanthogranulomatous pyelonephritis. *Br. J. Urol.* 65: 541–542.

65 Tiu, C.M., Chou, Y.H., Chiou, H.J. et al. (2001). Sonographic features of xanthogranulomatous pyelonephritis. *J. Clin. Ultrasound* 29: 279–285.

66 Zorzos, I., Moutzouris, V., Korakianitis, G., and Katsou, G. (2003). Analysis of 39 cases of xanthogranulomatous pyelonephritis with emphasis on CT findings. *Scand. J. Urol. Nephrol.* 37: 342–347.

67 Dunnick, N.R., Sandler, C.M., Amis, E.S., and Newhouse, J.H. (1997). Renal inflammatory disease. In: *Textbook of uroradiology*, 2e (eds. N.R. Dunnick, C.M. Sandler, E.S. Amis and J.H. Newhouse), 163–189. Baltimore: Williams & Wilkins.

68 Osca, J.M., Peiro, M.J., Rodrigo, M. et al. (1997). Focal xanthogranulomatous pyelonephritis: partial nephrectomy as definitive treatment. *Eur. Urol.* 32: 375–379.

69 Kim, J.C. (2001). US and CT findings of xanthogranulomatous pyelonephritis. *Clin. Imaging* 25: 118–121.

70 Zorzos, I., Moutzouris, V., Petraki, C., and Katsou, G. (2002). Xanthogranulomatous pyelonephritis—the "great imitator" justifies its name. *Scand. J. Urol. Nephrol.* 36: 74–76.

71 Parsons, M.A., Harris, S.C., Longstaff, A.J. et al. (1983). Xanthogranulomatous pyelonephritis: a pathological, clinical and aetiological analysis of 87 cases. *Diagn. Histopathol.* 6: 203–219.

72 Grainger, R.G., Longstaff, A.J., and Parsons, M.A. (1982). Xanthogranulomatous pyelonephritis: a reappraisal. *Lancet* 1: 1398–1401.

73 Gregg, C.R., Rogers, T.E., and Munford, R.S. (1999). Xanthogranulomatous Pyelonephritis. *Curr. Clin. Top. Infect. Dis.* 19: 287–304.

74 Tolia, B.M., Iloreta, A., Freed, S.Z. et al. (1981). Xanthogranulomatous pyelonephritis: detailed analysis of 29 cases and a brief discussion of atypical presentations. *J. Urol.* 126: 437–442.

75 Schoborg, T.W., Saffos, R.O., Urdaneta, L., and Lewis, C.E. (1980). Xanthogranulomatous pyelonephritis associated with renal carcinoma. *J. Urol.* 124: 125–127.

76 Hughes, P.M., Gupta, S.C., and Thomas, N.B. (1990). Case report: xanthogranulomatous pyelonephritis in childhood. *Clin. Radiol.* 41: 360–362.

77 Rosoff, J.S., Raman, J.D., and Del Pizzo, J.J. (2006). Feasibility of laparoscopic approach in management of xanthogranulomatous pyelonephritis. *Urology* 68: 711–714.

78 Guarino, N., Casamassima, M.G., Tadini, B. et al. (2005). Natural history of vesicoureteral reflux associated with kidney anomalies. *Urology* 65: 1208–1211.

79 Schechter, H., Leonard, C.D., and Scribner, B.H. (1971). Chronic pyelonephritis as a cause of renal failure in dialysis candidates. *JAMA* 216: 514–517.

80 Craig, W.D., Wagner, B.J., and Travis, M.D. (2008). Pyelonephritis: Radiologic-pathologic review. *Radiographics* 28: 255–277.

81 Kawashima, A., Sandler, C.M., Goldman, S.M. et al. (1997). CT of renal inflammatory disease. *Radiographics* 17: 851–866.

82 Majd, M., Blask, A.R.N., Markle, B.M. et al. (2001). Acute pyelonephritis: comparison of diagnosis with 99mTc-DMSA SPECT, spiral CT, MR imaging, and power Doppler US in an experimental pig model. *Radiology* 218: 101–108.

83 Araújo, C.B., Barroso, U. Jr., Barroso, V.A. et al. (2003). Comparative study between intravenous urography and renal scintigraphy with DMSA for the diagnosis of renal scars in children with vesicoureteral reflux. *Int. Braz. J. Urol.* 29: 535–539.

84 Noe, H.N. (1992). The long-term results of prospective sibling reflux screening. *J. Urol.* 148: 1739–1742.

85 Adachi, R.T. and Carter, R. (1969). Perinephric abscess: current concepts in diagnosis and management. *Am. Surg.* 35: 72–75.

86 Meng, M.V., Mario, A.L., and Mcaninch, J.W. (2002). Current treatment and outcomes of perinephric abscesses. *J. Urol.* 168: 1337–1340.

87 Coelho, R.F., Schneider-Monteiro, E.D., Mesquita, J.L. et al. (2007). Renal and perinephric abscesses: analysis of 65 consecutive cases. *World J. Surg.* 31: 431–436.

88 Thorley, J.D., Jones, S.R., and Sanford, J.P. (1974). Perinephric abscess. *Medicine (Baltimore)* 53: 441–451.

89 Papper, S. (1978). Interstitial nephritis: perinephric abscess. In: *Clinical Nephrology*, 2e, 273–274. Boston: Little, Brown.

90 Finegold, S.M. (1977). Perinephric abscess. In: *Infectious Diseases*, 2e (ed. P. Hoeprich), 474–478. Harper and Row: Hagerstown, MD.

91 Hotchkiss, R.S. (1953). Perinephric abscess. *Am. J. Surg.* 85: 471–483.

92 Parks, R.E. (1950). The radiographic diagnosis of perinephric abscess. *J. Urol.* 64: 555–563.

93 Malgieri, J.J., Kursh, E.D., and Persky, L. (1977). The changing clinicopathological pattern of abscesses in or adjacent to the kidney. *J. Urol.* 118: 230–232.

94 Salvatierra, O. Jr., Bucklew, W.B., and Morrow, J.W. (1967). Perinephric abscess: a report of 71 cases. *J. Urol.* 98: 296–302.

95 Anderson, K.A. and McAninch, J.W. (1980). Renal abscesses: classification and review of 40 cases. *Urology* 16: 333–338.

96 Sheinfeld, J., Erturk, E., Spataro, R.F. et al. (1987). Perinephric abscess: current concepts. *J. Urol.*: 137191–137194.

97 Plevin, S.N., Balodimos, M.C., and Bradley, R.F. (1970). Perinephric abscess in diabetic patients. *J. Urol.* 103: 539–543.

98 Freedman, L.R. (1979). Interstitial renal inflammation, including pyelonephritis and urinary tract infection. In: *Strauss and Welt's Diseases of the Kidney*, 3e, vol. 2 (eds. L.E. Earley and C.W. Gottschalk), 817–876. Boston: Little, Brown.

99 Simpkins, K.C. and Barraclough, N.C. (1973). Renal cortical abscess, perinephritis and perinephric abscess in diabetes. *Br. J. Radiol.* 46: 433–436.

100 Schiff, M., Glickman, M., Weiss et al. (1977). Antibiotic treatment of renal carbuncle. *Ann. Intern. Med.* 87: 305–308.

101 Lyons, R.W., Long, J.M., Lytton, B. et al. (1972). Arteriography anid antibiotic therapy of a renal carbuncle. *J. Urol.* 107: 524–526.

102 Schneider, M., Becker, J.A., Staiano, S. et al. (1976). Sonographic correlation of renal and perirenal infections. *Am. J. Roentgenol.* 127: 1007–1014.

103 Doolittle, K.R. and Taylor, J.N. (1963). Renal abscess in the differential diagnosis of mass in kidney. *J. Urol.* 89: 649–651.

104 Timmons, J.W. and Permutter, A.D. (1976). Renal abscess: a changing concept. *J. Urol.* 115: 299–301.

105 Hoverman, I.V., Gentry, L.O., Jones, D.W. et al. (1980). Intrarenal abscess: report of 14 cases. *Arch. Intern. Med.* 140: 914–916.

106 Graves, R.C. and Parkins, L.E. (1936). Carbuncle of the kidney. *J. Urol.* 35: 1–14.

107 Fair, W.R. and Higgins, M.H. (1970). Renal abscess. *J. Urol.* 104: 179–183.

108 Manjon, C.C., Sanchez, A.T., Lara, J.D.P. et al. (2003). Retroperitoneal abscesses—analysis of a series of 66 cases. *Scand. J. Urol. Nephrol.* 37: 139–144.

109 Smith, E.H. and Bartrum, R.J. Jr. (1974). Ultrasonically guided percutaneous aspiraticn of abscesses. *Am. J. Roentgenol. Radium Ther. Nucl. Med.* 122: 308–312.

110 Caldomone, A.A. and Frank, I.N. (1980). Percutaneous aspiration in the treatment of renal abscess. *J. Urol.* 123: 92–93.

111 Pitts, W.R., Kazam, E., Gershowitz, M. et al. (1975). A review of 100 renal and perinephric sonograms with anatomic diagnoses. *J. Urol.* 114: 21–26.

112 Hauser, M.F. and Alderson, P.O. (1978). Gallium-67 imaging in abdominal disease. *Semin. Nucl. Med.* 8: 251–270.

113 Coleman, R.E., Black, R.E., Welch, D.M. et al. (1980). Indium-lll labeled leukocytes in the evaluation of suspected abdominal abscesses. *Am. J. Surg.* 139: 99–104.

114 Dalla Palma, L., Pozzi-Mucelli, F., and Ene, V. (1999). Medical treatment ofrenal and perirenal abscesses: CT evaluation. *Clin. Radiol.* 54: 792–797.

115 Siegel, J.F., Smith, A., and Moldwin, R. (1996). Minimally invasive treatment of renal abscess. *J. Urol.* 155: 52–55.

116 Dembry, L.M. and Andriole, V.T. (1997). Renal and Perinephric abscesses. *Infect. Dis. Clin. North Am.* 11: 663–680.

117 Gibson, M.S., Puckett, M.L., and Shelly, M.E. (2004). Renal tuberculosis. *Radiographics* 24: 251–256.

118 Christensen, W.I. (1974). Genitourinary tuberculosis: Review of 102 cases. *Medicine (Baltimore)* 53: 377–390.

119 Narayana, A. (1982). Overview of renal tuberculosis. *Urology* 19: 231–237.

120 Simon, H.B., Weinstein, A.J., Pasternak, M.S. et al. (1977). Genitourinary tuberculosis. Clinical features in a general hospital population. *Am. J. Med.* 63: 410–420.

121 Krishnamoorthy, S. and Gopalakrishnan, G. (2008). Surgical management of renal tuberculosis. *Indian J Urol.* 24: 369–375.

122 Tonkin, A.K. and Witten, D.M. (1979). Genitourinary tuberculosis. *Semin. Roentgenol.* 14: 305–318.

123 Wise, G.J. (2009). Urinary tuberculosis: modern issues. *Curr. Urol. Rep.* 10: 313–318.

124 Merchant, S.A. (1993). Tuberculosis of the genitourinary system. *Indian J. Radiol. Imaging.* 3: 253–274.

125 Das, K.M., Indudhara, R., and Vaidyanathan, S. (1992). Sonographic features of genitourinary tuberculosis. *AJR Am. J. Roentgenol.* 158: 327–329.

126 Lamm, D.L. (1992). Complications of bacillus Calmette-Guérin immunotherapy. *Urol. Clin. North Am.* 19: 565–572.

127 Garcia, J.E., Thiel, D.D., and Broderick, G.A. (2007). BCG pyelonephritis following intravesical therapy for transitional cell carcinoma. *Can. J. Urol.* 14: 3523–3525.

128 Elkin, M. (1990). Urogenital tuberculosis. In: *Clinical Urography* (ed. H.M. Pollack), 1020–1052. Philadelphia: WB Saunders.

129 Daher Ede, F., Silva Júnior, G.B., Damasceno, R.T. et al. (2007). End-stage renal disease due to delayed diagnosis of renal tuberculosis: A fatal case report. *Braz. J. Infect. Dis.* 11: 169–171.

130 Wise, G.J. and Marella, V.K. (2003). Genitourinary manifestations of tuberculosis. *Urol. Clin. North Am.* 30: 111–121.

131 Moussa, O.M., Eraky, I., El-Far, M.A. et al. (2000). Rapid diagnosis of genitourinary tuberculosis by polymerase chain reaction and non-radioactive DNA hybridization. *J. Urol.* 164: 584–588.

132 Pang, Y., Shang, Y., Lu, J. et al. (2017). GeneXpert MTB/RIF assay in the diagnosis of urinary tuberculosis from urine specimens. *Sci. Rep.* 7: 6181.

133 Kenney, P.J. (1990). Imaging of chronic renal infections. *AJR Am. J. Roentgenol.* 155: 485–494.

134 Premkumar, A., Lattimer, J., and Newhouse, J.H. (1987). CT and sonography of advanced urinary tract tuberculosis. *AJR Am. J. Roentgenol.* 148: 65–69.

135 Kapoor, R., Ansari, M.S., Mandhani, A., and Gulia, A. (2008). Clinical presentation and diagnostic approach in cases of genitourinary tuberculosis. *Indian J Urol.* 24: 401–405.

136 Muttarak, M., Chiang Mai, W.N., and Lojanapiwat, B. (2005). Tuberculosis of the genitourinary tract: Imaging features with pathological correlation. *Singapore Med. J.* 46: 568–574.

137 Kulchavenya, E. (2013). Best practice in the diagnosis and management of urogenital tuberculosis. *Ther. Adv. Urol.* 5: 143–151.

4

Acute Kidney Stone Management

Justin S. Ahn[1] and Jonathan D. Harper[2]

[1] Department of Urology, UCSF School of Medicine, San Francisco, CA, USA
[2] Department of Urology, University of Washington School of Medicine, Seattle, WA, USA

Introduction

Acute renal colic from kidney stones is a common urologic emergency, with significant morbidity and potential mortality risk. Renal colic pain from kidney stones is colloquially described as more painful than childbirth and can result in associated nausea, vomiting, dehydration, and opioid use. Renal obstruction from a stone carries risk of transient or permanent renal injury, and in the setting of infection can prove highly morbid if not fatal. Kidney stone prevalence continues to rise and is estimated to affect 1 in 11 Americans in their lifetimes, with estimates as high as 50% recurrence rates [1, 2]. Stone prevalence, recurrence rate, as well as the unplanned acuity of symptoms requiring emergent evaluation and management, have resulted in kidney stones being the most costly benign urologic disease [3]. Emergency departments are commonly the initial sites of presentation for symptomatic kidney stones, with an estimated 1.2 million associated visits annually in the U.S. [4], resulting in roughly $5 billion in respective charges in 2009 [5]. The differential diagnosis of acute flank and abdominal pain is extensive (Table 4.1) and appropriate evaluation in the primary care or emergency department setting, with urologic consultation or referral, is essential to deliver efficient care and optimize patient outcomes.

History and Physical

Patients typically present with acute onset of sharp, unilateral abdominal, or flank pain that may radiate to the groin and is often described as the worst they have experienced. As stones migrate distally in the ureter, pain may be more focused in the lower abdomen, groin, scrotum, or labia. Location of pain may correspond to stone location within the ureter. Pain is classically intermittent but can be constant with episodic exacerbations. Patients in acute colic are often restless and unable to find a comfortable position in contrast to those with intra-peritoneal pathology such as appendicitis.

A Clinical Guide to Urologic Emergencies, First Edition. Edited by Hunter Wessells, Shigeo Horie, and Reynaldo G. Gómez.
© 2021 John Wiley & Sons Ltd. Published 2021 by John Wiley & Sons Ltd.
Companion website: www.wiley.com/go/wessells/urologic

Table 4.1 Differential diagnosis of renal colic.

Genitourinary

Urinary tract obstruction
   Intrinsic (stones, clot, stricture, neoplasm)
   Extrinsic (malignancy, retroperitoneal fibrosis, endometriosis)

Urinary tract inflammation/infection
   Pyelonephritis
   Cystitis

Retroperitoneal hemorrhage

Renal laceration

Renal malignancy

Ruptured, hemorrhagic, or enlarging renal cyst

Vascular

Aortic dissection

Abdominal aortic aneurysm

Abdominal organ ischemia

Gastrointestinal

Acute hepatitis

Appendicitis

Pancreatitis

Cholecystitis

Diverticulitis

Acute gastritis

Duodenal or gastric ulcer

Bowel obstruction or perforation

Constipation

Volvulus

Irritable bowel syndrome

Gynecologic

Ruptured ectopic pregnancy

Ovarian cyst

Ovulatory or menstrual pain

Ovarian torsion

Pelvic inflammatory disease

Musculoskeletal

Muscle strain

Rib or spine fracture

Ankylosing spondylitis

Table 4.1 (Continued)

Neurologic
Radiculopathy
Fibromyalgia
Endocrine
Adrenal crisis
Rheumatologic
Systemic lupus erythematosus
Other
Munchausen syndrome
Secondary gain

Adapted from Miller and Stoller [6]

Nausea and vomiting are common. Other findings may include gross hematuria; fevers and chills in the setting of systemic infection; or acute lower urinary tract symptoms such as urinary urgency and dysuria, which could be associated with concomitant UTI (urinary tract infection) or bladder irritation from a stone in the distal ureter. Stones that pass into the bladder can typically be easily expelled during urination. In rare circumstances, more likely seen with larger stones or urethral strictures, a stone could become trapped in the urethra.

Additional Relevant History

A pertinent urologic history should elicit prior nephrolithiasis episodes and stone type, associated surgeries or interventions, recent or recurrent UTIs, urinary tract reconstruction, or congenital urinary abnormalities. Patients with a known history of uric acid stones may be candidates for medical stone dissolution with urinary alkalization. To risk stratify patients, it is important to elicit comorbidities that may guide management decisions, such as frailty, immune compromised status, bleeding disorders or active anticoagulation, and cardiopulmonary disease. A patient's social situation can also factor into clinical decision-making, particularly those at risk for noncompliance, delayed follow-up, or limited access to healthcare. Patients should be queried as to any acute or chronic opioid use that may place them at risk for abuse. If there is any suspicion for opioid seeking behavior, many states in the United States have online registries, also known as prescription drug monitoring programs, that providers may use to screen prescription records throughout a state.

Physical Exam

Vital signs have a critical role in the management pathway. Signs of pyelonephritis or systemic infection require immediate attention and may include high-grade fevers (>38.5°C), hemodynamic instability in the form of hypotension with or without tachycardia, diaphoresis, rigors, or altered mental status. Tachycardia or hypertension may be caused by pain and improved with analgesics.

Costovertebral angle tenderness may be present in patients with acute renal colic. Abdominal exam findings may reveal localized tenderness on the ipsilateral upper or lower quadrant, without peritoneal signs. Diffuse abdominal tenderness may be present with pyelonephritis. Dry mucus membranes or poor skin turgor suggest dehydration. Genital exams are not typically warranted for renal colic evaluation, unless the patient notes focal genital or groin pain.

Diagnostic Evaluation

Laboratory

Urine – Urinalysis (UA) with reflexive culture should be performed in the acute management of stones. Microscopic hematuria is common. The presence of white blood cells or leukocyte esterase can suggest infection or urinary tract inflammation from a stone, while nitrites, or bacteriuria are more specific for UTI or colonization. Urine is ideally collected prior to administering antibiotics, since sterilization may occur within four hours of first dose. The absence of organism identification or antibiotic susceptibilities poses a challenge in appropriate treatment, particularly for patients with a history of recurrent urinary infections or multidrug resistant organisms. Patients with urease-producing organisms such as Proteus, Pseudomonas, Klebsiella, Staphylococcus, or Mycoplasma, may harbor bacteria-laden struvite (magnesium ammonium phosphate) stones and are prone to recurrent UTIs until the stone is removed.

Serum – A basic metabolic panel and complete blood count can assist providers in triaging patients presenting with renal colic. Creatinine elevation is seen in ureteral obstruction or dehydration and is more pronounced in patients with chronic kidney disease or a solitary kidney. If available, it is helpful to compare serum creatinine levels with prior known baseline values to look for a relative elevation, particularly in patients with preexisting chronic kidney disease. The presence of concomitant electrolyte abnormalities with creatinine elevation, particularly hyperkalemia or acidosis, should prompt concerns for evolving renal failure or uremia. Dehydration secondary to vomiting or oral intolerance may manifest as a hypokalemic, hypochloremic metabolic alkalosis. Acute hyponatremia, acidosis, or coagulopathy can suggest sepsis.

Leukocytosis may be secondary to infection or stress response. Coagulation studies (platelets, international normalized ratio (INR), prothrombin time (PT)/partial prothrombin time (PTT) are not routinely necessary, unless being considered for acute percutaneous interventions such as nephrostomy tube drainage. Blood cultures from two separate draw sites are recommended if there is concern for sepsis.

Imaging

Imaging plays an essential role in evaluation of acute renal colic, with the primary goal of looking for stone presence, size, location, and hydronephrosis. Kidney stones that pass into the ureter are most often found at three sites of physiological narrowing: the ureteropelvic junction, the crossing over the iliac vessels, and the ureterovesical junction. Approximately 20% of patients that undergo imaging for flank pain will be diagnosed with a stone [7]. There are several options for imaging, each with their respective advantages and

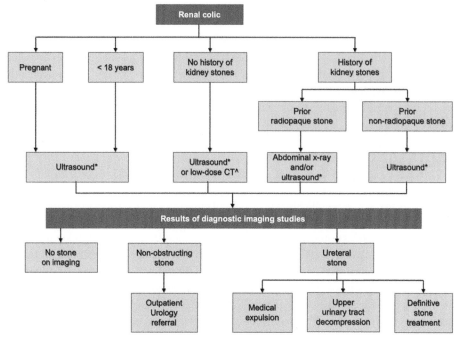

* If incomplete or equivocal results on ultrasound (e.g. hydronephrosis without a visible stone, poor visualization, etc), consider low-dose CT KUB.
^ Consider standard-dose CT for patients with body mass index (BMI) ≥ 40 kg/m².

Figure 4.1 Suggested algorithm for diagnostic imaging for acute renal colic. Adapted from Miller and Stoller [6]

disadvantages. Imaging practices may also be partly determined by healthcare system resources and availability. Providers should consider these factors when deciding on appropriate imaging. Figure 4.1 details a suggested algorithm of imaging evaluation; a comparison of imaging modalities is listed in Table 4.2.

The gold standard remains non-contrast computed tomography (CT) of the abdomen and pelvis (CT KUB), with a median sensitivity and specificity of 98 and 97% respectively [8]. In the acute setting, CT (Figure 4.2) is ideal for assessing for other intra-abdominal pathology, defining urinary tract anatomy and stone location, and measuring stone burden. The cumulative radiation exposure risk to kidney stone patients is significant and should be considered when deciding on CT imaging. A 2019 national study revealed that patients with active kidney stone disease received nearly 10× as many CT scans as non-kidney stone patients over a three-year period [9]. The use of low radiation dose CT KUB (<4 mSv) is strongly encouraged if nephrolithiasis is high in the differential diagnosis, allowing for comparable sensitivity and specificity for stone detection compared to standard dose CT, with significantly less radiation exposure [10]. Despite concerns for compromise in imaging resolution with lower dose, a 2018 study using low dose CT at an effective dose average of 1.9 mSv in patients with suspected nephrolithiasis found excellent sensitivity and specificity (92 and 96% respectively) for the detection of alternative non-stone diagnoses (ex: UTIs, appendicitis, diverticulitis, etc.) [11]. Many hospital radiology departments now offer dedicated low dose or even ultra-low dose (<2 mSv) CT scan protocols if

Table 4.2 Comparison of imaging modalities for renal colic.

Imaging modality	Sensitivity/ specificity for stone detection (%)	Radiation (mSv)	Cost[a]	Advantages	Disadvantages
Plain film (abdominal x-ray)	57/76	0.7	1	• Low cost • Identifies radiopaque stones • Can trend stone size and location	• Poor sensitivity • Limited by intestinal gas and body habitus • No information regarding obstruction
Renal ultrasound	61/97	0	5	• Identifies hydronephrosis and obstruction • Can trend stone burden • No ionizing radiation	• Poor sensitivity • Overestimates stone size • Limited by body habitus • Provides limited anatomy • Provides limited assessment of stone burden • Operator dependent • Poor visualization of ureter
CT KUB	98/97	10	10	• Gold standard for stone diagnosis	• Cost • Radiation
Low-dose CT KUB	94/86	3	10	• Less radiation than standard-dose CT • High sensitivity and specificity	• Limited in obese patients with body mass index $\geq 40\,kg/m^2$
CT Abd/Pelvis with IV contrast (2-phase)	98/97	15	20	• Provides detailed abdominopelvic anatomy	• Contrast required • Radiation • Not recommended for routine stone workup
CT intravenous pyelogram (IVP) or Urogram (3-phase)	98/97	20	20	• Gold standard for evaluation of unexplained hematuria	• Contrast required • Highest radiation • Not recommended for routine stone workup

[a] Cost units compared to plain film (abdominal x-ray), per 2012 CMS data.

specifically requested. It is important to note that CT urogram or the use of IV contrast is not routinely indicated for nephrolithiasis evaluation, as contrast in the kidney and upper urinary tract may obscure stone visualization. These multi-phase studies also expose the patients to superfluous radiation. Contrast can yield information about renal function and excretion and is useful for evaluating renal masses, gross hematuria, and upper urinary

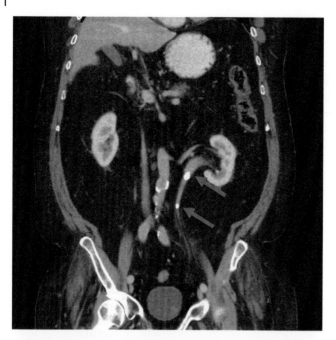

Figure 4.2 CT KUB demonstrating two ureteral stones (arrows) within the left proximal ureter with associated hydroureteronephrosis. *Source:* courtesy of Jonathan D. Harper, MD.

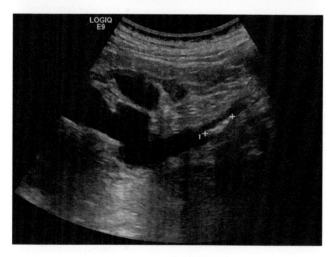

Figure 4.3 Renal ultrasound shows a proximal ureteral stone (yellow cross marks) with associated hydroureteronephrosis. *Source:* courtesy of Jonathan D. Harper, MD.

tract anatomy. If kidney stones are high on the differential diagnosis, a non-contrast phase CT is generally sufficient.

Renal Ultrasound (US) (Figure 4.3) remains particularly useful as a point of care, cost-effective, screening modality for upper urinary tract obstruction or nephrolithiasis without ionizing radiation. It is considered first-line imaging for pediatric or pregnant patients and should be strongly considered in adults with a known history of stones and prior CT imaging [12]. Although ureteral stones outside the ureteropelvic and ureterovesical junction may be difficult to identify with US, hydronephrosis secondary to obstruction can be readily seen, even in obese patients, which may guide management and help patients to avoid CT imaging. US is

Figure 4.4 Plain film abdominal x-ray demonstrates a large radiopaque left proximal ureteral stone (arrow) and two small distal ureteral stones versus vascular phleboliths (arrowhead). *Source:* courtesy of Jonathan D. Harper, MD.

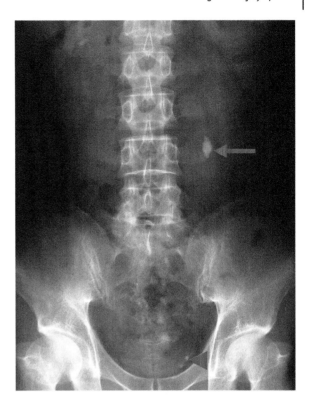

estimated to cost half that of a CT scan. As US utilization and technology improve, there is an increasing role for US in the primary evaluation of acute renal colic patients. A large multicenter study randomized non-obese patients presenting to tertiary emergency departments with suspected nephrolithiasis to receive initial US versus CT KUB. Those undergoing initial US had significantly lower cumulative radiation exposure over six months, without a difference in complications, adverse events, pain scores, return Emergency Department (ED) visits, or hospitalizations [13].

Abdominal plain films or "x-rays" (XR) (Figure 4.4) can serve as an adjunct imaging modality in the acute setting to image radiopaque stones. It is not typically recommended alone, as initial evaluation of renal colic patients, due to its inability to assess for obstruction. However, it may be used to monitor for movement or passage of a known radiopaque stone, seen on former XR or CT scout images. XR can also be used in combination with US to increase diagnostic sensitivity and accuracy. In combination, XR and US allows for improved assessment of urinary tract dilation, stone size, and location compared to either alone.

Management of Symptoms

Pain from renal colic is classically addressed with nonsteroidal anti-inflammatories (NSAIDs), opiates, and alpha-adrenergic receptor blockers. Providers should consider oral or parenteral NSAIDs for first-line pain relief, as studies have shown them to be at least as effective as opioids [14]. NSAIDs provide directed analgesia with a relatively low side effect profile via prostaglandin inhibition, resulting in vasoconstriction of the afferent renal arterioles and direct relaxation of the ureter [15]. The reduced glomerular blood flow results in reduced urine production and can decrease distension of upper urinary tract and its associated pain. NSAIDs should be used with caution if taken for prolonged periods or at high doses. They should be avoided in patients with renal insufficiency or risk of gastrointestinal bleed. High dose acetaminophen (1 g IV or PO), has similar mechanisms of action against prostaglandins, though with less potency [16]. It can serve as an alternative for patients with NSAID contraindications, but should be avoided in those with hepatic dysfunction.

Parenteral and oral opiates provide potent pain relief when NSAIDs are contraindicated or ineffective. In the wake of the opioid epidemic, opioid prescriptions for renal colic patients should be limited and prescribed judiciously on an as-needed basis. To minimize or avoid the need for opioids, providers should consider multimodal non-opioid pain regimens. Scheduled maximum dose acetaminophen and ibuprofen is an example. Other medications that can supplement and provide benefit via alternative pharmacological pathways include gabapentin or tramadol. If opioids are prescribed, care should be taken to educate patients on potential side effects and the need to avoid driving or operating heavy machinery while taking the medication. Physician–patient pain contracts can also be considered up front, particularly in those with a history of chronic pain or opioid use, to define boundaries and criteria, and should be coordinated with other physicians involved in the patient's care. Stool softeners should be prescribed concomitantly to prevent constipation.

Alpha-1 adrenergic receptor blockers (tamsulosin, alfuzosin), which are often used for medical expulsive therapy (MET), can supplement renal colic analgesia via ureteral smooth muscle relaxation. Nausea is often relieved with control of pain, although antiemetic therapy may be required. Nonpharmacologic therapies have also shown benefit, such as heat compresses or acupuncture to the flank or abdomen [17, 18]. Transcutaneous ultrasonic propulsion is under investigation as a noninvasive way to reposition stones and perhaps relieve pain and obstruction [19]. This remains experimental.

Trial of Stone Passage/Medical Expulsion Therapy

Patients with ureteral stones without an indication for urgent intervention (Table 4.3) should be considered for MET. Stones <5 mm are estimated to have a 77% passage rate, and 23% intervention rate, while those >5 mm are estimated at 46 and 54% respectively [20]. Distal ureteral calculi (71%) are more likely to pass than proximal stones (22%) [21]. Four to

Table 4.3 Indications for urgent decompression, via ureteral stenting or placement of percutaneous nephrostomy tube (PCN).

Obstructing stone in the presence of any of the following:
Infection
Compromised Renal Function
Solitary kidney or Bilateral Ureteral Stones
Intolerable Refractory Symptoms

Table 4.4 Estimated spontaneous passage rate and time-to-passage, by stone width.

Stone width	Spontaneous passage rate[a]	Mean passage time[a]
1–4 mm	85%	10 days
5–7 mm	50%	16 days
7–9 mm	15%	25 days
>9 mm	< 10%	Not reported

[a] Estimates based on averages of multiple studies.

six weeks may be allowed for trial of passage if patient symptoms are tolerable. XR (if the stone is radiopaque), US, or low dose CT KUB may be used to check for stone position or passage. Interval renal function labs should be considered in patients with acute kidney injury or preexisting chronic kidney disease. Table 4.4 reflects composite averages of stone passage rate and time based on stone size [22–25].

Ideal patients for MET are those with larger distal ureteral stones of 5–10 mm with well-controlled symptoms, adequate renal functional reserve, and without signs of systemic infection. Alpha blockers such as tamsulosin may relax ureteral wall smooth muscle and improve chances of successful stone passage by up to 20%. More contemporary data suggests this benefit is primarily for stones >5 mm found in the distal third of the ureter at diagnosis [26]. Alpha blocker therapy has also been shown to reduce pain scores and the time to expulsion [27]. Patients receiving these medications should be advised of an approximate 1 in 10 chance of dizziness or hypotension, and in men, retrograde ejaculation. They should be avoided in patients with chronic hypotension or at risk for falls. Given the potential benefits and limited side effect profile of selective alpha-1 receptor blockers, it is reasonable to consider their use in the majority of patients undergoing MET.

Calcium channel blockers (nifedipine) are an alternative option but thought to be inferior to alpha blockers [28]. Efficacy is attributed to ureteral smooth muscle dilation.

A course of low-dose oral corticosteroids can be considered in combination with alpha blockers. Their use may help reduce inflammation and edema of the ureteral wall. Although a decreased passage time by two days has been reported, there was no difference in ultimate stone expulsion rate, analgesic use, lost workdays, and delayed hospitalizations when compared with alpha blocker alone [29]. The side-effect profile with corticosteroids is limited at low doses and when using short therapy durations.

While there is no substantial evidence of the role of hydration with stone passage rates, adequate fluid intake is recommended and may help with expulsion, while mitigating risk of future stone formation. General recommendations for stone prevention are 2–3 l of fluid intake for a goal urine output of over 2 l/day [30].

Medical Dissolution Therapy

Uric acid stones are radiolucent on XR and are typically under 500 Hounsfield Units on CT imaging. Urine pH is typically less than 5.5 in these cases. Patients with a known history of uric acid stones can be considered for medical dissolution therapy with urinary alkalization. By making the urine more alkaline (pH >6–6.5 ideally), uric acid stones can decrease in size or even dissolve completely back into solution [31]. Urinary alkalinization is usually accomplished with oral potassium citrate or sodium-based alkali. Patients started on therapy should be allowed four to six weeks minimum until repeat imaging and should have early follow-up for electrolyte and urine pH checks.

Elevated serum uric acid levels can increase the risk for uric acid or calcium oxalate stone formation primarily based on urine pH. Hyperuricemia is not present in most stone formers, including those with uric acid stones. Concurrent hyperuricemia in patients with kidney stones should be considered for correction, for example, with medication such as allopurinol. Patients may have a history of obesity, gout, myelogenous or lymphocytic proliferative disorders, recent chemotherapy, alcoholism, or excess purine intake.

Acute Procedural Intervention

Indications

The most important determination is whether a patient needs urgent intervention (Table 4.3). After a thorough evaluation, the decision for urgent intervention versus outpatient management hinges on the presence or absence of ureteral obstruction with infection, compromised renal function, patient symptoms, and social considerations.

Infectious symptoms in a patient with an obstructing kidney stone are considered a urologic emergency and should prompt immediate management and urologic consultation. Infectious symptoms can include fever, rigors, tachycardia, hypotension, tachypnea, altered mental status, or any combination. Similar to an abscess, an obstructed system will have limited response to antibiotics and carries significant time-sensitive morbidity and mortality risk. These patients can decline rather quickly, particularly in those with less functional reserve or immunocompromised status. In the presence of evolving sepsis or hemodynamic instability, fluid resuscitation, lab work including blood and urine cultures, as well as broad-spectrum antibiotics should be administered without delay, while concurrently arranging for emergent upper urinary tract decompression.

In contrast to the above situation, patients with a non-obstructing renal stone and UTI symptoms do not require urgent procedural intervention and can be considered for antibiotic therapy alone. Patients with ureteral stones without infectious symptoms, but inconclusive UA, should be managed based on clinical suspicion and risk assessment. A healthy patient with a ureteral stone and inconclusive UA could be managed with or without empiric outpatient antibiotics and urine culture. Meanwhile, an inconclusive UA in a high-risk patient (e.g. elderly, pregnant, diabetic, or immunocompromised) should be managed with more caution with options of decompression, inpatient observation on antibiotics, or prioritized outpatient stone treatment.

An obstructing stone with renal function compromise or renal failure is another indication for urgent upper urinary tract decompression. Patients at highest risk include those with a solitary or transplant kidney, bilateral obstructing stones, or chronic kidney disease. In rare cases of fulminant uremia, urgent upper urinary tract decompression and hemodialysis should be carefully coordinated with a nephrologist. An acutely elevated creatinine could also be attributed to hypovolemia secondary to oral intolerance and vomiting. For these suspected patients without other indications for acute drainage, one may consider symptom control and intravenous or oral fluid replacement, observation and recheck of renal function.

Patients with intolerable renal colic symptoms (e.g. pain, nausea, vomiting, anorexia) that cannot be mitigated with outpatient oral medications, also warrant urgent intervention. Refractory renal colic symptoms usually require hospital admission for intravenous analgesics and hydration and are alleviated with upper urinary tract decompression or stone removal, which should be performed expeditiously to minimize length of hospitalization and polypharmacy. In our experience, these patients tend to have an increased likelihood of impacted stones with higher grades of obstruction.

Patients with prolonged obstruction due to a ureteral stone, greater than four to six weeks, should receive priority for definitive stone treatment or urgent decompression if definitive management cannot be performed in the near future. The same consideration should apply for patients with large ureteral stones >10 mm that are likely to fail trial of passage. Patients presenting with a chronically obstructing stone may demonstrate renal deterioration on imaging with calyceal blunting and renal parenchymal atrophy. In cases of high-grade or complete obstruction, irreversible renal injury can begin to occur within a few weeks [32].

Patient social elements may factor into relative indications for intervention. This includes those at risk for noncompliance, poor follow-up, or limited access to healthcare (e.g. homelessness, living in remote area), as well as patients who cannot afford the risk of complications while on MET or awaiting definitive stone treatment (ex: international traveling, high-stake work obligations such as commercial pilots).

Upper Urinary Tract Decompression

Upper urinary tract decompression is accomplished by placement of either an endoscopic ureteral stent (Figure 4.5) or percutaneous nephrostomy tube (PCN). Urinary drainage with either of these methods can alleviate renal colic symptoms, promote recovery from acute renal injury or infection, and facilitate future stone treatment. By alleviating the comorbidities associated with acute stone presentation, urinary decompression can temporize patients until urologic follow-up and definitive management.

Ureteral stents are hollow plastic tubes, typically 5–7 Fr diameter, with pigtail curls on each end. The stent runs the length of the ureter with the curls deployed in the bladder and renal pelvis for fixation. It is not uncommon for ureteral stones to be pushed back into the kidney at the time of placement, though most often the ureter dilates to accommodate both the stone and stent. It is rare for a stone to pass alongside the stent and as such, a definitive stone treatment is expected after the acute episode resolves. A string may be left attached that exits out of the urethra to facilitate stent removal; however, this is usually not done in the acute stone setting since a stone removal procedure may still be required. If no string is left, the stent is removed by performing an office cystoscopy.

The stent's primary advantage is that it is completely internalized and facilitates drainage by augmenting the pre-existing natural urine passage. Although typically placed under general anesthesia with fluoroscopic guidance, ureteral stents can also be placed in amenable patients under local anesthesia at the bedside [33]. Point-of-care US could improve this

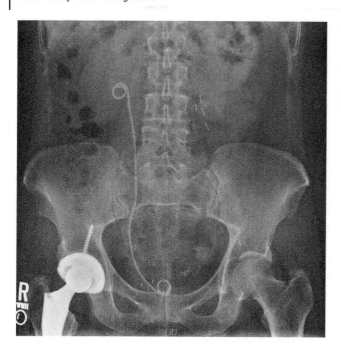

Figure 4.5 Plain film abdominal x-ray demonstrates a right ureteral stent in appropriate position, with proximal curl within renal pelvis and distal curl within the bladder. *Source:* courtesy of Jonathan D. Harper, MD.

technique in the absence of portable fluoroscopy. Ureteral stents have notable stent-associated symptoms. Stent irritation of the upper urinary tract and bladder can result in hematuria, spasms of abdominal and flank pain, as well as bothersome lower urinary tract symptoms such as urgency, frequency, and dysuria. Stent-associated symptoms can range from absent to severe, with the majority of patients falling in between. Because ureteral stents are completely internalized, they are at risk for being left *in situ* for prolonged periods and encrusting if a patient fails to follow-up for removal. Patients need to be counseled appropriately about need for removal. Retained encrusted stents can contribute to loss of kidney and be very challenging to remove.

PCNs are typically pigtail-type catheters that are placed directly through the patient's flank into the renal collecting system. They are deployed with image guidance, most often renal US or fluoroscopy, using a Seldinger technique, and are secured in place with an external suture at the skin level and a separate suture within the tube that maintains the pigtail curl. They can be easily removed with little discomfort by cutting the two fixation sutures. Common tube sizes are around 8–10 Fr. In the acute setting, they are placed using local anesthesia with or without sedation, which makes them advantageous for hemodynamically unstable patients to avoid the hypotensive effects of general anesthesia induction. PCNs are contraindicated in patients with underlying coagulopathy or on therapeutic anticoagulation. Morbid obesity, abnormal renal anatomy, lack of hydronephrosis, and patient difficulty lying prone can make percutaneous interventions more challenging but are not contraindications. PCNs are typically placed by Interventional Radiologists in the United States with a minority of Urologists performing the procedure for acute stone disease. The tube is connected to a urinary drainage bag, which is a common source of burden for patients. Furthermore, placement of the tube through the flank can make it uncomfortable for patients to lay on that side.

Ureteral stents and PCNs have their respective advantages and disadvantages, which patients should be counseled about. When comparing outcomes, they are both effective at upper urinary tract decompression and have similarly rare complication rates [34]. From a quality of life perspective, PCNs may be slightly better tolerated than ureteral stents and require less analgesic use [35]. Although the patient's clinical picture and preferences are important to consider when deciding on drainage options, there are additional relevant factors, including shortest time to decompression, availability of hospital resources and urologic or interventional radiologic staff, physician preference, future surgical stone treatment approach, and cost. After carefully taking into account the aforementioned variables, providers can decide on the best drainage option for the patient.

Stone Treatment

If urgent intervention is warranted, immediate definitive stone treatment in the form of lithotripsy or stone extraction may be considered in lieu of isolated drainage. Patients must be infection free and clinically stable to prevent risks of exacerbating their infection or clinical status with additional urinary tract manipulation or anesthesia time. This option may be considered for patients with isolated refractory renal colic symptoms, mild acute kidney injury, or in those that are not good candidates for MET (ex: large stone, patient preference). Even if the patient is a candidate for immediate definitive management, it is common for hospital workflow and resource availability to ultimately dictate when the procedure may take place. Furthermore, it is possible that attempting definitive stone management acutely may prove difficult due to acute inflammation, edema, and ureteral stone impaction. If these findings arise intra-operatively, switching to drainage alone and surgical deferral are recommended.

The primary stone treatment options are ureteroscopy with stone extraction or laser lithotripsy, extracorporeal shockwave lithotripsy, or percutaneous nephrolithotomy. All procedures are typically performed under general anesthesia on an outpatient basis, with the exception of percutaneous nephrolithotomy, which often involves overnight inpatient hospitalization. Generally, a stone burden <1.5 cm is managed with ureteroscopy or extracorporeal shockwave lithotripsy. For stones >2 cm, percutaneous nephrolithotomy is the treatment of choice.

Prognosis

Renal colic patients proceeding with MET should receive appropriate discharge instructions and follow-up arrangements. Patients should receive a urine strainer if available and be instructed to strain their urine to monitor for visual confirmation of stone passage. Stone capture will allow for stone analysis and eliminate unnecessary repeat imaging or surgery. Patients should be counseled regarding return precautions to the emergency department, in particular fever >38.5°C, intractable pain or nausea not responsive to oral medications, or oral intolerance.

Regardless of a patient's initial disposition (MET, drainage, stone treatment), patients should have close follow-up with a urologist, ideally within two to four weeks if not sooner. Urologic follow-up accomplishes several goals: (i) to confirm stone clearance with symptom screening and possible interval imaging; (ii) to plan for stone and drain removal, if still present, in a timely fashion; iii) to offer counseling and metabolic evaluation for stone prevention; and (iv) to plan surveillance imaging for recurrence monitoring. Many academic hospital centers have dedicated centers or urologists specializing in kidney stones that may be preferable if available locally, but the majority of general urologists manage routine nephrolithiasis.

It is important that renal colic patients managed as outpatients have follow-up regardless of symptom resolution. Patients that pass and capture their stone with complete resolution of symptoms typically do not require additional follow-up imaging to check for passage; however, patients that have resolution of symptoms, but do not clearly visualize their stone are at risk for a retained ureteral stone. It is possible that patients visualize some debris or small blood clot in the toilet that they mistake for their stone and do not capture. Retained ureteral stones over time can cause chronic irritation of the ureteral wall and result in associated scarring and stricture. An initially painful ureteral stone may remain in place but become less painful over time, if not asymptomatic. The resulting process, also known as "silent hydronephrosis" though reportedly rare among patients with ureteral stones, approximately 1% [36], is likely underreported, and can lead to long-term kidney damage or even failure if it remains undetected.

Special Considerations

Pregnant Patients

Acute renal colic is the most common non-obstetric cause of hospital admission during pregnancy [37] and doubles the risk of preterm delivery. [38] Management is similar to the general population, though with some unique considerations. To minimize radiation exposure, US should be considered as first-line imaging. For equivocal cases, assessing for ureteral jet and measurement of renal resistive indices can increase sensitivity of stone diagnosis. Transvaginal US can also be used for suspected distal ureteral stone if not seen with transabdominal US. In cases of non-diagnostic US imaging, MRI (Magnetic Resonance Imaging), or ultra-low-dose CT (outside the 1st trimester if possible), can be considered with appropriate counseling of lower sensitivity and ionizing radiation risk, respectively [39].

Fifty to eighty percent of symptomatic stones during pregnancy will pass spontaneously with appropriate hydration and analgesia [14]. There is limited data suggesting that tamsulosin can be safely taken for MET during pregnancy; however, caution is recommended, especially in the 1st trimester during organogenesis. [40, 41] Asymptomatic bacteriuria should be treated in this patient population, given elevated risk of pyelonephritis and fetal complications.

Ureteral stents or PCN tubes can be placed for decompression; however, they are prone to faster rates of tube encrustation and require exchanges every four to six weeks. Ureteroscopy with laser lithotripsy or stone extraction under general anesthesia may be performed relatively safely in the 2nd or 3rd trimester as an alternative to serial drain exchanges. Shockwave lithotripsy is contraindicated in pregnancy and percutaneous neph-rolithotomy is generally avoided. Coordination with an obstetrician is prudent prior to any procedural intervention to appropriately plan for fetal monitoring or other precautions.

Pediatric Patients

Evaluation and management of acute kidney stones in children is generally similar to that of adult patients with few exceptions. US should be considered as first-line imaging in this population to avoid radiation exposure and due to generally superior visualization of anat-omy, compared to adults. If CT KUB must be performed, low, or ultra-low dose imaging should be ensured. Urologic follow-up in this patient population is highly recommended due to the life-long elevated risk for stone recurrence, as well as the relatively higher rates of metabolic or urinary tract abnormalities, compared to adults.

Conclusion

Management of the acute kidney stone patient can be simplified to stone recognition and triage. Imaging evaluation should attempt to limit radiation exposure through the use of low-dose CT scans or US. Infection in the setting of an obstructing stone is time sensitive, potentially life-threatening, and warrants immediate decompression with a ureteral stent or PCN. Other indications for decompression are an obstructing stone with renal compro-mise, or intractable renal colic symptoms. Immediate lithotripsy or stone removal can be performed in clinically stable patients without infection. Effective decision-making and coordination between front-line providers (Emergency Medicine, Family Medicine, Internal Medicine) and specialists (Urology, Interventional Radiology) is required to achieve the best patient outcomes. Urologic follow-up is recommended, regardless of acute outcomes, for future stone prevention counseling.

References

1 Scales, C.D. Jr., Smith, A.C., Hanley, J.M., Saigal, C.S. Urologic Diseases in America Project. (2012). Prevalence of kidney stones in the United States. Eur. Urol. 62 (1): 160–165

2 Uribarri, J., Oh, M.S., and Carroll, H.J. (1989). The first kidney stone. *Ann. Intern. Med.* 111 (12): 1006–1009.

3 Litwin, M.S. and Saigal, C.S. (2012). *Urologic Diseases in America. Table 14–46: Economic Impact of Urologic Disease.* Washington, DC: Urologic Diseases in America, National Institute of Diabetes and Digestive and Kidney Diseases, National Institutes of Health, Public Health Service, US Department of Health and Human Services NIH publication 12-7865.

4 Eaton, S.H., Cashy, J., Pearl, J.A. et al. (2013). Admission rates and costs associated with emergency presentation of urolithiasis: analysis of the Nationwide Emergent Sample 2006–2009. *J. Endourol.* 27 (12): 1535–1538.

5 Ghani, K.R., Roghmann, F., Sammon, J.D. et al. (2014). Emergency department visits in the United States for upper urinary tract stones: trends in hospitalization and charges. *J. Urol.* 191 (1): 90–96.

6 Miller, J. and Stoller, M. (2013). Renal colic and obstructing kidney stones: diagnosis and management. In: *Urological Emergencies* (ed. H. Wessells), 221–238. New York: Humana Press.

7 Hyams, E.S., Korley, F.K., Pham, J.C., and Matlaga, B.R. (2011). Trends in imaging use during the emergency department evaluation of flank pain. *J. Urol.* 186 (6): 2270–2274.

8 Fulgham, P.F., Assimos, D.G., Pearle, M.S., and Preminger, G.M. (2012). American Urologic Association Guideline: American Urologic Association. Available from: https://www.auanet.org/education/imaging-for-ureteral-calculous-disease.cfm.

9 Dai, J.C., Chang, H.C., Holt, S.K., and Harper, J.D. (2019). National Trends in CT Utilization and Estimated CT-related Radiation Exposure in the Evaluation and Follow-up of Stone Patients. *Urology.* 133:50-56..

10 Poletti, P.A., Platon, A., Rutschmann, O.T. et al. (2007). Low-dose versus standard-dose CT protocol in patients with clinically suspected renal colic. *AJR Am. J. Roentgenol.* 188 (4): 927–933.

11 Weinrich, J.M., Bannas, P., Regier, M. et al. (2018). Low-dose CT for evaluation of suspected Urolithiasis: diagnostic yield for assessment off alternative diagnoses. *AJR Am. J. Roentgenol.* 210 (3): 557–563.

12 Passerotti, C., Chow, J.S., Silva, A. et al. (2009). Ultrasound versus computerized tomography for evaluating urolithiasis. *J. Urol.* 182 (4 Suppl): 1829–1834.

13 Smith-Bindman, R., Aubin, C., Bailitz, J. et al. (2014). Ultrasonography versus computed tomography for suspected nephrolithiasis. *N. Engl. J. Med.* 371 (12): 1100–1110.

14 Pathan, S.A., Mitra, B., and Cameron, P.A. (2018). A systematic review and meta-analysis comparing the efficacy of nonsteroidal anti-inflammatory drugs, opioids, and paracetamol in the treatment of acute renal colic. *Eur. Urol.* 73 (4): 583–595.

15 Chaignat, V., Danuser, H., Stoffel, M.H. et al. (2008). Effects of a non-selective COX inhibitor and selective COX-2 inhibitors on contractility of human and porcine ureters *in vitro* and *in vivo*. *Br. J. Pharmacol.* 154 (6): 1297–1307.

16 Graham, G.G., Davies, M.J., Ray, R.O. et al. (2013). The modern pharmacology of paracetamol: therapeutic actions, mechanism of action, metabolism, toxicity and recent pharmacological findings. *Inflammopharmacology* 21 (3): 201–232.

17 Kober, A., Dobrovits, M., Djavan, B. et al. (2003). Local active warming: an effective treatment for pain, anxiety and nausea caused by renal colic. *J. Urol.* 170 (3): 741–744.

18 Lee, Y.H., Lee, W.C., Chen, M.T. et al. (1992). Acupuncture in the treatment of renal colic. *J. Urol.* 147 (1): 16–18.

19 Harper, J.D., Cunitz, B.W., Dunmire, B. et al. (2016). First in human clinical trial of ultrasonic propulsion of kidney stones. *J. Urol.* 195 (40): 956–964.

20 Leavitt, D.A., de la Rosette, J.J.M.C.H., and Hoenig, D.M. (2016). Strategies for nonmedical management of upper urinary tract calculi. In: *Campbell-Walsh Urology*, 11e, Chapter 53, vol. 2 (eds. A.J. Wein, L.R. Kavoussi, A.C. Novick, et al.), 1235–1259. Philadelphia: Elsevier, Inc.

21 Morse, R.M. and Resnick, M.I. (1991). Ureteral calculi: natural history and treatment in an era of advanced technology. *J. Urol.* 145 (2): 263–265.

22 Ueno, A., Kawamura, T., Ogawa, A., and Takayasu, H. (1977). Relation of spontaneous passage of ureteral calculi to size. *Urology* 10 (6): 544–546.

23 Coll, D.M., Varanelli, M.J., and Smith, R.C. (2002). Relationship of spontaneous passage of ureteral calculi to stone size and location as revealed by unenhanced helical CT. *AJR Am. J. Roentgenol.* 178 (1): 101–103.

24 Dong-Un, T., Yun, S.H., Won, T.K. et al. (2011). Expectant management of ureter stones: outcome and clinical factors of spontaneous passage in a single institution's experience. *Korean J. Urol.* 52 (12): 847–851.

25 Miller, O.F. and Kane, C.J. (1999). Time to stone passage for observed ureteral calculi: a guide for patient education. *J. Urol.* 162 (3 Pt 1): 688–690; discussion 690–1.

26 Ye, Z., Zeng, G., Yang, H. et al. (2018). Efficacy and safety of Tamsulosin in medical expulsive therapy for distal ureteral stones with renal colic: a multicenter, randomized, double-blind, placebo-controlled trial. *Eur Urol.* 73 (3): 385–391.

27 Cui, Y., Chen, J., Zeng, F. et al. (2019). Tamsulosin as a medical expulsive therapy for ureteral stones: a systematic review and meta-analysis of randomized controlled trials. *J. Urol.* 201 (5): 950–955.

28 Preminger, G.M., Tiselius, H.G., Assimos, D.G. et al. (2007). EAU/AUA Nephrolithiasis Guideline Panel. 2007 guideline for the management of ureteral calculi. *J. Urol.* 178 (6): 2418–2434.

29 Dellabella, M., Milanese, G., and Muzzonigro, G. (2005). Medical-expulsive therapy for distal ureterolithiasis: randomized prospective study on role of corticosteroids used in combination with tamsulosin-simplied treatment regimen and health-related quality of life. *Urology* 66 (4): 712–715.

30 Pearle, M.S., Goldfarb, D.S., Assimos, D.G. et al. (2014). Medical Management of Kidney Stones: American Urologic Association Guideline American Urologic Association. Available from: https://www.auanet.org/education/guidelines/management-kidney-stones.cfm.

31 Maalouf, N.M., Cameron, M.A., Moe, O.W., and Sakhaee, K. (2004). Novel insights into the pathogenesis of uric acid nephrolithiasis. *Curr. Opin. Nephrol. Hypertens.* 13 (2): 181–189.

32 Vaughan, E.D. Jr. and Gillenwater, J.Y. (1971). Recovery following complete chronic unilateral ureteral occlusion: functional, radiographic and pathologic alterations. *J. Urol.* 106 (1): 27–35.

33 Nourparvar, P., Leung, A., Shrewsberry, A.B. et al. (2016). Safety and efficacy of ureteral stent placement at the bedside using local anesthesia. *J. Urol.* 195 (6): 1886–1890.

34 Weltings, S., Schout, B.M.A., Roshani, H. et al. (2019). Lessons from literature: nephrostomy versus double J ureteral catheterization in patients with obstructive urolithiasis-which method is superior? *J. Endourol.* 33 (10): 777–786.

35 De Sousa, M.N., Pereira, J.P., Mota, P. et al. (2019). Percutaneous nephrostomy vs ureteral stent for hydronephrosis secondary to ureteric calculi: impact on spontaneous stone passage and health-related quality of life-a prospective study. *Urolithiasis* 47 (6): 567–573.

36 Wimpissinger, F., Turk, C., Kheyfets, O., and Stackl, W. (2007). The silence of the stones: asymptomatic ureteral calculi. *J. Urol.* 178 (4 Pt 1): 1341–1344.

37 Strong, D.W., Murchison, R.J., and Lynch, D.F. (1978). The management of ureteral calculi during pregnancy. *Surg. Gynecol. Obstet.* 146 (4): 604–608.

38 Swartz, M.A., Lydon-Rochelle, M.T., and Simon, D.e.a. (2007). Admission for nephrolithiasis in pregnancy and risk of adverse birth outcomes. *Obstet. Gynecol.* 109 (5): 1099–1104.

39 Brisbane, W., Bailey, M.R., and Sorensen, M.D. (2016). An overview of kidney stone imaging techniques. *Nat. Rev. Urol.* 13 (11): 654–662.

40 Bailey, G., Vaughan, L., Rose, C., and Krambeck, A. (2016). Perinatal outcomes with Tamsulosin therapy for symptomatic Urolithiasis. *J. Urol.* 195 (1): 99–103.

41 Abbott, J.E. and Sur, R.L. (2016). When is a urology drug safe enough for pregnancy. *J. Urol.* 195 (1): 13–14.

5

Traumatic Adrenal Hemorrhage

Hong Truong[1] and Bradley D. Figler[2]

[1] *Department of Urology, Thomas Jefferson University Hospital, Philadelphia, PA, USA*
[2] *Department of Urology, University of North Carolina-Chapel Hill, Chapel Hill, NC, USA*

Introduction

Traumatic adrenal injury is rare, occurring in an estimated 0.15–2.4% of adult and pediatric trauma patients [1–4]. Adrenal injury in the blunt trauma patient is typically an incidental finding with little clinical significance, but can occasionally result in life-threatening complications such as hemorrhage or adrenal insufficiency. Historically, adrenal injury after blunt trauma was considered a marker of severe injury, though that relationship may no longer exist, as modern computed tomography (CT) allows for the detection of less significant adrenal injuries [5].

Adrenal hemorrhage is typically managed conservatively; when intervention is required, angio-embolization is preferred to adrenalectomy. Bilateral adrenal injury is rare, but when this occurs, adrenal insufficiency should be considered as a cause of shock and managed appropriately. While little data exist regarding long-term outcomes after adrenal injury, there is no known association with adrenal insufficiency.

Relevant Anatomy

The adrenal glands are paired organs located deep in the retroperitoneum, superior and medial to the upper pole of the kidney. Both glands are enclosed in the perirenal (Gerota's) fascia and are separated from the upper pole of the kidneys by perirenal fat. The adrenal glands are not visible upon direct inspection of the retroperitoneum. Thus, the identification of the adrenal glands requires dissection and mobilization of adjacent structures and surrounding adipose tissue. The adrenal cortex is differentiated from its surrounding adipose tissue by its darker yellow color, finely granular surface, and firm consistency. The adult adrenal glands are 3–5 cm in the greatest transverse dimension and weigh between 4 and 6 g.

The left adrenal gland has a semi-lunar shape. Its borders include the stomach, the tail of the pancreas, and the splenic vein and artery inferiorly. The right adrenal gland is pyramidal in shape. Its borders include the liver, the duodenum, and the inferior vena cava (IVC). The right adrenal gland often has a retrocaval extension. Both adrenal glands are in contact with the diaphragm posteriorly.

The adrenal glands receive rich blood supply from three sources: the superior adrenal artery, a branch of the inferior phrenic arteries; the middle adrenal artery arising directly from the aorta; and the inferior adrenal arteries derived from the ipsilateral renal artery. Each adrenal gland has one vein. The left adrenal vein is approximately 2–3 cm in length, and typically drains into the left renal vein, which empties into the IVC. The right adrenal vein is less than 1 cm in length and drains directly into the IVC at a 45° angle. The short length and direct course of the right adrenal vein into the IVC poses a challenge during adrenal surgery and may explain the greater incidence of adrenal injury on the right [6].

Etiology

Blunt Trauma

Blunt mechanism of injury accounts for the majority of traumatic adrenal injury [7]. Several mechanisms have been proposed for adrenal injury resulting from blunt trauma and relate to the unique vascular anatomy of the gland (Figure 5.1). Direct compression of the adrenal gland against the spine may occur, and is typically associated with rib fracture,

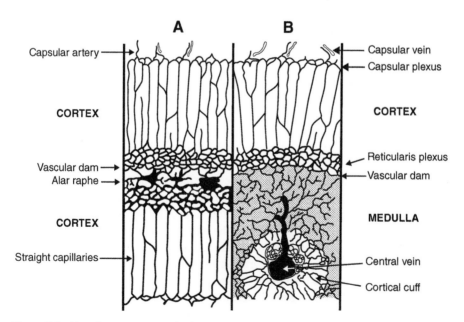

Figure 5.1 Vascular arrangement in the tail (A) and head/body (B) of the adrenal gland, demonstrating abrupt transition from arterial to venous circulation ("vascular dam"). (*Source:* from Ref. [28], with permission.)

reflecting the amount of force transmitted directly to the adrenal gland. These injuries are typically ipsilateral to the major source of trauma [6, 8].

Transient increases in intra-adrenal venous pressure due to compression of the IVC during blunt trauma may also result in adrenal injury. This occurs because the vascular architecture of the adrenal gland creates a relative vascular dam where all the blood supply is drained into relatively few venules and a single adrenal vein in each side (Figure 5.1). The small adrenal venules cannot accommodate the acute rise in the adrenal vein pressure and are vulnerable to rupture. This mechanism is thought to account for the greater incidence of right-sided injuries, since the very short right adrenal vein communicates directly with the IVC [8].

Rapid deceleration has also been implicated in blunt trauma adrenal injury and is thought to result from shearing of small sinusoids and venules in the adrenal medulla and juxtamedullary cortex (Figure 5.1) [6]. Rarely, avulsion of the right adrenal vein has been reported [9].

Penetrating Trauma

Penetrating injury is a rare cause of traumatic adrenal hemorrhage, accounting for up to 18.6% of traumatic adrenal injury in adults [7] and 4% in the pediatric population [4, 10]. Nearly all penetrating adrenal injuries are associated with injuries to surrounding structures such as the spleen, kidney, paraspinal muscles, pancreas, liver, diaphragm, great vessels, and stomach [8].

Staging

The Organ Injury Scaling (OIS) Committee of the American Association for the Surgery of Trauma (AAST) devised injury severity scores for individual organs to facility clinical risk stratification and outcome research. The OIS classification scheme for adrenal injury (Table 5.1) was published in 1996 [11] and has not undergone any formal reclassification since its original publication. The OIS grades I to V represent increasingly severe injuries

Table 5.1 The American Association for the Surgery of Trauma (AAST) organ injury scaling for the adrenal injury [11].

Grade[a]	Description of Injury
I	Contusion
II	Laceration involving only cortex (<2 cm)
III	Laceration extending into medulla (≥2 cm)
IV	>50% parenchymal destruction
V	Total parenchymal destruction (including massive intraparenchymal hemorrhage) Avulsion from blood supply

[a]Advance one grade for bilateral lesions up to grade V.

based on potential threat to the patient's life. Unlike in renal trauma, there is currently no guideline on the management of adrenal trauma based on AAST OIS grades [12].

Presentation

Since isolated traumatic adrenal injury is extremely rare, patients with adrenal trauma often present with nonspecific signs and symptoms of multi-organ trauma. Organs commonly injured in association with adrenal trauma include the liver (57.8–63.1%), ribs (42.1–50.9%), kidney (46.2–41.3%), spleen (32.9–34.4%), diaphragm (22%), pancreas (19%), and bowel (24%) [1, 7, 13, 14]. Over half of patients have tender abdomen, contusion, abrasion, seatbelt signs, and hematuria; about one-third of patients present with thoracic injuries, including pulmonary contusion, pneumothorax, hemothorax, or back tenderness; and hemodynamic instability occurs in 11.4–30.7% of cases [7, 14]. Laboratory evaluation of patients with traumatic adrenal hemorrhage may be normal or indicate anemia or electrolyte disturbances consistent with adrenal insufficiency.

Primary adrenal insufficiency is a rare finding in patients with bilateral adrenal injury, and may not occur until 90% or more of adrenal tissue is affected [14–19]. Nonetheless, these patients should be monitored for symptoms and signs of adrenal insufficiency, which include abdominal pain, nausea, altered mental status, hypotension, hyponatremia, hyperkalemia, and acidosis [20]. The diagnosis of adrenal insufficiency requires a high index of clinical suspicion and can be confirmed with serum cortisol and adrenocorticotropic hormone (ACTH) stress test.

Imaging

There is no clinical indication for adrenal imaging in the setting of blunt or penetrating trauma. As a result, adrenal injury is often discovered incidentally on CT imaging following trauma. Typical CT findings of traumatic adrenal injury includes focal adrenal hematoma (30–83%), diffuse irregular hemorrhage obliterating the gland (9–17.1%), adrenal gland swelling (4.9–18%), periadrenal fat stranding (11–93%), diffuse hemorrhage in the adjacent retroperitoneum (9.8–22%), and compression of the adrenal gland by adjacent traumatic injuries (3.7%). In rare cases, adrenal gland rupture and active extravasation of contrast material from ruptured adrenal arteries and veins is demonstrated on CT (Figure 5.2) [21–23].

It can be challenging to distinguish adrenal hemorrhage from adenoma and malignancy. Adrenal injury typically appears as a hyper-attenuating (40–90 HU), homogenous, non-enhancing adrenal mass (Figure 5.3). Periadrenal fat stranding is a characteristic feature that is more typical of adrenal trauma and uncommon in adrenal adenoma and malignancy. Over time, adrenal hematomas may calcify and typically decrease in size or resolve completely [22, 23].

Clinically insignificant adrenal adenomas are typically small (<4 cm), hypo-attenuating (<10 HU), homogenous, enhancing, demonstrate rapid washout (>50% contrast wash-out

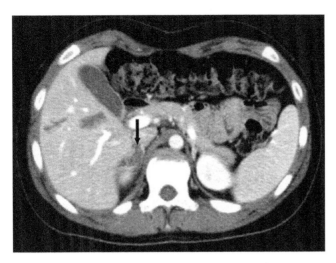

Figure 5.2 Contrast enhanced axial abdominal CT image demonstrating right adrenal gland rupture (arrow). (*Source:* from Ref. [21], with permission.)

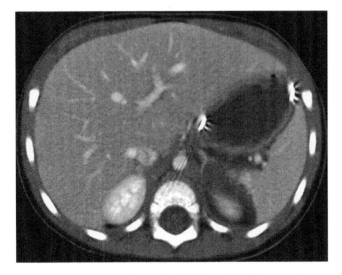

Figure 5.3 Contrast enhanced axial abdominal CT image of a two-year-old patient who suffered left adrenal gland trauma and traumatic brain injury as a result of a motor vehicle collision. The image reveals a hypodense region in the left adrenal gland with stranding of the periadrenal fat, consistent with left adrenal hematoma. The hyperdense structure in the stomach represents feeding tube. (*Source:* from Ref. [4], with permission.)

on 10-minute delay), and remain stable in size over time. In contrast, adrenal malignancies vary in size, attenuation, homogeneity, and often increase in size over time. The characteristic feature of adrenal malignancy is contrast enhancement and retention, with <50% washout after 10 minutes. If the nature of an adrenal mass cannot be clearly determined on a CT scan, a follow-up study two to four months later is recommended [23].

Other imaging modalities, including ultrasound, magnetic resonance imaging (MRI), and angiography, are poorly studied in the context of acute adrenal injury, limiting their utility. Sonography may be helpful in monitoring adrenal hematomas over time, particularly in children [24].

Management

Traumatic adrenal injury, while often discovered incidentally, is associated with high injury severity in multiple organs. Trauma patients who sustain adrenal injury have up to five times higher mortality rates compared to patients who do not suffer from adrenal injury [9]. The complications and deaths of patients with traumatic adrenal hemorrhage are largely due to concomitant injuries rather than from the adrenal trauma itself. Thus, the initial management of patients with traumatic adrenal injury is directed at controlling associated injuries such as liver laceration, pulmonary contusion, and renal trauma.

The general approach is governed by the extent of adrenal cortical injury, the status of the contralateral adrenal gland, the patient's hemodynamic stability, electrolyte abnormalities, and associated injuries.

Patients who are hemodynamically stable after adrenal injury can be safely observed. In modern trauma series, nearly all patients with adrenal trauma have been effectively managed non-operatively [4, 7, 13, 14].

Relative indications for operative intervention include high-grade adrenal injury with extensive parenchymal damage in the context of intraperitoneal injuries that require exploration. Surgical options include total adrenalectomy in patients with preserved contralateral gland or partial adrenalectomy and adrenal gland repair to preserve adrenal function and prevent adrenal insufficiency in patients who require bilateral adrenal resection. Successful angio-embolization of massive unilateral traumatic adrenal hemorrhage has been reported [25, 26] and is the preferred management strategy for isolated adrenal hemorrhage requiring intervention. Because of the redundant vascular supply, selective angio-embolization is unlikely to result in adrenal insufficiency.

Adrenal insufficiency following bilateral traumatic adrenal hemorrhage is treated similarly to acute adrenal insufficiency from other causes. Goals of medical management are: replace cortisol deficiency; treat hypotension, preferably with volume resuscitation; and reverse electrolyte abnormalities, i.e. hyponatremia and hyperkalemia. Parenteral bolus of 100 mg (or 50 mg/m^2 for children) hydrocortisone can be given immediately, followed by 200 mg (50–100 mg/m^2 for children) hydrocortisone given continuously over 24 hours or divided into four 6-hourly injections. Once patients are more stable, glucocorticoid replacement can be administered in two to three daily oral doses (e.g. 15–25 mg hydrocortisone TID, to correspond with physiological pulsatile cortisol secretion). Mineralocorticoid replacement (e.g. 0.05–0.1 mg oral fludrocortisone daily morning dose) is also required in patients with primary adrenal insufficiency. Dose adjustment should be based on clinical parameters, such as blood pressure, salt craving, and serum electrolyte levels rather than serum cortisol levels [27]. Patients with primary adrenal insufficiency should follow-up with an endocrinologist every three to four months during the first year and annually until symptoms of adrenal insufficiency resolve or patients are stable on treatment regimen [27].

Complications of Adrenal Trauma

Long-term sequelae of adrenal trauma are minimal. All reported cases of primary adrenal insufficiency following traumatic injury requiring corticosteroid therapy were recoverable without need for long-term medical management [14–19].

Conclusion

Traumatic adrenal injury is rare because of its protected location in the retroperitoneum. Abdominal CT is essential for accurately diagnosis and staging. While adrenal hemorrhage is typically managed conservatively, intervention in the form of angio-embolization, partial adrenalectomy, or adrenalectomy may be necessary. Patients with bilateral adrenal injury should be monitored for adrenal insufficiency and treated appropriately.

References

1 Rana, A.I., Kenney, P.J., Lockhart, M.E. et al. (2004). Adrenal gland hematomas in trauma patients. *Radiology* 230 (3): 669–675.

2 Burks, D.W., Mirvis, S.E., Shanmuganargan, K. et al. (1992). Acute adrenal injury after blunt abdominal trauma: CT findings. *AJR. American Journal of Roentgenology* 158 (3): 503–507.

3 Gabal-Shehab, L. and Alagiri, M. (2005). Traumatic adrenal injuries. *The Journal of Urology* 173 (4): 1330–1331.

4 Figler, B.D., Webman, R., Ramey, C. et al. (2011). Pediatric adrenal trauma in the 21st century: Children's Hospital of Atlanta experience. *The Journal of Urology* 186 (1): 248–251.

5 DiGiacomo, J.C., Gerber, N., Angus, L.D.G. et al. (2019). Blunt adrenal injury: results of a state trauma registry review. *The American Surgeon* 85 (4): 390–396.

6 Sevitt, S. (1955). Post-traumatic adrenal apoplexy. *Journal of Clinical Pathology* 8 (3): 185.

7 Stawicki, S.P., Hoey, B.A., Grossman, M.D. et al. (2003). Adrenal gland trauma is associated with high injury severity and mortality. *Current Surgery* 60 (4): 431–436.

8 Gómez, R.G., McAninch, J.W., Carroll, P.R. et al. (1993). Adrenal gland trauma: diagnosis and management. *The Journal of Trauma* 35 (6): 870–874.

9 Feliciano, D.V. (1990). Management of traumatic retroperitoneal hematoma. *Annals of Surgery* 211 (2): 109.

10 Sivit, C., Ingram, J.D., Taylor, G.A. et al. (1992). Posttraumatic adrenal hemorrhage in children: CT findings in 34 patients. *AJR. American Journal of Roentgenology* 158 (6): 1299–1302.

11 Moore, E.E., Malangoni, M.A., Cogbill, T.H. et al. (1996). Organ injury scaling VII: cervical vascular, peripheral vascular, adrenal, penis, testis, and scrotum. *Journal of Trauma and Acute Care Surgery* 41 (3): 523–524.

12 Morey, A.F., Brandes, S., Dugi, D.D. 3rd et al. (2014). Urotrauma: AUA guideline. *The Journal of Urology* 192 (2): 327–335.

13 Mehrazin, R., Derweesh, I.H., Kincade, M.C. et al. (2007). Adrenal trauma: Elvis Presley Memorial Trauma Center experience. *Urology* 70 (5): 851–855.

14 Alsayali, M.M., Atkin, C., Rahim, R. et al. (2010). Traumatic adrenal gland injury: epidemiology and outcomes in a major Australian trauma center. *European Journal of Trauma and Emergency Surgery* 36 (6): 567–572.

15 Rao, R.H., Vagnucci, A.H., Amico, J.A. et al. (1989). Bilateral massive adrenal hemorrhage: early recognition and treatment. *Annals of Internal Medicine* 110 (3): 227–235.

16 Feuerstein, B. and Streeten, D.H. (1991). Recovery of adrenal function after failure resulting from traumatic bilateral adrenal hemorrhages. *Annals of Internal Medicine* 115 (10): 785–786.

17 Lewis, J.V. (1994). Bilateral adrenal hemorrhage after blunt trauma: diagnosis by computed tomography. *Southern Medical Journal* 87 (12): 1269–1271.

18 Udobi, K.F. and Childs, E.W. (2001). Adrenal crisis after traumatic bilateral adrenal hemorrhage. *Journal of Trauma and Acute Care Surgery* 51 (3): 597–600.

19 Francque, S.M., Schwagten, V.M., Ysebaert, D.K. et al. (2004). Bilateral adrenal haemorrhage and acute adrenal insufficiency in a blunt abdominal trauma: a case-report and literature review. *European Journal of Emergency Medicine* 11 (3): 164–167.

20 Bouillon, R. (2006). Acute adrenal insufficiency. *Endocrinology and Metabolism Clinics* 35 (4): 767–775.

21 Pinto, A., Scaglione, M., Guidi, G. et al. (2006). Role of multidetector row computed tomography in the assessment of adrenal gland injuries. *European Journal of Radiology* 59 (3): 355–358.

22 Pinto, A., Scaglione, M., Pinto, F. et al. (2003). Adrenal injuries: spectrum of CT findings. *Emergency Radiology* 10 (1): 30–33.

23 Sinelnikov, A.O., Abujudeh, H.H., Chan, D. et al. (2007). CT manifestations of adrenal trauma: experience with 73 cases. *Emergency Radiology* 13 (6): 313–318.

24 Simon, D.R. and Palese, M.A. (2009). Clinical update on the management of adrenal hemorrhage. *Current Urology Reports* 10 (1): 78–83.

25 Igwilo, O.C., Sulkowski, R.J., Shah, M.R. et al. (1999). Embolization of traumatic adrenal hemorrhage. *Journal of Trauma and Acute Care Surgery* 47 (6): 1153–1155.

26 Ikeda, O., Urata, J., Araki, Y. et al. (2007). Acute adrenal hemorrhage after blunt trauma. *Abdominal Imaging* 32 (2): 248–252.

27 Bornstein, S.R., Allolio, B., Arlt, W. et al. (2016). Diagnosis and treatment of primary adrenal insufficiency: an endocrine society clinical practice guideline. *The Journal of Clinical Endocrinology & Metabolism* 101 (2): 364–389.

28 Symington, T. (1969). *Functional Pathology of the Human Adrenal Gland*. Edinburgh: Livingstone.

6

External Ureteral Trauma

Humberto G. Villarreal[1] and Steven J. Hudak[2]

[1] *Loma Linda University Medical Center, Loma Linda, CA, USA*
[2] *UT Southwestern Medical Center, Dallas, TX, USA*

Introduction

Trauma is a frequent cause of death and disability. Injuries were the third most common causes of death worldwide, accounting for approximately 9% of mortalities in 2012 [1]. In 2013, the Center for Disease Control data reported "unintentional injury" as the fourth leading cause of death for all age groups in the U.S. and injury-specific mechanisms represented the top three causes of mortality for ages 15–34 [2]. Genitourinary injuries are identified in 10% of hospitalized trauma patients [3], typically in the context of complex polytraumatic injuries [4]. However, traumatic ureteral injuries are relatively rare, representing less than 1% of all genitourinary injuries in historical studies [5, 6]. Recent work by Siram et al. demonstrated a higher rate of traumatic ureteral injury at 2.5% in a retrospective analysis of almost 23 000 genitourinary injuries identified in the National Trauma Database from 2002–2006 [7]. The greater frequency of traumatic ureteral injury is believed to be secondary to enhanced imaging techniques and improved trauma outcomes resulting in a larger proportion of patients surviving from point of injury to higher-level care.

Anatomical Considerations

Located in the retroperitoneum, the ureters are narrow in caliber and well protected by surrounding organs and musculoskeletal structures. The proximal ureter begins at the ureteropelvic junction and transitions to the mid ureter as it crosses the sacroiliac joint. The middle ureter spans the sacro-iliac region to become the distal ureter as it enters the true pelvis. The ureters course anterior to the posterior abdominal wall musculature and are in closest proximity to the quadratus lumborum, psoas muscles, and the iliacus as they enter the bony pelvis. The lumbar spine is medial and posterior to the abdominal portion of the ureter. The "pelvic ureter" begins as it crosses the common iliac

A Clinical Guide to Urologic Emergencies, First Edition. Edited by Hunter Wessells, Shigeo Horie, and Reynaldo G. Gómez.

vessels and is associated with the ilium posteriolaterally and the sacrum posteriomedially. Abdominal and pelvic organs overlie the ureter throughout its course. While its location explains the high rate of iatrogenic ureteral injury during colorectal, gynecological, and vascular surgical procedures, the deep, well-protected nature of the ureter likely explains its lower vulnerability to violent trauma when compared to other genitourinary organs.

Mechanisms of Injury

Penetrating ureteral trauma is the most common mechanism of injury across multiple single-institution case series and retrospective reviews [5, 6, 8, 9]. It is noteworthy that the preponderance of ureteral trauma literature reports mostly on penetrating trauma, with most studies focusing on gunshot wounds (GSW) alone, potentially overestimating the incidence of gunshot-related ureteral injuries [6]. While ureteral injuries occur in only 2–4% of abdominal GSWs [10, 11], GSW injuries are nonetheless predominant in the penetrating ureteral trauma literature.

Due to points of fixation at the ureteropelvic and ureterovesical junctions, the ureter is susceptible to avulsion injury as a result of rapid deceleration or violent motor vehicle trauma [12]. Additionally, severe distraction of skeletal structures can lacerate or avulse the ureter. Whereas historical studies estimated blunt ureteral trauma to comprise only 4–6% of all traumatic ureteral injuries [6, 9], the National Trauma Data Bank (NTDB) series reported a much higher frequency of 38% [7]. Another key finding of this study was the significant difference in Injury Severity Score (ISS) for blunt (21.5) versus penetrating (16.0) injuries, further highlighting the severity of trauma associated with blunt ureteral injury.

Concomitant Injuries

Approximately 90% of traumatic ureteral injuries occur in the setting of polytrauma [13]. Associated injuries are not surprising given the ureter's anatomical proximity to intra-abdominal, retroperitoneal, vascular, and skeletal structures. The American Association for the Surgery of Trauma (AAST) grades ureteral injuries based on the presence and size of the laceration/transection, as well as the presence and size of associated devascularization adjacent to the transection (Table 6.1) [14]. This classification scheme has been previously validated and demonstrated to correlate with the complexity of ureteral repair and number of associated injuries [9]. Bowel injuries are the most common injuries associated with ureteral trauma. In the largest single-institution series on GSWs to the ureter, bowel injuries represented 56% of all observed concomitant injuries [15]. While penetrating ureteral injuries are commonly associated with bowel and vascular injuries, blunt ureteral injuries are more likely to be associated with pelvic and/or vertebral fractures. Additionally, blunt trauma is more frequently associated with arterial injury compared to the venous injuries more common to penetrating trauma (Table 6.2). In fact, the 38% incidence of vascular injury in the NTDB series is more than twice the previously reported incidence of the largest single-institution series [15].

Table 6.1 AAST organ injury scale: ureter.

Grade[a]	Injury Type	Description of Injury
I	Hematoma	Contusion or hematoma without devascularization
II	Laceration	<50% transection
III	Laceration	>50% transection
IV	Laceration	Complete transection with 2 cm devascularization
V	Laceration	Avulsion with >2 cm devascularization

[a]Advance one grade if multiple lesions exist *Source:* adapted from Moore et al. [14].

Table 6.2 Ureteral trauma: patterns and mechanism of injury.

Associated Injuries	% Blunt (n = 224)	% Penetrating (n = 358)
Vascular		
Artery	9	17
Vein	5	27
Hollow viscus		
Small intestines	3	46
Colon and appendix	7	44
Rectum	1	7
Bony Injuries		
Pelvic fracture	20	1
Vertebral fracture	3	<1

Source: adapted from Siram et al. [7].

Diagnosis

Immediate signs and symptoms of traumatic ureteral injury are largely non-specific. In penetrating trauma, the trajectory of the missile or stab wound may be the first indication of a ureteral injury during the primary trauma survey. Physical examination findings for blunt trauma are less reliable, though flank ecchymosis or a "seatbelt sign" might raise suspicion for renal, ureteral, and/or bladder injury. Hematuria is absent in 15–56% of ureteral injuries and this absence may be a factor in delayed diagnosis of traumatic ureteral injuries [13, 15, 16]. The presence of hematuria warrants thorough evaluation, either pre-operative or intra-operative, depending on the specific clinical condition of each patient.

Diagnostic Imaging

The sensitivity of radiographic testing in the setting of ureteral injury has been reported as low as 20% [17]. Intravenous urography (IVU) has an unacceptably high non-diagnostic rate with an estimated cumulative sensitivity of 51% [18]. An explanation for the high false-negative rate of IVU is the possibility that some of the studies performed might not reflect a "complete IVU," with the requisite scout, serial images at 5–20 minutes, oblique views, bladder, and post-void images. Nonetheless, the "complete IVU" was considered in 2004 by experts to be a reliable and accurate modality in stable patients [19]. Thus, when CT (computed tomograpy) is not available, IVU findings suggestive of traumatic ureteral injury include frank extravasation of contrast, non-visualization of the affected system, hydronephrosis and medial deviation of the ureter [15]. Finally, despite its high accuracy, retrograde pyelography is cumbersome and time-consuming and thus not typically appropriate in the acute trauma setting.

Well-established clinical practice guidelines from the American Urological Association (AUA) and the European Association of Urology (EAU) recommend intravenous (IV) contrast enhanced abdominal/pelvic CT with 10 minute delayed imaging for stable trauma patients with suspected ureteral injuries [20, 21]. Ureteral injuries should be suspected based on the clinical criteria discussed above (high energy blunt trauma, penetrating abdominopelvic injuries). Findings suggestive of traumatic ureteral injury include contrast extravasation (Figure 6.1), ipsilateral delayed pyelogram/hydronephrosis (Figure 6.2), and lack of contrast in the ureter distal to the suspected injury. When contrast is not given or

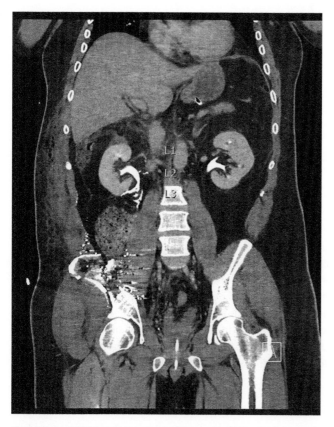

Figure 6.1 Right proximal ureteral injury after GSW. Note contrast extravasation. *Source:* courtesy of Steven J. Hudak, MD.

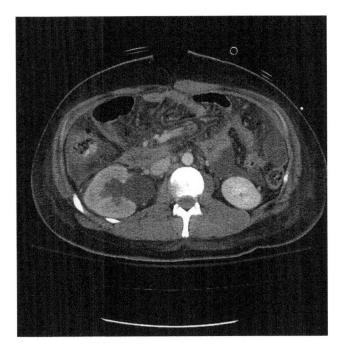

Figure 6.2 Delayed nephrogram and hydronephrosis associated with right ureteral injury after GSW. *Source:* courtesy of Steven J. Hudak, MD.

10-minute delayed images are not obtained, findings are less specific, including subtle perinephric stranding, low-density retroperitoneal fluid, ureteral dilation/deviation, or bladder displacement [7, 22].

Intra-operative Diagnosis

A significant proportion of patients with traumatic ureteral injuries will proceed directly to the operating room for exploratory laparotomy prior to radiographic evaluation, due to patient instability or mechanism of injury. International series on traumatic ureteral injuries report rates of intra-operative diagnosis of 40–85% in patients without pre-operative imaging [23, 24]. The sensitivity of intra-operative identification was reported at 88.9% on a meta-analysis [16] of the traumatic ureteral injury literature, with a range of 63–95% in selected series [5, 25]. Hence, intra-operative diagnosis remains the most common and reliable means of identifying traumatic ureteral injuries. During exploratory laparotomy, identification of a retroperitoneal hematoma or fluid collection combined with organ injuries in the vicinity of the ureter raises the suspicion of traumatic ureteral injury.

The AUA Urotrauma Guideline states that direct ureteral inspection during laparotomy is necessary for all patients with suspected ureteral injury without pre-operative imaging [20]. Various adjunctive techniques can be utilized to aid in detection of these injuries at the time of operative exploration. Intravenous methylene blue or indigo carmine may aid in detection of transecting ureteral injuries, but will not identify ureteral contusions and may be less reliable for the hypotensive patient with poor perfusion and thus low urine output. The same dyes can be injected into the renal pelvis or ureter, but care must be taken to avoid spillage as this can obscure the operative field. Retrograde instillation of dyes or contrast can also be performed via cystoscopic or open cannulation of the ureters, but this approach may also miss significant ureteral contusions. Placing each individual injury pattern in the context of the stability of the patient (see next section) will help the surgeon decide how extensive the intra-operative process to diagnose a suspected traumatic ureteral injury should be. Finally, the intra-operative "one-shot" intravenous pyelogram (IVP) does not reliably exclude traumatic ureteral injuries and thus should not be used for this purpose [19].

Delayed Diagnosis

Unfortunately, a significant number of ureteral injuries are not recognized at the time of initial laparotomy. The rate of missed ureteral injury varies greatly across single-institution series but is on average 38% [13]. Kunkle et al. cited patient intra-operative factors germane to the complex polytrauma patient such as bleeding, hypotension, coagulopathy, and hypothermia contributing to missed ureteral injuries. Surgeon-specific factors include inadequate retroperitoneal exploration and inappropriately low index of suspicion for ureteral injury. Proximal ureteral injuries are more prone to delayed recognition due to their less accessible location and greater potential to be confounded by the presence of a perinephric hematoma when a concomitant renal laceration is present [16, 17]. Finally, some traumatic ureteral injuries may be dynamic in their manifestation, particularly when caused by GSWs or high-energy blast mechanisms. Cass reported on a series of 12 patients with ureteral contusions secondary to GSWs. Two injuries were repaired primarily at initial exploration due to intra-operative appearance of the ureter, while the remaining 10 injuries were observed, of which two eventually developed urinary fistula [26].

The eventual diagnosis of missed ureteral injuries presents unique management challenges in the short and long term. Signs and symptoms may be nonspecific, including flank or abdominal pain, anorexia, ileus, fever, and in severe cases of ongoing urinary extravasation, peritonitis and/or sepsis. Elevated serum creatinine can be indicative of peritoneal absorption of extravasated urine, while more specific findings include urinary drainage from surgical drains or urinary-cutaneous fistula. Urinary leak is confirmed by sending the effluent for creatinine. Management is discussed below, but in all cases begins with urinary diversion (with nephrostomy tube or ureteral stent), urinoma drainage, and appropriate treatment of the associated infection (Figure 6.3).

Diagnostic Endoscopy and Urography

Endoscopic evaluation and treatment may be required at different stages in the evaluation and management of traumatic ureteral injuries. Due to trauma acuity, endoscopic evaluation may not always be possible or practical at initial presentation or laparotomy. Many modern trauma operating rooms now have combined fluoroscopic capabilities, which would allow urologists to incorporate these interventions earlier in their management of complex polytrauma patients. Retrograde or antegrade urography may be necessary when CT or IVU findings are equivocal or in the delayed detection and management of suspected

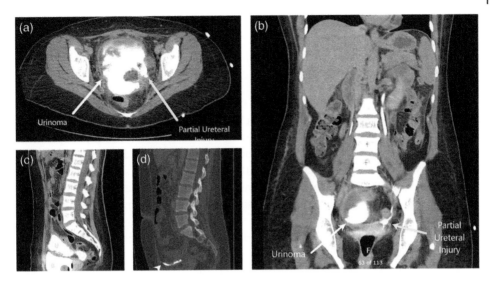

Figure 6.3 Missed distal ureteral injury detection and management. (a) Partial Ureteral Injury (yellow arrow) and urinoma (white arrow). (b) Partial Ureteral Injury (yellow arrow) and urinoma (white arrow). (c) Urinoma (U) and Bladder (B). (d) Percutaneous drain (arrowhead). *Source:* courtesy of Steven J. Hudak, MD.

injuries. Finally, diagnostic endoscopy and urography is a useful adjunct in surgical planning for definitive reconstruction in the later stages of damage control surgery.

Management

Advanced Trauma and Life Support (ATLS) guidelines dictate initial evaluation and treatment of all trauma patients and genitourinary injuries must be managed without violating ATLS and damage control surgical principles. Coexisting life-threatening injuries take precedence and patient physiology may further influence the ability to assess for traumatic ureteral injury in an acute versus a delayed setting. In the exploratory surgical setting, careful attention must be paid to location of ureteral injury along with degree of tissue devitalization. Furthermore, in penetrating trauma secondary to GSWs, ballistic effects of the missile must be well understood, as direct and indirect cavitary forces can have immediate and potentially delayed tissue effects. Santucci et al. have thoroughly examined the wound ballistics literature and report on several accepted fallacies of gunshot injuries. Specifically, their review highlights the difference between high- and low-velocity ballistics in terms of tissue effect and explains how the effects of high-velocity missiles are overestimated and misrepresented in the literature. Further attention is given to the quality of the missile (jacketed vs. unjacketed), as experimental studies and clinical correlates clearly demonstrate the profound tissue effects of unjacketed projectiles. The collective evidence presented as part of their review challenges the dogmatic recommendation for wide excision of tissue in high velocity wounds in favor of judicious debridement to limit the extent of iatrogenic injury at the time of surgical exploration [27]. An added benefit of a staged, "damage control" approach may allow time for certain blast or contusive injuries to declare themselves (further discussed below).

Ureteral Contusions

Ureteral contusions are the least severe of the traumatic injuries; however, their evaluation and management require a certain degree of clinical intuition and vigilance. There is controversy regarding optimal management of these injuries. Potential treatment options in the intra-operative setting include observation, excision, and debridement with uretero-ureterostomy or endoscopic management with indwelling ureteral stent. The decision to employ any of these options is based upon clinical assessment of tissue compromise and as previously discussed, even "normal" appearing ureters at exploration may eventually manifest delayed complications such as urinary extravasation and/or ureteral stricture. It is noteworthy that in the ureteral contusion series by Cass, only two injuries were repaired primarily and none of the remaining injuries were treated with ureteral stenting. It is the expert opinion of the AUA Urotrauma panel that all ureteral contusions diagnosed at laparotomy should be treated with either ureteral stenting or resection with primary repair based on ureteral viability and clinical scenario [20]. There is no reported recommendation for duration of indwelling stent and choice of follow-up imaging is at the discretion of the clinician. The authors' practice is to stent ureteral contusions when surgical exploration confirms intact ureteral mucosa. Unless complications arise or the patient's status prohibits, the stent is removed in two to four weeks and a renal ultrasound is performed one month later. Symptomatic patients and/or the finding of hydronephrosis on ultrasound are usually managed with temporary nephrostomy tube drainage followed by definitive ureteral reconstruction three to six months later, depending on the overall clinical scenario.

Surgical Principles

The extent of tissue devitalization and the level of the ureteral injury will influence the plan for ureteral reconstruction. In stable patients, it is recommended that traumatic ureteral lacerations be repaired at the time of laparotomy. The AUA Urotrauma Guideline further recommends that injuries proximal to the iliac vessels be repaired primarily over a ureteral stent, whereas injuries distal to the iliac vessels should be treated with ureteral reimplantation or primary repair over a stent whenever possible [20]. Depending on the length of ureteral loss, primary ureteral repair or reimplantation may be challenging, if not impossible. Techniques such as bladder mobilization and downward nephropexy have been described in ureteral reconstruction and may be used alone or in conjunction with other accepted ureteral reimplantation techniques such as bladder hitch or flap [28]. Careful ureteral mobilization should aim to preserve the adventitial blood supply. After judicious debridement of non-viable tissue, a widely spatulated, tension-free and watertight anastomosis should be performed in order to optimize the success of the reconstruction. Simple penetrating ureteral trauma (from stab injury or low velocity projectile) rarely requires extensive debridement, whereas blast injuries should be considered in the context of trauma to the surrounding tissues. Questionable ureteral viability may necessitate temporizing urinary drainage and a second operative look in accordance with damage control

Figure 6.4 Antegrade nephrostogram after prior ureteral ligation due to major concomitant vascular injury and colonic injury. *Source:* courtesy of Steven J. Hudak, MD.

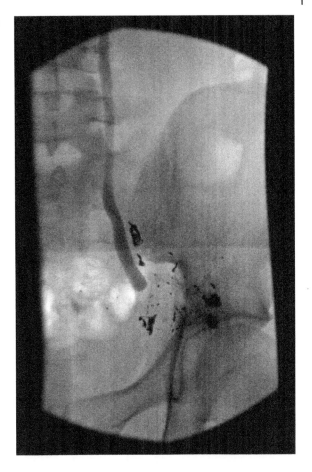

surgical principles. In situations of extensive ureteral loss, transureteroureterostomy can be performed but is rarely reported in the setting of acute trauma; ileal interposition is strongly discouraged in the acute trauma setting due to the need for bowel preparation and contraindication in the setting of impaired renal function [29]. In such cases, where complex reconstruction is needed, a patient would be better managed with temporary urinary drainage followed by delayed definitive repair [20]. Buccal mucosal graft augmented ureteral reconstruction is being performed more frequently and can be considered in repairs of proximal and mid-ureteral injuries in an onlay or augmented anastomotic fashion (Figure 6.4). Ureteral repairs may be retroperitonealized or wrapped with omentum to reduce the risk of leakage and improve vascularity [28]. Passive or closed-suction drains can be placed in the area of the repair and may be of diagnostic value in identifying delayed necrosis leading to anastomotic failure and urine leak. Given the association of ureteral trauma with hollow viscus injuries and intra-abdominal contamination, there may be hesitation to undertake definitive ureteral reconstructions in this setting. Azimuddin et al. refute this notion and provide evidence for reconstructive success, even in the setting of gross intra-abdominal contamination, with the repair failures in this series not correlated with the degree of intra-abdominal soilage [25]. Ultimately, proper assessment of the severity of ureteral injury along with meticulous surgical technique results in successful repairs reported at approximately 80% across multiple series [10, 15, 30].

Damage Control Surgery

Over the past 25 years, the principle of damage control surgery has evolved to include applications for multiple surgical subspecialties in the care of the complex polytrauma patient. Basic tenets of damage control surgery include abbreviated laparotomy with control of life-threatening injuries and contamination (phase 1) followed by correction of coagulopathy, metabolic derangements, and normalization of body temperature (phase 2). Usually by 72 hours, the third phase of damage control surgery typically involves multiple definitive surgeries in preparation for prolonged critical care support or eventual recovery [31]. In their validation of the AAST classification for ureteral injuries, Best at al. established the association between traumatic ureteral injuries and overall severity of trauma, as indicated by mean ISS >15 (major trauma) [9]. Initial applications of damage control principles in urologic trauma included exteriorization of the transected ureter as a "tube ureterostomy" or management with stenting of partial injuries [25]. Smith et al. describe the utilization of "single J" stents for tube ureterostomy and secure the stent to the proximal end of the ureteral defect with a permanent suture to prevent dislodgement. Pediatric feeding tubes can be used in a similar manner when urinary stents are not available. Tube ureterostomy prevents urinary extravasation while facilitating ureteral reconstruction during a subsequent laparotomy once the patient has been stabilized. When patient instability, concomitant injuries, and/or the degree of ureteral loss prohibit reconstruction in the acute phase, the ureter should be ligated at the proximal end of the defect (Figure 6.5). A percutaneous

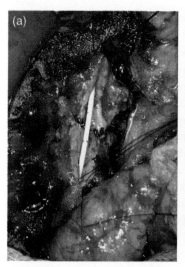 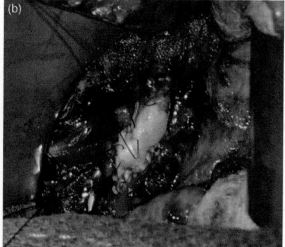

Figure 6.5 Augmented anastomotic buccal ureteroplasty. (a) Viable ureteral ends anastomosed dorsally. (b) 4-cm buccal graft anastomosed ventrally. (Ureteroureterostomy would not have been possible due to long segment of ureteral compromise and undue tension.) *Source:* courtesy of Humberto G. Villarreal, MD.

nephrostomy tube is then placed which will facilitate urinary drainage until reconstruction (or nephrectomy) is performed after initial recovery and rehabilitation.

Delayed Management of Injuries

Whether missed on pre-operative or intra-operative evaluation or manifested in a delayed fashion due to ballistic effects on tissue or failed primary repair, a proportion of ureteral injuries will be recognized well beyond the acute phase of resuscitation or surgery. The AUA Urotrauma Guideline recommends attempts at ureteral stenting for incomplete ureteral injuries diagnosed post-operatively or in a delayed setting, with use of percutaneous nephrostomy and delayed reconstruction when needed [20]. In many cases, late diagnosis of ureteral injury is prompted by complications related to urinary obstruction and/or extravasation at or above the level of the missed injury. In such cases, percutaneous drainage of any associated urinoma/abscess facilitates infection control and resolution of urinary leakage at the site of injury.

Complications

Due to the association of traumatic ureteral injuries with complex polytrauma, patients with these injuries are subject to significant morbidity and complications, at times resulting in prolonged convalescence or mortality. While the increased incidence of traumatic ureteral injuries likely reflects improved survivability due to advances in trauma and critical care, the morbidity secondary to ureteral injuries can be mitigated by timely recognition and treatment. Most of the morbidity and reported complications of traumatic ureteral injury can be attributed to delayed recognition [15, 29]. The severity of morbidity related to these injuries can range from urinary tract infection to sepsis, peritonitis, urinary fistula, ureteral stricture, or renal loss. Early-case series report nephrectomy rates as high as 44% for ureteral injuries diagnosed in a delayed setting [32]. More contemporary studies estimate the rate of nephrectomy for delayed diagnosed injuries at 18.4% compared to 2.4% for those recognized early [16]. Delayed diagnosis ultimately results in a prolonged hospital course. NTDB analysis revealed an average length of hospitalization of 17.2 days for penetrating trauma compared to 13.5 days for blunt mechanisms, in spite of lower median ISSs for penetrating trauma [7]. These length of hospitalization estimates are lower than the previously reported 19 days for immediately recognized injuries and further emphasize the significance of delayed detection of injuries with a mean length of hospitalization of 36.6 days on meta-analysis [16]. Finally, the current impact of traumatic ureteral injuries can be assessed through analysis of resource utilization and cost, which in our current healthcare climate, likely eclipses the previously estimated costs of $25 000 for treating a single ureteral injury [15].

Failed repairs or complications thereof may also contribute significantly to the morbidity of traumatic ureteral injuries. The rate of complications related to traumatic ureteral injuries is variable in single-institution series but was reported at 36.2% by Pereira et al. [13]. The clinical impact of the high complication rate is uncertain given inconsistent reporting and the potentially broad range of possible complications. Fraga et al. reported a 55% rate of complications with factors such as shock on admission, ISS > 25, colonic injuries, and delayed diagnosis of ureteral injury, as factors contributing to complications [23].

However, the true impact of ureteral injury on mortality is unclear as it is rarely reported and most likely related to life-threatening associated injuries and the potential complications of their respective treatment. All-cause mortality in traumatic ureteral injury literature is variable. Siram et al. reported a 9% mortality for blunt and a 6% rate for penetrating trauma based on NTDB data. The traumatic ureteral injury literature reports an associated 17% mortality [13] in patients with these injuries, while Kunkle et al. further stratified mortality rates at 6.1 and 13.2% for early-diagnosed and missed ureteral injuries respectively [16].

Conclusions

Ureteral injuries due to external trauma are rare, but their association with complex polytrauma and propensity to be detected in a delayed fashion pose significant diagnostic and therapeutic challenges. A high index of suspicion for ureteral injury must be maintained, especially for high-energy blunt abdominal trauma and penetrating injuries in the vicinity of the ureter. Stable trauma patients not proceeding directly to laparotomy can be imaged without significant interruption to acute care. Evaluation should include contrast enhanced CT with delayed phase imaging to appropriately assess for ureteral injury. Intra-operative detection of traumatic ureteral injury is highly sensitive and prompt repair of detected ureteral injuries should be undertaken whenever possible. When needed, damage-control principles are applicable to urologic trauma and can help optimize conditions for eventual repair of recognized injuries. With improved detection, management, and vigilance for potential complications of traumatic ureteral injuries, the morbidity, cost, and potential mortality of these injuries can be decreased and lead to improved patient outcomes.

References

1 WHO (2014). *The top 10 causes of death*, in *Fact Sheet*. World Health Organization.
2 CDC (2013). *10 Leading Causes of Death by Age Group, United States – 2013*. Center for Disease Control and Prevention.
3 McGeady, J.B. and Breyer, B.N. (2013). Current epidemio0logy of genitourinary trauma. *Urol. Clin. North Am.* 40 (3): 323–334.
4 Tezval, H., Terzal, M., von Klot, C. et al. (2007). Urinary tract injuries in patients with multiple trauma. *World J. Urol.* 25 (2): 177–184.
5 Presti, J.C. Jr., Carroll, P.R., and McAninch, J.W. (1989). Ureteral and renal pelvic injuries from external trauma: diagnosis and management. *J. Trauma* 29 (3): 370–374.
6 Elliott, S.P. and McAninch, J.W. (2003). Ureteral injuries from external violence: the 25-year experience at San Francisco General Hospital. *J. Urol.* 170 (4 Pt 1): 1213–1216.
7 Siram, S.M., Gerald, S.Z., Greene, W.R. et al. (2010). Ureteral trauma: patterns and mechanisms of injury of an uncommon condition. *Am. J. Surg.* 199 (4): 566–570.

8 Ghali, A.M., El Malik, E.M., Ibrahim, A.I. et al. (1999). Ureteric injuries: diagnosis, management, and outcome. *J. Trauma* 46 (1): 150–158.

9 Best, C.D., Petrone, P., Buscarini, M. et al. (2005). Traumatic ureteral injuries: a single institution experience validating the American Association for the Surgery of Trauma-Organ Injury Scale grading scale. *J. Urol.* 173 (4): 1202–1205.

10 Holden, S., Hicks, C.C., O'Brien, D.P. et al. (1976). Gunshot wounds of the ureter: a 15-year review of 63 consecutive cases. *J. Urol.* 116 (5): 562–564.

11 Rober, P.E., Smith, J.B., and Pierce, J.M. Jr. (1990). Gunshot injuries of the ureter. *J. Trauma* 30 (1): 83–86.

12 Elliott, S.P. and McAninch, J.W. (2006). Ureteral injuries: external and iatrogenic. *Urol. Clin. North Am.* 33 (1): 55–66, vi.

13 Pereira, B.M., Ogilvie, M.P., Gomez-Rodriguez, J.C. et al. (2010). A review of ureteral injuries after external trauma. *Scand. J. Trauma Resusc. Emerg. Med.* 18: 6.

14 Moore, E.E., Cogbill, T.H., Jurkovich, G.J. et al. (1992). Organ injury scaling. III: chest wall, abdominal vascular, ureter, bladder, and urethra. *J. Trauma* 33 (3): 337–339.

15 Perez-Brayfield, M.R., Keane, T.E., Krishnan, A. et al. (2001). Gunshot wounds to the ureter: a 40-year experience at Grady Memorial Hospital. *J. Urol.* 166 (1): 119–121.

16 Kunkle, D.A., Kansas, B.T., Pathak, A. et al. (2006). Delayed diagnosis of traumatic ureteral injuries. *J. Urol.* 176 (6 Pt 1): 2503–2507.

17 Medina, D., Lavery, R., Ross, S.E. et al. (1998). Ureteral trauma: preoperative studies neither predict injury nor prevent missed injuries. *J. Am. Coll. Surg.* 186 (6): 641–644.

18 Digiacomo, J.C., Frankel, H., Rotondo, M.F. et al. (2001). Preoperative radiographic staging for ureteral injuries is not warranted in patients undergoing celiotomy for trauma. *Am. Surg.* 67 (10): 969–973.

19 Brandes, S., Coburn, M., Armenakas, N. et al. (2004). Diagnosis and management of ureteric injury: an evidence-based analysis. *BJU Int.* 94 (3): 277–289.

20 Morey, A.F., Brandes, S., Dugi, D.D. 3rd et al. (2014). Urotrauma: AUA guideline. *J. Urol.* 192 (2): 327–335.

21 Serafetinides, E., Kitrey, N.D., Diakovic, N. et al. (2015). Review of the current management of upper urinary tract injuries by the EAU Trauma Guidelines Panel. *Eur. Urol.* 67 (5): 930–936.

22 Ortega, S.J., Netto, F.S., Hamilton, P. et al. (2008). CT scanning for diagnosing blunt ureteral and ureteropelvic junction injuries. *BMC Urol.* 8: 3.

23 Fraga, G.P., Borges, G.M., Mantovani, M. et al. (2007). Penetrating ureteral trauma. *Int. Braz J Urol* 33 (2): 142–148, discussion 149-50.

24 Abid, A.F. and Hashem, H.L. (2010). Ureteral injuries from gunshots and shells of explosive devices. *Urol. Ann.* 2 (1): 17–20.

25 Azimuddin, K., Milanesa, D., Ivatury, R. et al. (1998). Penetrating ureteric injuries. *Injury* 29 (5): 363–367.

26 Cass, A.S. (1984). Ureteral contusion with gunshot wounds. *J. Trauma* 24 (1): 59–60.

27 Santucci, R.A. and Chang, Y.J. (2004). Ballistics for physicians: myths about wound ballistics and gunshot injuries. *J. Urol.* 171 (4): 1408–1414.

28 Knight, R.B., Hudak, S.J., and Morey, A.F. (2013). Strategies for open reconstruction of upper ureteral strictures. *Urol. Clin. North Am.* 40 (3): 351–361.

29 Armenakas, N.A. (1999). Current methods of diagnosis and management of ureteral injuries. *World J. Urol.* 17 (2): 78–83.

30 Palmer, L.S., Rosenbaum, R.R., Gershbaum, M.D. et al. (1999). Penetrating ureteral trauma at an urban trauma center: 10-year experience. *Urology* 54 (1): 34–36.

31 Chovanes, J., Cannon, J.W., and Nunez, T.C. (2012). The evolution of damage control surgery. *Surg. Clin. North Am.* 92 (4): 859–875, vii–viii.

32 McGinty, D.M. and Mendez, R. (1977). Traumatic ureteral injuries with delayed recognition. *Urology* 10 (2): 115–117.

7

Iatrogenic Ureteral Injury

Haruaki Kato, Kazuyoshi Iijima, Tomohiko Oguchi, and Seiji Yano

Department of Urology, Nagano Municipal Hospital, Nagano, Japan

Introduction

The structure of the ureter is delicate and can be vulnerable to surgical injury, especially when deviated from the normal anatomical course by adhesion due to previous surgery, tumor, or by involvement with the tumor itself. Additionally, traditional hemostasis by mass ligation may inadvertently involve the ureter; recently developed sealing devices can also easily damage the ureter along with other tissue during the dissection. Finally, current endoscopic surgery for ureteral stones or tumors carry a potential risk of severe mucosal injury or ureteral disruption. Therefore, urologists have to keep in mind how to repair the injured ureter during the initial surgery (intra-operative injury), as well as how to manage the condition when the ureteral injury only becomes evident in a delayed fashion post-operatively.

Etiology

Iatrogenic ureteral injuries during surgery occur rarely, ranging from 0.02 to 6% of cases [1]. However, it is more commonly seen during gynecological surgery, especially during transabdominal hysterectomy in cases complicated by infection, previous surgery, or an enlarged uterus with malignancy [2]. Probable causes of injury are a partial or complete inclusion of the ureter with a pedicle ligature or a hemostatic suture, a crush injury by hemostatic clamp, a segmental excision with the resected specimen, or thermal injury by sealing devices [3]. The most common site of injury is near the uterosacral ligaments [4].

Other procedures contributing to ureteral injuries include colorectal surgeries, vascular surgeries, and large retroperitoneal tumor resections. The causes of the ureteral injury might be similar to those of gynecological surgeries. Additionally, an excessively aggressive dissection or skeletonization, ignoring the vascular supply of the ureter, might cause ischemic change of the ureteral wall, which results in either delayed presentation of a leak or as stricture formation.

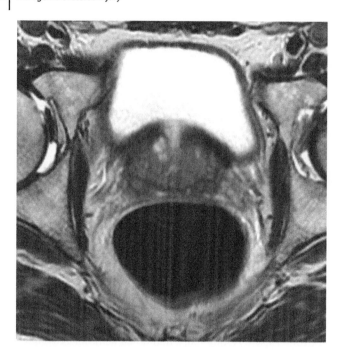

Figure 7.1 Pre-operative MRI of the prostate demonstrating a small cystic lesion on the right side. Post-operative enhanced CT showed division of the ectopic ureter into the prostate. *Source:* courtesy of Haruaki Kato, M.D.

The field of urology is not immune to this type of complication. Ureteral transection by a hemostatic sealing device during partial nephrectomy may occur due to extensive perinephric fat; misidentifying a thin ureter for the gonadal vein during retroperitoneal lymph node dissection for testicular cancer may also lead to injury. Overconfidence and overuse of a sealing device might contribute to these types of injuries.

With the development of endoscopic ureteral surgery, iatrogenic ureteral injury during biopsy or resection of mucosal lesions and treatment of urolithiasis are fortunately uncommon. However, ureteral avulsion or circumferential mucosal injury can occur rarely, especially during ureteroscopic stone removal in a forcible or an inadvertent manner.

Finally, inadvertent division of a pelvic ectopic ureter can occur during robotic-assisted radical prostatectomy, if the ureter enters into the prostatic urethra in cases with complete ureteral duplication. In an illustrative case, the pre-operative magnetic resonance imaging (MRI) showed only a small cystic lesion in the prostate (Figure 7.1). Complete duplicated ureter with an ectopic insertion into the prostatic urethra is very uncommon and MRI could usually detect an evident cystic lesion in the prostate [5]. Careful pre-operative investigations are very important to avoid an unnecessary iatrogenic ureteral injury.

Management

Iatrogenic ureteral injury should be repaired immediately intra-operatively during the initial surgery (Figure 7.2). Unfortunately, the recognition of ureteral injury or obstruction may only be accomplished after the surgery, as is the case in the majority of iatrogenic ureteral injuries [1].

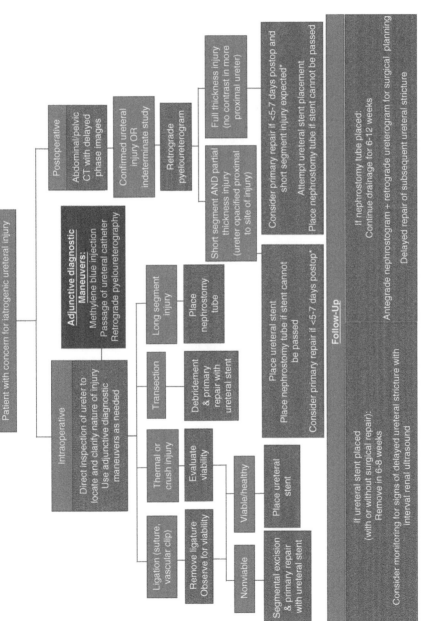

Figure 7.2 Algorithm for the evaluation and management of iatrogenic ureteral injury detected intra-operatively and post-operatively. *Source:* courtesy Alexander Skokan, MD, University of Washington.

* If there is evidence of a heavily contaminated field (e.g. locoregional infection, large urinoma), primary repair should not be attempted. Nephrostomy tube drainage of the kidney +/– percutaneous drainage of any periureteral collections should be pursued.

The following text appears within the figure:

Patient with concern for iatrogenic ureteral injury

Intraoperative
Direct inspection of ureter to locate and clarify nature of injury
Use adjunctive diagnostic maneuvers as needed

Postoperative
Abdominal/pelvic CT with delayed phase images
Confirmed ureteral injury OR indeterminate study
Retrograde pyeloureterogram

Adjunctive diagnostic Maneuvers:
Methylene blue injection
Passage of ureteral catheter
Retrograde pyeloureterography

Ligation (suture, vascular clip)
Remove ligature
Observe for viability

Thermal or crush injury
Evaluate viability

Transection
Debridement & primary repair with ureteral stent

Long segment injury
Place nephrostomy tube

Nonviable
Segmental excision & primary repair with ureteral stent

Viable/healthy
Place ureteral stent

Place ureteral stent
Place nephrostomy tube if stent cannot be passed
Consider primary repair if <5-7 days postop*

Short segment AND partial thickness injury (ureter opacified proximal to site of injury)
Consider primary repair if <5-7 days postop and short segment injury expected*
Attempt ureteral stent placement
Place nephrostomy tube if stent cannot be passed

Full thickness injury (no contrast in more proximal ureter)

Follow-Up

If ureteral stent placed (with or without surgical repair):
Remove in 6-8 weeks
Consider monitoring for signs of delayed ureteral stricture with interval renal ultrasound

If nephrostomy tube placed:
Continue drainage for 6-12 weeks
Antegrade nephrostogram + retrograde ureterogram for surgical planning
Delayed repair of subsequent ureteral stricture

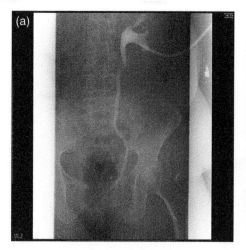 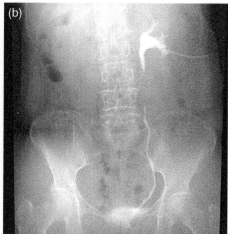

Figure 7.3 (a) Nephrostogram showing complete obstruction of the left ureter detected after hysterectomy. A percutaneous nephrostomy was inserted. (b) Three months after nephrostomy, the obstructive part of the ureter was spontaneously re-canalized, demonstrating free flow of contrast into the bladder. *Source:* courtesy of Haruaki Kato, M.D.

In the acute intra-operative setting, surgeons should use direct ureteral inspection or adjunctive diagnostic maneuvers such as dye injection, catheter passage, or retrograde pyeloureterography. The type of management depends on injury mechanism and severity. Ligations should be removed when identified. In such cases, and with thermal or crush injuries, the ureter is observed for viability. If viable, retrograde ureteral catheterization is the best choice for diagnosis and management initially. If a guidewire is passable at the injured site, a ureteral stent should be placed temporally for at least six weeks. If resection is indicated, or a complete transection is found, primary repair over a ureteral stent should be performed (see below). For long segment injuries, in which reimplantation or primary repair cannot bridge the gap, nephrostomy tube placement is indicated.

Most iatrogenic injuries are discovered post-operatively, and present with pain, leakage of urine, urinoma formation, or acute kidney injury. Contrast enhanced computed tomography (CT) (see Figure 7.2) with delayed images is recommended. In such cases, the overall patient status requires consideration. If uninfected and stable, retrograde ureteropyelography is appropriate with attempted stenting for ligation and partial injuries. If a wire cannot be negotiated into the renal pelvis or complete obstruction is detected, insertion of a percutaneous nephrostomy tube is the next step for appropriate management. Definitive surgery may be considered immediately, if within a five- to seven-day window of the initial iatrogenic injury (see next section). Alternatively, in such patients, the repair of the ureter should be performed at the appropriate interval after the surgery. We have occasionally observed cases of spontaneous restoration of ureteral continuity two to three months after gynecological surgery among patients with complete obstruction managed by a nephrostomy tube (Figure 7.3). The presumed reason for resolution is that an absorbable suture used for ligation was reabsorbed without occlusion of the lumen.

Timing of Repair

Immediate repair remains the best choice for the iatrogenic ureteral injury when the injury is obviously identified during an open surgery (see Figure 7.2). However, when the injury is identified post-operatively, or during an endoscopic or ureteroscopic surgery, stenting with ureteral catheter or nephrostomy and deferred repair seem to be better solutions, since these strategies successfully resolve urinary leakage and allow subsequent identification of healthy or unhealthy ureteral tissue later. If neither procedure (ureteral stenting and nephrostomy construction) successfully diverts the urinary tract, immediate open or endoscopic repair should be considered.

Similarly, cases with active sepsis, infected urinoma, bowel complications, or other complicating factors should consider appropriate nephrostomy and percutaneous drainage of any collections before considering definitive repair.

We usually remove the ureteral stent about six weeks after its placement and observe whether progressive hydronephrosis develops. If obstruction becomes evident, then repair of the stricture should be undertaken. In cases managed with nephrostomy, combined antegrade pyeloureterography and retrograde ureterography will delineate complete obstruction or stricture of the ureter, which also necessitates a delayed reconstruction of the damaged ureter.

Surgical Technique

A variety of surgical procedures have been described for the treatment of iatrogenic ureteral injury. However, the choice is usually simple, dependent on the site of the injury, the extent of the lesion, renal functional reserve, and the condition of the para-injured site in relation to inflammation, fibrosis, scar tissue, tumor, or irradiation.

1) Uretero-ureterostomy, Uretero-pyelostomy:
   Damaged segments or defects of the ureter that are short, in the mid- or upper ureter, can be appropriately repaired by uretero-ureterostomy or uretero-pyelostomy. As long as the proximal and distal part of the ureter are healthy and vascularized and can be mobilized, excision of the damaged site is performed for easy anastomosis with minimum tension. After excision of the damaged segment, the proximal and distal ends of the ureter are spatulated and overlapping mucosa-to-mucosa anastomosis should be performed with placement of a ureteral stent. When the defect of the ureter is relatively long in the upper ureter, full mobilization of the kidney and downward nephropexy to the psoas muscle might be required (Figure 7.4). If the vascularization of the ureter is questionable, wrapping a pedicled omental flap around the anastomotic site might enhance the healing process (Figure 7.5).

2) Uretero-calicostomy:
   Considered in a broad sense as an iatrogenic ureteral injury, stricture after pyeloplasty or percutaneous treatment of stone disease in the renal pelvis is included in this chapter as an iatrogenic cause. In these cases, an anastomosis between the renal pelvic and the upper ureteral is usually difficult, since fibrotic tissue and scar form around the stricture segment and the renal hilus. Therefore, uretero-calicostomy is a solution favored for these strictures near the ureteropelvic junction (UPJ). The distal ureter is fully mobilized to the level near the common iliac artery and the spatulated ureteral end is

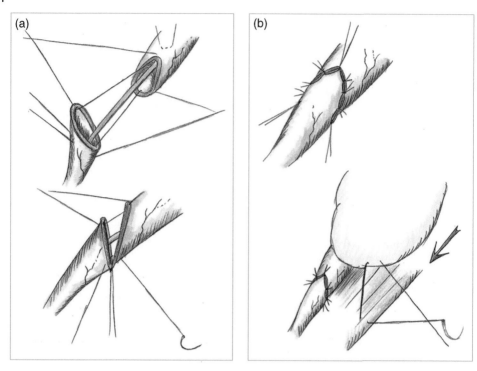

Figure 7.4 Uretero-ureterostomy. Spatulated, tension-free, mucosa-to-mucosa anastomosis with stent placement is a key to success for uretero-ureterostomy. Nephropexy can be used to reduce tension on upper ureteral anastomosis. *Source:* courtesy of Haruaki Kato, M.D.

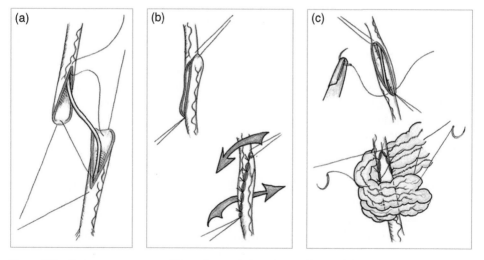

Figure 7.5 Uretero-ureterostomy. When the repair is performed intra-abdominally, an omental flap wrapped around the repair ensures healing. *Source:* courtesy of Haruaki Kato, M.D.

(a)

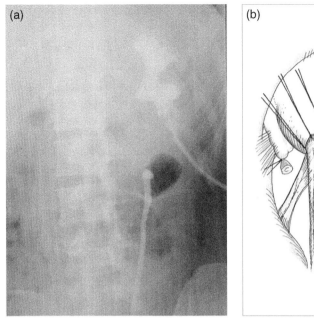

(b)

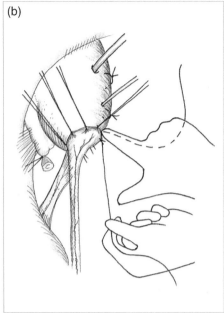

(c)

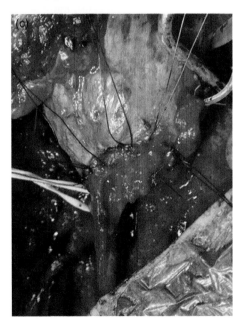

Figure 7.6 Uretero-calicostomy. The fully mobilized distal spatulated ureter is anastomosed to the lower calyces in a case of a long upper ureteral defect. Note nephrostomy tube and ureteral stent exiting renal parenchyma above the anastomosis. *Source:* courtesy of Haruaki Kato, M.D.

anastomosed to the dependent part of the renal lower calyces after wedge resection of the renal parenchymal tissue with stenting (Figure 7.6). Excellent results can be obtained easily when the lower pole parenchymal tissue is thin due to hydronephrosis.

The lower ureter is the most common site of vulnerability to iatrogenic gynecological or pelvic surgical injury. In cases with lower ureteric injury, the proximal ureter should be implanted directly into the bladder with or without submucosal implantation technique, which is more effective and safer than primary uretero-ureterostomy. The reasons for this relate to questionable vascularization of the distal ureter due to involvement of branches of the internal iliac artery with hemostatic ligation, extravasation of urine in the early post-operative phase, and finally, the distal part of the ureter is buried in fibrotic tissue or in dense scar tissue in the late post-operative phase. Therefore, uretero-neocystostomy is an effective and safe procedure when the bladder has adequate capacity and vascularization.

1) Direct uretero-neocystostomy:

   After preparing the distal part of the ureter for implantation into the bladder wall, a direct uretero-neocystostomy is preferred when the length of the mobilized ureter is long enough to reach the bladder [6]. Implantation with refluxing or anti-refluxing is a matter of surgeon preference, but a spacious submucosal tunnel should be created in the bladder wall to prevent obstruction when choosing anti-refluxing style. The re-stricture or re-obstruction of the anastomosis will cause more deterioration of renal function than reflux. A point of controversy is whether the site of re-implantation into the bladder is better on the posterior or anterior dome than on the lateral aspects, because re-implantation of the ureter into the lateral wall of the bladder is prone to kinking with filling of the bladder [7]. In our practice, the appropriate or suitable site for the ureteral implantation is determined after mobilization of the bladder from the retropubic space and the lateral aspects of pelvis, and instillation of about 200 ml saline into the bladder.

2) Psoas hitch procedure:

   The psoas hitch procedure is a reliable procedure for repair of injuries to the lower third of the ureter, with a high success rate [8]. Mobilization of the bladder and fixation to the psoas muscle above the level of the iliac vessels allows tension-free uretero-vesical-anastomosis with or without a submucosal tunnel to prevent reflux. The implantation site is immobilized, which prevents kinking of the ureter during filling and emptying of the bladder. However, thickening of the wall of a contracted bladder or history of pelvic irradiation are contraindications for this procedure. The ureter is secured above the injured site extraperitoneally; after being divided, the proximal ureter is further mobilized cranially with careful preservation of its blood supply. In general, after mobilization from the retropubic space, lateral pelvic wall, and peritoneum, the bladder is opened with an approximate 5-cm incision, which is oriented almost perpendicular to the ureteral course. An index finger is inserted into the bladder from the cystotomy, and the cephalic part of the bladder wall is brought up to the intended part of the psoas muscle and is fixed to the muscle with two to three sutures avoiding the genitofemoral nerve. Then the ureter is implanted into the submucosal tunnel created in the dorsal part of the bladder. If the bladder is very capacious after mobilization, we usually fix the dome of the bladder to the psoas muscle and implant the ureter into a suitable site on the anterior aspect of the bladder with submucosal tunnel technique (Figure 7.7). Care

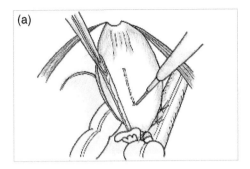 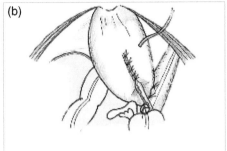

Figure 7.7 Modified psoas hitch procedure. The fully mobilized bladder dome is fixed to the psoas muscle. Then the ureteral end is anastomosed to the suitable anterior aspect of the bladder wall. *Source:* courtesy of Haruaki Kato, M.D.

should be taken not to take a deep stitch in the psoas muscle for fixation, since cases of femoral nerve neuropathy after the psoas hitch procedure have been reported [9]. This complication spoils the result of excellent repair of an iatrogenic ureteral injury. Suture for fixation to the psoas muscle should be superficial and preferably not exceed a depth of 3 mm [10].

3) Boari flap procedure:

When the lower ureteral defect is too long to allow a bladder psoas hitch, a pedicle flap of the anterior bladder wall is swung cranially to be anastomosed with or without antirefluxing tunnel, and finally tubularized, and the bladder defect is closed continuously. In general, the Boari flap procedure is a creative technique producing good results and can bridge a significant defect. However, this procedure carries an inherent risk of ischemia in its tubularized portion, which may result in anastomotic stricture or reduction of bladder capacity post-operatively.

4) Trans-uretero-ureterostomy:

Trans-uretero-ureterostomy is not indicated for most short iatrogenic ureteral injuries and is seldom used. However, in a distal ureter that is not suitable for primary ureteroureterostomy (i.e. irradiated, buried in frozen pelvis), or when implantation of the proximal ureter into the bladder is contraindicated (i.e. contracted, irradiated, thickened bladder), then trans-uretero-ureterostomy might be a viable option. Since there is a potential risk of bilateral obstruction, care should be taken to create a tension-free anastomosis from a well vascularized and fully mobilized donor ureter into a healthy recipient ureter in end-to-side fashion.

The indications for trans-uretero-ureterostomy are limited; we thus would consider using intestinal segments to bridge large gaps between the proximal end of the ureter and the bladder (see below).

Complete Ureteral Loss

As a consequence of a major iatrogenic injury or failed multiple attempts at ureteral repair, an entire ureter might be lost. In these cases, auto-transplantation of the kidney or ureteral substitution using an intestinal segment should be considered before nephrectomy. Autotransplantation can overcome any defect, but requires special expertise in a referral center.

1) Auto-transplantation:

   As a final option for a long ureteral loss due to iatrogenic injury, renal auto-transplantation is described for solving this type of complication in any textbook. However, renal auto-transplantation is rarely applicable in contemporary urologic practice, especially in an acute setting. Furthermore, an inflammatory effect due to previous surgery or extravasation of urine around the renal hilum might preclude dissection of the renal vessels, and the damaged renal pelvis or short proximal ureter may be difficult to anastomose directly to the distal ureteral stump or a tubularized bladder flap. For these reasons, we prefer to apply substitution ureteroplasty using bowel segments rather than try to perform renal auto-transplantation.

2) Substitution ureteroplasty using bowel segments:

   Substitution ureteroplasty seems to be an attractive means for bridging a long defect of the ureter, since the bowel segments usually are intact, even in patients with severe iatrogenic ureteral injuries. Ureteral substitution using bowel segments is usually applied for a delayed repair, especially when the defect is too long for successful ureteral reimplantation with a Boari flap or psoas hitch. Bowel segments have been obtained from the ileum, colon, appendix, and stomach. Despite absorption of urine and secretion of mucus, interposition of an intact ileal segment has been popularized and produces favorable results in the long term [11, 12], when the renal reserve is sufficient. However, ileal dilatation due to urinary stasis with ileo-renal reflux and absorption of urine from the ileal mucosa might deteriorate the renal function. Therefore, several techniques were devised to prevent the ileo-renal reflux with a proximal anti-refluxing technique [13, 14] and were assessed clinically by Xu et al. [15]. For relatively short defects, as with the appendix in the middle part of the right side, the Yang-Monti tube [16, 17] from the ileal segment is always available to any part of the ureter. The surface of the ileal mucosa is minimized in the Yang-Monti tube, to prevent dilatation of the tube and minimize urine absorption. To bridge a longer ureteral defect, multiple Yang-Monti tubes created from ileum are connected [18], or a Yang-Monti tube is created from a single or a double colonic segment [19, 20]. These procedures are advantageous to use in patients with impaired renal function. We also construct a continent transverse-colon pouch and totally replace the ureter using a transversally reconfigured colonic segment (Yang-Monti tube) [21].

Outcomes and Complications

In the early post-injury period, urinary ascites, urinoma formation, fistula, or ureteral obstruction may complicate iatrogenic ureteral injury, particularly when unrecognized intra-operatively. In addition to prompt drainage, appropriate treatment of urinary or wound infection and hemodynamic stabilization are essential. Stricture formation, fistula, and renal loss represent the most significant long-term complications of ureteral injury from any cause. Success rates for endoscopic management of iatrogenic ureteral injuries have not been established to the same degree as surgical reconstruction. As with initial injury management, treatment of complications depends on mechanism and location. Short strictures and small fistulae may respond to endoscopic management [1]. Conversely, longer strictures and persistent large urinary fistulae necessitate reoperation and may

Table 7.1 Outcomes of ureteral reconstruction for injury[a]

Repair type	Stricture free rates
Uretero-ureterostomy	96%
Reimplantation	97%
Boari Flap	81–88%
Ureteral replacement	>95%
Autotransplantation	>80–95%[b]

[a] Adapted from information from Roupret et al. (2015) [22].
[b] Major complication is graft loss.

require more complex repairs as outlined above. Outcomes of the delayed reconstruction of ureteral injuries, as outlined in Table 7.1, reflect the evidence review of the European Association of Urology (EAU) Guidelines Panel, with the caveat that outcomes for iatrogenic injury may be different than for other causes [22].

Conclusions

Prevention or careful recognition of iatrogenic ureteral injuries during surgery is of critical importance, and immediate recognition and optimal management may reduce the damage and the defect created by the injury. However, once severe injuries are recognized, repair should be undertaken considering the timing of recognition, extent and site of the injury. Therefore, urologic surgeons should always bear in mind several surgical options for repairing the injuries, acknowledging the expertise required for each surgical technique.

References

1 Summerton, D.J., Kitrey, N.D., Lumen, N. et al. (2012). European Association of Urology: EAU guidelines on iatrogenic trauma. *Eur. Urol.* 62 (4): 628–639.
2 Elliott, S. and McAninch, J. (2006). Ureteral injuries: external and iatrogenic. *Urol. Clin. North Am.* 33: 55–66.
3 Turner-Warwick, R. and Chapple, C. Ureteral injuries and fistulae. In: Functional Reconstruction of the Urinary Tract and Gynaeco-Urology (eds. R. Turner-Warwick and C. Chapple), 611–628. Blackwell.
4 Grainger, D., Soderstom, R., Schiff, S. et al. (1990). *Obstet. Gynecol.* 75: 839–843.
5 Marien, T.P., Shapiro, E., Melamed, J. et al. (2008). *Rev. Urol.* 10: 297–303.
6 Manoharan, M. and Tunuguntla, H.S. (2005). Standard reconstruction techniques: techniques of ureteroneostomy during urinary diversion. *Surg. Oncol. Clin. North Am.* 14: 367–379.
7 Hensle, T., Berdon, W., Baker, D., and Goldstein, H. (1982). The ureteral "J" sign: radiographic demonstration of iatrogenic distal ureteral obstruction after ureteral reimplantation. *J. Urol.* 127: 766–768.

8 Riedmiller, H., Becht, E., Jacobi, G., and Hohenfellner, R. (1984). Psoas-hitch ureteroneocystostomy: experience with 181 cases. *Eur. Urol.* 10: 145–150.

9 Maldonado, P.A., Slocum, M.D., Chin, K., and Corton, M.M. (2014). Anatomical relationships of psoas muscle: clinical applications to psoas hitch ureteral implantation. *Am. J. Obstet. Gynecol.* 211: 563.e1–6.

10 Pinto, A.C., Macea, J.R., and Pecoraro, M.T. (2012). Femoral nerve neuropathy after the psoas hitch procedure. *Einstein* 10: 371–373.

11 Boxer, R.J., Fritzsche, P., Skinner, D.G., and Kaufman, J.J. (1979). Replacement of the ureter by small intestine: clinical application and results of the ileal ureter in 89 patients. *J. Urol.* 121: 728–731.

12 Waldner, M., Hertle, L., and Roth, S. (1999). Ileal ureteral substitution in reconstructive urological surgery: is an antireflux procedure necessary? *J. Urol.* 162: 323–326.

13 Kato, H., Abol-Enein, H., Igawa, Y. et al. (1999). A case of ileal ureter with proximal antireflux system. *Int. J. Urol.* 6: 320–323.

14 Kato, H., Kiyokawa, H., Igawa, Y., and Nishizawa, O. (2001). The serous-lined tunnel principle for urinary reconstruction: a more rational method. *BJU Int.* 87: 783–788.

15 Xu, Y.M., Qian, L., Qiao, Y. et al. (2008). Ileal ureteric replacement with an ileo-psoas muscle tunnel antirefluxing technique for the treatment of long segment ureteric strictures. *BJU Int.* 102: 1452–1456.

16 Yang, W.H. (1993). Yang needle tunneling technique in creating antireflux and continent mechanism. *J. Urol.* 150: 830–834.

17 Monti, P.R., Lara, R.C., Dutra, M.A., and De Carvalho, J.R. (1997). New technique for construction of efferent conduit based on the Mitrofanoff principle. *Urology* 49: 112–115.

18 Ali-el-Dein, B. and Ghoneim, M.A. (2003). Bridging long ureteral defects using the Yang-Monti principle. *J. Urol.* 169: 1074–1077.

19 Pope, J. and Kock, M.O. (1996). Ureteral replacement with reconfigured colon substitute. *J. Urol.* 155: 1693–1695.

20 Lazica, D.A., Ubrig, B., Brandt, A.S. et al. (2012). Ureteral substitution with reconfigured colon: long-term followup. *J. Urol.* 187: 542–548.

21 Kato, H., Igawa, Y., and Nishizawa, O. (1999). Transverse colon pouch with total replacement of the ureter by reconfigured colon segment. *J. Urol.* 161: 1902–1903.

22 Roupret, M., Babjuk, M., Comperat, E. et al. (2015). European Association of Urology guidelines on upper urinary tract urothelial cell carcinoma: 2015 update. *Eur. Urol.* 68 (5): 868–879.

Section II

Lower Urinary Tract

8

Bladder Injuries
Yosuke Nakajima

Kawasaki Municipal Ida Hospital, Kawasaki, Japan

Introduction

Bladder injuries are broadly classified by etiology: external trauma (e.g. traffic injuries, penetrating injuries), or iatrogenic trauma (e.g. pelvic or transurethral surgery). Incidence of bladder injuries is relatively low, and bladder rupture *per se* is not fatal, although missed injuries or inappropriate non-operative management of complex cases may cause significant complications. Furthermore, coexisting injuries frequently require prompt and appropriate treatments to avoid long-term disability and improve post-operative patients' quality of life.

Etiology

1) Bladder injuries by external trauma:
   Road traffic accidents are the leading cause of bladder injuries, followed by falls; most are associated with pelvic bony fracture or internal organ injuries [1–7]. Sixty to ninety percent of external trauma-induced bladder blunt injuries accompany pelvic fractures [8]. Although bladder injury itself is not fatal, it most often occurs as a part of multi-organ injuries as a consequence of high-energy trauma; mortality rate is as high as 20% due to coexisting severe head, thoracic, and abdominal injuries [4]. Meanwhile, only a small percentage of pelvic fractures overall have an accompany bladder injury [5]. By contrast, penetrating injuries by stab or gunshot wounds to the bladder are relatively rare [9].

   Classification: Bladder injuries are broadly divided into contusion and rupture, with the latter being clinically important. Bladder ruptures are divided into three types: extraperitoneal (EP), intraperitoneal (IP), and combined intra-EP bladder ruptures. Among them, EP bladder rupture is the most common type, with the IP type ranks second [2, 6, 8]. Coexisting urethral injuries are seen in 4.1–15% of cases [5, 6]. The American Association for the

A Clinical Guide to Urologic Emergencies, First Edition. Edited by Hunter Wessells, Shigeo Horie, and Reynaldo G. Gómez.
© 2021 John Wiley & Sons Ltd. Published 2021 by John Wiley & Sons Ltd.
Companion website: www.wiley.com/go/wessells/urologic

Surgery of Trauma (AAST) created an Organ Injury Scale for bladder injuries, in which location and size of the bladder laceration confers gradations of severity.

Most EP ruptures are induced by pelvic fractures in which bladders are exposed to severe shearing force [2, 7]. EP ruptures comprise the following several types: a simple case in which extravasation of urine is confined to the pelvic cavity (Figures 8.1a and b), bladder neck injuries, existence of fractured bone debris in the bladder wall [6], concurrent rectal injuries, and complicated cases with penetrating injuries [4]. On the other hand, IP bladder ruptures are induced by a sudden rise in intra-abdominal pressure due to a blunt external force such as the one caused by a seat belt, although the bladder may rupture with seemingly low impact blunt trauma. Fully distended bladders are especially prone to this type of pressure rise, and the most fragile part, the bladder dome, is most likely to rupture [2, 4, 6, 10] (Figure 8.1c). Therefore, bladder distension is one of the risk factors for IP bladder

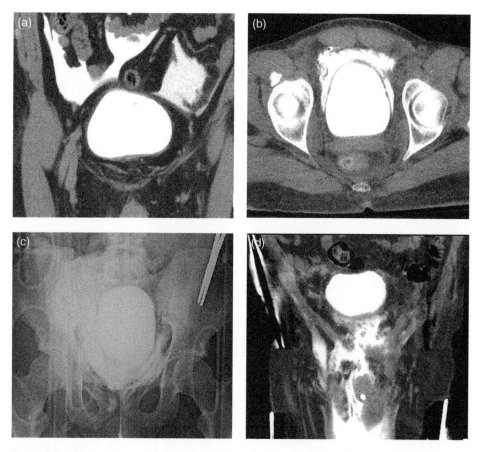

Figure 8.1. CT and fluoroscopic imaging of bladder rupture including: (a) coronal view of CT cystogram showing an intraperitoneal (IP) rupture with extravasated contrast outlining loops of bowel; (b) axial view of CT cystogram showing an EP bladder rupture with molar tooth extravasation pattern; (c) fluoroscopic cystogram showing an EP rupture with extravasation into the soft tissues of the pelvis; and (d): coronal view of CT cystogram showing an EP rupture with extensive extravasation tracking into the scrotum.

rupture [6]. The least frequent combined type is often seen in impalement injuries, such as open and penetrating injuries caused by stakes or iron bars.

2) Iatrogenic bladder injuries:

Among all the urogenital organs, the bladder is the most susceptible organ to iatrogenic injuries [11]. Iatrogenic bladder injuries can occur as a complication of several surgical procedures, such as hysterectomy, Cesarean section [12–15], colon cancer surgery, inguinal surgery [6, 12, 16], transurethral resection (TUR) of bladder tumor, holmium laser enucleation of prostate [12, 17, 18], and sling surgery for urinary incontinence [19]. In some cases, a ruptured wall is immediately recognizable, but in other cases, they are detected by abnormal signs, such as extravasation of urine, a sudden increase in hematuria, or presence of pneumoperitoneal gas getting into urine collection bag [6].

Clinical Symptoms and Imaging Diagnoses

Because treatment of concurrent severe injuries of other organs tends to be prioritized, bladder injuries may be diagnosed in a delayed manner, or even get overlooked [4]. Gross hematuria is a major symptom of bladder injuries [6], and in cases of pelvic fractures, bladder injuries most likely coexist in the presence of gross hematuria [1, 2, 20]. The combination of these two symptoms is an absolute indication for cystography [1, 2, 20]. Aside from gross hematuria, abdominal tenderness, urinary retention, and bruises over the upper part of pelvic bone [6] are important signs to suspect bladder injuries. Specifically, tremendous abdominal tenderness, peritoneal irritation sign, anuria, and no urinary flow through a catheter are important signs of IP bladder rupture [2]. Furthermore, extravasation of urine extending beyond perineum and thighs indicates the existence of EP bladder rupture (Figure 8.1d). Bleeding per the external urethral meatus indicates a high likelihood of urethral trauma. Thus, in such a case, retrograde urethrography should be performed prior to cystography, as outlined below.

Cystography, or computed tomography (CT) cystography, is required to make a diagnosis of bladder injuries. Both diagnostic imaging techniques have high sensitivity (90–95%) and high specificity (100%) [2, 7]. The following considerations are needed when performing these imaging techniques.

Plain Film Cystography (Figure 8.1b):

First, a standard or "Scout Film" Kidney, Ureter, Bladder (KUB) static radiograph should be taken following placement of an indwelling urethral catheter in order to assess the status of the bony pelvis, the presence of bone debris, and the existence of dislocation. Next, slowly instill at least 350 ml [2, 3] of dilute contrast medium into the bladder via gravity from a height of 40 cm above the bladder. Then, the anteroposterior view and the oblique view are taken. Because insufficient instillation of contrast media may cause injuries to be missed, full distention of the bladder is important. Of note, since some injuries are detectable only after discharge of contrast media, images after bladder filling as well as post-drainage are imperative with plain film cystography [3], so that even the smallest amount of extravasation can be detected. Interpretation of the radiogram after fluoroscopic imaging during cystography also requires special attention. Occasionally, collection of contrast media under the diaphragm or beside the liver leads to a diagnosis, so inclusion of upper abdominal areas in the KUB radiography is recommended. In IP bladder ruptures, the outline of colon loops or liver becomes enhanced [6]. Flame-shaped contrast extravasation around the bladder is a well-known sign for EP bladder ruptures [6].

CT cystography:

CT cystography involves retrograde instillation of contrast agent into bladders similar to that described above, with subsequent abdominopelvic CT imaging [2, 3]. CT cystography with its improved detection of extravasation does not require scout or post drainage films, and nowadays CT cystography is often preferred over conventional cystography [21]. Due to the comprehensive detection ability of CT, CT cystography also allows us to diagnose other injuries or make a differential diagnosis for abdominal pain [6].

Other methods of diagnostic imaging, abdominal ultrasound, and cystography in which urethral catheter is clamped at the excretory phase of contrast-enhanced CT or intravenous pyelogram (IVP), have been reported [2] (Figure 8.1a). However, they may be insufficiently sensitive and specific for accurate diagnosis [2]. For the detection of iatrogenic bladder injuries after sling surgery or complex pelvic surgery, routinely conducting cystoscopy at the end of the case is recommended [2].

Treatment of Bladder Injuries

Importantly, the severity and type of rupture influences the course of treatment.

EP bladder rupture due to blunt trauma, irrespective of its mechanism, can be effectively treated with drainage by indwelling urethral catheters only [2, 4, 6, 20]. Successful management requires a larger (e.g. 18 - 20Fr.) caliber Foley catheter to ensure adequate drainage and avoid blockage by clots. Cystography is performed between 7 and 14 days of catheter placement. If there is no detectable contrast extravasation, the catheter can be removed. Persistence of contrast extravasation requires continued catheter drainage, and the same procedure is repeated after an additional seven days [10, 22].

Conversely, surgical repair is indicated for IP ruptures, combined ruptures, and complicated EP ruptures (indentation of bone debris into the bladder, bladder neck injuries, coexisting rectal or vaginal injuries), and bladder injuries caused by penetrating trauma [2, 4, 9, 20]. Bladder exploration may be undertaken via an intra- or EP approach through a midline or Pfannenstiel incision. Close communication with the primary trauma surgery team and orthopedics is essential to ensure coordination of different surgical interventions. Standard surgical repair usually involves two-layered closure of the mucosa/submucosa and muscle layer with absorbable suture (2-0 or 3-0) [6]. Bladder neck injuries require a specific mention. Because of the risk of incontinence, anatomical proximity to the fractured bony pelvis, and likely failure of non-operative approaches, recognition, and prompt surgical repair are essential. Exposure may be difficult and close coordination with the orthopedic surgeon should be sought. Laparoscopic surgical repair has been described to treat hemodynamically stable IP ruptures without coexisting injuries [7]. In simple and typical IP ruptures, urethral catheters can be removed after 7–10 days of surgical repair without cystography. For more complicated and severe ruptures treated surgically, cystography should be performed prior to catheter removal. In addition, an indwelling urethral catheter is sufficient for urine drainage, thus suprapubic cystostomy is not necessary [20].

Regarding iatrogenic bladder ruptures, immediate surgical repair would be optimal, provided the injury is detected during the primary operation [2]. Similar to non-iatrogenic bladder ruptures, the course of treatment depends on type of rupture when the injuries are only found post-operatively. EP bladder ruptures can be treated with conservative medical management with drainage by indwelling urethral catheters. Meanwhile, surgical repair is usually necessary for IP bladder ruptures [2]. Especially in the case of IP bladder ruptures caused by transurethral resection (TUR) of bladder tumor, careful inspection would be needed during the operation to determine whether concurrent bowel injuries occurred or not [2].

Long-term Consequences

Complicated EP bladder ruptures should be surgically repaired to avoid long-term sequelae from the injury, as mentioned above. Concurrent rectal or vaginal lacerations may lead to fistula formation to the ruptured bladder, and in this setting the EP bladder rupture should be repaired. Bladder neck injuries may not heal with catheter drainage alone and repair should be considered to avoid incontinence [1].

Complications

Complications of bladder injuries include urinary ascites due to IP rupture, infection including sepsis, persistent hematuria, incontinence, and fistula.

Foley catheter drainage alone has become routine management for EP bladder ruptures in many medical centers, and few reports address treatment failures with this approach. Of those patients managed non-operatively, 74% had spontaneous healing within 10–14 days; however, 26% had significant complications, including delayed healing, vesicocutaneous fistula, septic events, bladder calculi, or death. Patients with multiple pelvic fractures seem to be at high risk [23]. With bladder neck involvement, surgical exploration and repair are required to limit incontinence.

Conclusion

Because the bladder is well protected within the pelvis, the vast majority of injuries are associated with pelvic fractures. Bladder injuries are EP in approximately 60%, IP in approximately 30%, and the remaining injuries are both IP and EP ruptures [24]. Gross hematuria is the most common sign, present in 77–100% of injuries [1]. Retrograde cystography (CT or conventional) is critical, as it can determine the presence of an injury and whether it is IP or EP. Clinicians manage most EP bladder ruptures non-operatively with catheter drainage, while IP ruptures are surgically repaired [6].

References

1 Morey, A.F., Iverson, A.J., Swan, A. et al. (2001). Bladder rupture after blunt trauma: guidelines for diagnostic imaging. *J. Trauma* 51 (4): 683–686.

2 Summerton, D.J., Djakovic, N., Kitrey, N.D. et al. (2015). Guidelines on Urological Trauma. 22–27. Available from: http://uroweb.org/wp-content/uploads/EAU-Guidelines-Urological-Trauma-2015-v2.pdf (Access on 2015-8-28)

3 Ramchandani, P. and Buckler, P.M. (2009). Imaging of genitourinary trauma. *AJR Am. J. Roentgenol.* 192 (6): 1514–1523.

4 Pereira, B.M., de Campos, C.C., Calderan, T.R. et al. (2013). Bladder injuries after external trauma: 20 years experience report in a population-based cross-sectional view. *World J. Urol.* 31 (4): 913–917.

5 Bjurlin, M.A., Fantus, R.J., Mellett, M.M., and Goble, S.M. (2009). Genitourinary injuries in pelvic fracture morbidity and mortality using the National Trauma Data Bank. *J. Trauma* 67 (5): 1033–1039.

6 Gomez, R.G., Ceballos, L., Coburn, M. et al. (2004). Consensus statement on bladder injuries. *BJU Int.* 94 (1): 27–32.

7 Wirth, G.J., Peter, R., Poletti, P.A., and Iselin, C.E. (2010). Advances in the management of blunt traumatic bladder rupture: experience with 36 cases. *BJU Int.* 106 (9): 1344–1349.

8 Deibert, C.M. and Spencer, B.A. (2011). The association between operative repair of bladder injury and improved survival: results from the National Trauma Data Bank. *J. Urol.* 186 (1): 151–155.

9 Cinman, N.M., McAninch, J.W., Porten, S.P. et al. (2013). Gunshot wounds to the lower urinary tract: a single-institution experience. *J. Trauma Acute Care Surg.* 74 (3): 725–730; discussion 730-1.

10 Nakajima, Y. (2006). Urological trauma: bladder trauma, urethral trauma. *Urol. View* 4 (5): 26–30.

11 Cordon, B.H., Fracchia, J.A., and Armenakas, N.A. (2014). Iatrogenic nonendoscopic bladder injuries over 24 years: 127 cases at a single institution. *Urology* 84 (1): 222–226.

12 Armenakas, N.A., Pareek, G., and Fracchia, J.A. (2004). Iatrogenic bladder perforations: longterm followup of 65 patients. *J. Am. Coll. Surg.* 198 (1): 78–82.

13 Rahman, M.S., Gasem, T., Al Suleiman, S.A. et al. (2009). Bladder injuries during cesarean section in a University Hospital: a 25-year review. *Arch. Gynecol. Obstet.* 279 (3): 349–352.

14 Donnez, O., Jadoul, P., Squifflet, J., and Donnez, J. (2009). A series of 3190 laparoscopic hysterectomies for benign disease from 1990 to 2006: evaluation of complications compared with vaginal and abdominal procedures. *BJOG* 116 (4): 492–500.

15 Vakili, B., Chesson, R.R., Kyle, B.L. et al. (2005). The incidence of urinary tract injury during hysterectomy: a prospective analysis based on universal cystoscopy. *Am. J. Obstet. Gynecol.* 192 (5): 1599–1604.

16 Honore, C., Souadka, A., Goere, D. et al. (2012). HIPEC for peritoneal carcinomatosis: does an associated urologic procedure increase morbidity? *Ann. Surg. Oncol.* 19 (1): 104–109.

17 Balbay, M.D., Cimentepe, E., Unsal, A. et al. (2005). The actual incidence of bladder perforation following transurethral bladder surgery. *J. Urol.* 174 (6): 2260–2262; discussion 2262-3.

18 Nieder, A.M., Meinbach, D.S., Kim, S.S., and Soloway, M.S. (2005). Transurethral bladder tumor resection: intraoperative and postoperative complications in a residency setting. *J. Urol.* 174 (6): 2307–2309.

19 Novara, G., Artibani, W., Barber, M.D. et al. (2010). Updated systematic review and meta-analysis of the comparative data on colposuspensions, pubovaginal slings, and midurethral tapes in the surgical treatment of female stress urinary incontinence. *Eur. Urol.* 58 (2): 218–238.

20 Morey, A.F., Brandes, S., Dugi, D.D. 3rd et al. (2014). Urotrauma: AUA Guideline. *J. Urol.* 192 (2): 327–335.

21 ACR Appropriateness Criteria® blunt abdominal trauma. Available from: http://www.guideline.gov/content.aspx?id=37927 (Access on 2015-8-28)

22 Inaba, K., McKenney, M., Munera, F. et al. (2006). Cystogram follow-up in the management of traumatic bladder disruption. *J. Trauma* 60 (1): 23–28.

23 Kotkin, L. and Koch, M.O. (1995). Morbidity associated with nonoperative management of extraperitoneal bladder injuries. *J. Trauma* 38 (6): 895–898.

24 Brandes, S. and Borrelli, J. Jr. (2001). Pelvic fracture and associated urologic injuries. *World J. Surg.* 25 (12): 1578–1587.

9

Traumatic Urethral Injuries

Laura G. Velarde and Reynaldo G. Gómez

Urology Service, Hospital del Trabajador, Santiago, Chile

Introduction

Injuries to the urethra are not frequent, and usually happen in the context of a polytrauma patient, with severe associated injuries, among which pelvic fracture stands out.

Initial management is appropriately focused on life-threatening injuries, with the unintended consequence that the urethral injury could initially go unnoticed, potentially increasing management complexity and morbidity.

Moreover, in the context of a pelvic fracture, urethral and bladder injuries can coexist, so it is important to have a clear initial diagnostic protocol, which allows for proper and timely management. The key to success is a high index of suspicion of injuries, making the diagnosis on time, and performing early treatment.

Initial Management of Suspected Trauma to the Lower Urinary Tract

Faced with a polytraumatized patient in critical condition, the initial management will be determined by the patient's general condition, hemodynamic status, and associated injuries. In this situation, occasionally, urinary injuries may go unnoticed. For this reason, the evaluation must be carried out by a multidisciplinary and experienced team, capable of timely diagnosis of all injuries and establishment of treatment priorities [1].

Of greatest importance for the diagnosis of traumatic injuries of the lower urinary tract (bladder and urethra) is appropriate stratification of risk. Hematuria and pelvic fracture are the main indicators of risk.

The most relevant diagnostic elements are urethral bleeding (blood in the urethral meatus), hematuria (microscopic or gross), inability to urinate with or without bladder distention, low or diffuse abdominal pain, non-palpable prostate at the digital rectal

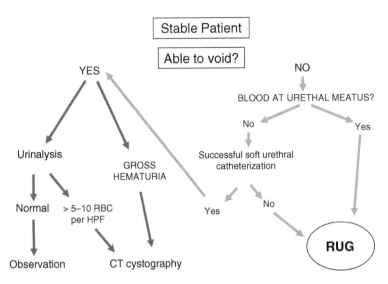

Figure 9.1 Initial management in a stable patient with suspected lower urinary tract injury. CT: computed tomography. RUG: retrograde urethrogram.

examination, and inability to pass a urethral catheter. It is also essential to rule out associated injuries to the rectum and the vagina.

Fractures that compromise the anterior and posterior pelvic rings impart the greatest odds of urethral and bladder injury. In this acute phase of injury, the patient must be evaluated by a urologist [2].

High-energy mechanism of injury with a pelvic fracture (traffic accidents, falls from height, run over by a car) as well as genital and/or perineal injuries (fall astride, motorcycle accident) require in-depth assessment to rule out a urethral and/or a bladder injury [3, 4].

The proposed initial diagnostic protocol shown in Figure 9.1 highlights the defining role of the patient's hemodynamic condition.

Hemodynamically unstable patients are often taken directly to the operating room without the opportunity to conduct imaging studies. In these cases, if there is suspicion of urethral injury, a retrograde urethrogram (RUG) can be performed on the operating table using a C-arm fluoroscopy unit. Conversely, hemodynamically stable patients afford time to carry out a programmed evaluation. In general, if the patient manages to urinate spontaneously and easily, a urethral lesion can be ruled out. However, if there is gross hematuria (or more than 5–10 red blood cells per high-power field in microscopic examination of urine), a study with intravenous contrast is required (see Chapter 8: Bladder Injuries) [5].

When there is blood in the meatus, a urethral injury can be expected, so urethral catheterization is contraindicated without first obtaining a RUG, since blind catheterization may aggravate the urethral lesion [3, 4]. Retrograde urethrography should be performed in a patient with a pelvic fracture and blood in the urethral meatus [4].

On the other hand, if the patient has not been able to urinate and has no blood in the meatus, a gentle urethral catheterization by a trained operator can be attempted with a 14–16 Fr well-lubricated soft rubber catheter. If catheterization is successful and there is also suspicion of bladder injury (hematuria, e.g.), computed tomography (CT) should be

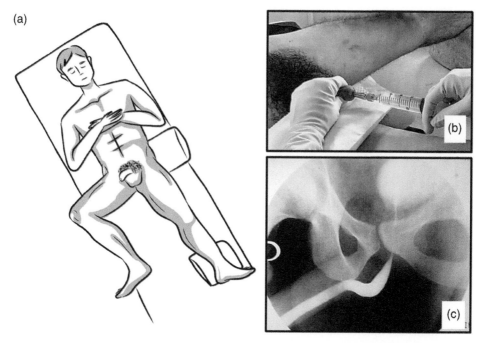

Figure 9.2 Retrograde urethrography: (a) Patient positioning. (b) Cone-tip syringe injecting the urethra. (c) Normal RUG, penile, bulbar, and posterior urethra demonstrated without extravasation; note elongation of the posterior urethra and bladder displaced by peri-vesical hematoma.

complemented with formal CT cystography, because no more than 15% of bladder ruptures are diagnosed on passive bladder filling with contrast enhanced CT (see Chapter 8: Bladder Injuries). For this reason, if the patient is stable, cystography filling of the bladder with up to 350–400 ml with dilute contrast should be done [4, 6]. If there is even a minimal difficulty in passing the catheter, it is advised not to insist, but to obtain a RUG to rule out a urethral injury.

RUG is typically performed supine in anterior oblique position, with the hip disprojected. This is achieved by placing the patient with one leg straight and the other with external rotation of the hip and knee flexion. A cushion is placed lo elevate the contralateral hemipelvis. This position allows imaging of the entire urethra without bone interpositions (Figure 9.2). In polytrauma patients with multiple long bone or pelvic fractures, this position is limited, and generally only anteroposterior images can be obtained (see below). In these cases, it is useful to tilt the x-ray beam cranially about 30° (Figure 9.3). The urethra is imaged by retrograde injecting of 50% diluted contrast medium with saline solution, using a syringe with a cone-tip inserted into the meatus. The urethra must be stretched to avoid kinks, and air bubbles avoided, so as to obtain clear images. The minimum amount of contrast necessary to define the diagnosis is injected, avoiding large extravasations that obscure the location of the lesion and potentially increase the risk of infection.

RUG may show elongation of the urethra without interruption of the submucosa and without extravasation of contrast (urethral contusion), extravasation with contrast passage to the bladder (partial urethral rupture), or extravasation without contrast passage to the

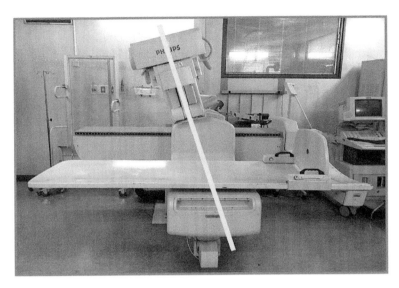

Figure 9.3 Thirty degree cranial tilt of x-ray beam.

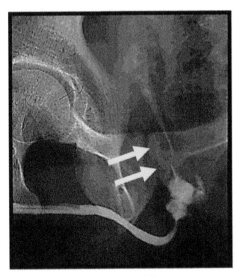

Partial urethral injury

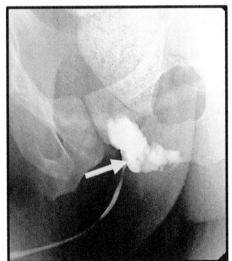

Total urethral injury

Figure 9.4 Partial and complete urethral injury: appearance on retrograde urethrogram.

bladder (complete urethral disruption) [7] (Figure 9.4). Sometimes this differentiation can be equivocal, since the contraction of the external sphincter may prevent the passage of contrast toward the prostate, leading to false diagnosis of a complete injury [8]. If RUG does not show urethral injury, a Foley catheter can be inserted.

When it is not possible to perform RUG under the conditions described, such as in patients with pelvic fracture managed with an external fixator or pelvic belt, the RUG can be carried out in the supine position as described above, or in the operating room in coordination with pelvic fracture fixation.

Patients transferred from another center may arrive with the urethral catheter already inserted, without prior RUG or information about urethral injury status. It is therefore essential to verify that the catheter is in the right position with the balloon inflated inside the bladder. The fact that it was possible to pass the catheter does not exclude a urethral injury; prior to removing this catheter, a peri-catheter urethrogram should be performed to identify any undiagnosed injury. For this, a 16–18G IV cannula is inserted between the catheter and the meatus and contrast is injected alongside the catheter (peri-catheter RUG). If extravasation is observed, a urethral injury is confirmed, and the catheter must remain in place for two to three more weeks.

Urethral Trauma

Urethral injuries do not constitute a life-threatening emergency by themselves. However, the importance of establishing prompt bladder drainage for monitoring of urine output in the polytrauma patient cannot be overstated. At the same time, to ensure the best long-term outcomes of urethral injury it is mandatory not to miss the diagnosis in the acute phase, to determine the type of injury suffered, and to decide about immediate or delayed treatment.

Urethral trauma is divided into trauma of the posterior and anterior urethra. For clarity, we will briefly describe the anatomy of the urethra and the characteristics of each of its divisions.

Urethral Anatomy

Male Urethra

The male urethra extends from the bladder neck to the urethral meatus, with an approximate length of 18 cm and a diameter of 9 mm during urination, being greater in the prostate, bulbar, and navicularis fossa segments. The urogenital diaphragm (aponeurotic muscle plane of the perineum) divides the urethra into posterior (proximal) and anterior (distal) segments [9] (Figure 9.5):

- *Sphincter complex*: Urinary continence depends on the sphincter complex that is formed by the internal and external sphincter, anatomically related to the posterior urethra. Each component has particular characteristics, but they act together to maintain urinary continence: the external sphincter is responsible for active continence and the internal sphincter of passive continence. Both can function independently, so that if one is injured, the other will be able to maintain continence [10].
- *Vascularization*: The arterial supply of the posterior urethra depends on the inferior vesical and rectal arteries, while the anterior urethra depends on inflow from the paired common penile arteries, branches of the internal pudendal artery. The anterior urethra has antegrade arterial supply (through the bulbourethral arteries) as well as a retrograde blood supply through the corpus spongiosum, which is irrigated by the dorsal, cavernous, urethral, and circumflex arteries. Urethral venous drainage occurs through Santorini's plexus and pudendal veins.
- *Innervation*: The urethra has autonomic and somatic innervation. The autonomic innervation depends on the inferior hypogastric plexus and the somatic from the pudendal nerve.

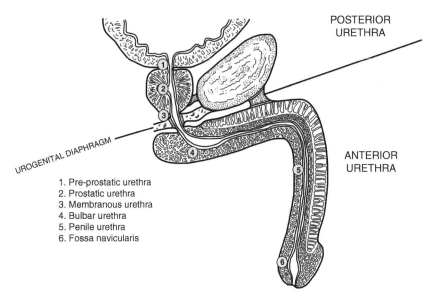

POSTERIOR
URETHRA

UROGENITAL DIAPHRAGM

ANTERIOR
URETHRA

1. Pre-prostatic urethra
2. Prostatic urethra
3. Membranous urethra
4. Bulbar urethra
5. Penile urethra
6. Fossa navicularis

Figure 9.5 Anatomy of the male urethra.

The **posterior urethra** measures about 4–5 cm from the bladder neck to the bulbo-membranous junction and is subdivided into pre-prostatic, prostatic, and membranous. The **pre-prostatic urethra** measures approximately 1 cm from the bladder neck to the prostate; at this level the periurethral glands and the internal sphincter (also called smooth sphincter or involuntary sphincter) are located. The **prostatic urethra**, measuring 3–4 cm, crosses the prostate at an angle of about 35° ventrally, emerging in front of the prostate apex and its most distal part is anchored to the back of the pubis by the pubo-prostatic ligaments, giving it firmness and immobility. The **membranous urethra**, measuring 1.5–2 cm, from the prostate apex, crosses the urogenital diaphragm in its anterior part, anterolaterally surrounded by the external urethral sphincter (also called striated sphincter or voluntary sphincter) and continuing to become the bulbar urethra.

The **Anterior Urethra** measures about 13 cm from the bulbo-membranous junction to the external urethral meatus. Subdivided into bulbar, penile, navicularis fossa, and urethral meatus, it is surrounded by the corpus spongiosum throughout its length, which is more developed at the level of the bulbar urethra. The **bulbar urethra** extends from the urogenital diaphragm to the peno-scrotal junction; it is located in the perineal region and is surrounded by the bulb of the corpus spongiosum, which in turn is covered by the bulbospongiosus muscle. The bulbar urethra includes the bulbo-urethral glands. The **penile urethra** is mobile and accompanies the corpora cavernosa during erection. On its way, the **navicularis fossa** crosses the glans and presents a pre-meatal dilation. The usual anatomical location of the **urethral meatus** is in the mid-apical part of the glans.

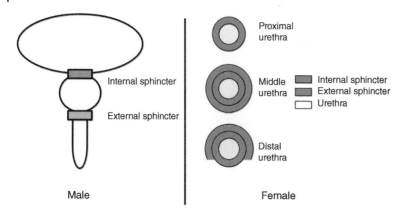

Figure 9.6 Schematic anatomy of male and female urinary sphincter complex.

Female Urethra

The female urethra has an approximate length of 3–5 cm. It is divided by the urogenital diaphragm into posterior segment (proximal) and distal segment (distal) to it. The posterior segment contains the proximal two-thirds and the distal segment the rest of the urethra [11]

- *Sphincter complex:* The internal sphincter is comprised of two layers of smooth muscle (a longitudinal inner layer and an outer circumferential layer, both continuation of the detrusor musculature), ending distally in a thick fibrous ring at the meatus. The external striated sphincter lies above the smooth muscle along the entire length of the urethra and is dorsally absent in the most distal part, adopting an omega shape (Figure 9.6).
- *Vascularization:* Arterial supply depends on the internal pudendal artery and venous drainage is performed through the pelvic plexus.
- *Innervation:* The female urethra has autonomic and somatic innervation similar to the male.

Urethral Trauma Classification

Numerous schema for classification of urethral injuries have been proposed, including that of the American Association for the Surgery of Trauma (AAST) and another more recently proposed by the European Association of Urology (EAU) [6]. The main difference in the two classifications relates to the differential stratification between anterior and posterior urethral complete rupture. The comparisons are shown in Table 9.1.

Unfortunately, due to the difficulty in establishing an accurate admission diagnosis of urethral injury, and the lack of close correlation of imaging and anatomical findings, this classification and others that have been proposed have not found practical clinical application.

According to the mechanism of injury, urethral trauma can be [1, 12]:

- *Blunt trauma:* In the posterior urethra, the most frequent mechanism is bulbomembranous disruption due to a pelvic fracture. In the anterior urethra, the most frequent mechanism is due to a direct blow in the perineal region, fall astride injury or a sports accident, causing the rupture of the bulbar urethra.

Table 9.1 Classification of urethral injuries.

American Association for the Surgery of Trauma (AAST)	European Association of Urology (EAU)
• Type 1: Contusion • Type 2: Stretch injury (elongation) • Type 3: Partial disruption • Type 4: Complete disruption with urethral separation of <2 cm • Type 5: Complete disruption with urethral separation of >2 cm or extension of injury into the prostate or vagina	• Type 1: Stretch injury (elongation) • Type 2: Contusion • Type 3: Partial rupture • Type 4: Complete rupture of the anterior urethra • Type 5: Complete rupture of the posterior urethra • Type 6: Partial or complete rupture of the posterior urethra associated with a tear of the bladder neck or vagina

Adapted from References 6 and 36.

- *Penetrating trauma*: Caused by a stab wound, firearm, projectile, or fragmentation devices such as mines and improvised explosive devices (IED).
- *Trauma during sexual activity*: Cavernous body rupture occurs due to forced flexion of the erect penis and in 10–20% of cases is associated with urethral rupture [13].
- *Internal trauma*: Due to iatrogenic instrumentation or introduction of foreign bodies, for sexual gratification or in psychiatric patients.

Trauma to the Posterior Urethra

Injuries to the posterior urethra are usually secondary to high-kinetic energy mechanisms: 90% of injuries to the posterior urethra are associated with a fractured pelvis; in turn, approximately 10% (3–25%) of pelvic fractures have an associated urethral injury, being more frequent in more severe unstable fractures. For this reason, a urethral injury should be directly ruled out in all patients with a pelvic fracture [2, 3, 6, 7].

Female urethral lesions associated with pelvic fractures are very rare (0.7%) [14]. However, they may be frequently associated with bladder neck injury and also vaginal and/ or rectal injury, requiring acute operative repair. These patients are at risk for significant sexual and lower urinary tract dysfunction [15].

In developed countries, the most frequent cause of this type of injury is motor vehicle collisions and falls, while in developing countries, bicycle and motorcycle collisions predominate. The severity and complexity are greater in developing countries and this seems to be related to poor management in the acute phase, since the first care is provided by emergency physicians rather than by specialized urologists [7].

The posterior urethra is more vulnerable to injury because it is attached to the posterior aspect of the pubis by the pubo-prostatic ligaments. Furthermore, the membranous urethra is the least elastic portion, and is not protected by the prostate or the corpus spongiosum [1, 7]. This anatomical relationship with the anterior arch of the bone pelvis explains why a disruption of the pelvic ring can injure the urethra at the membranous level. The urethral injury can occur distal, proximal or through the urogenital diaphragm, but It has been shown that 70–75% of lesions occur just distal to the external sphincter at the

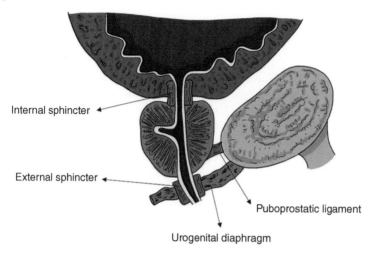

Internal sphincter

External sphincter

Puboprostatic ligament

Urogenital diaphragm

Figure 9.7 Anatomical relationships of the posterior urethra.

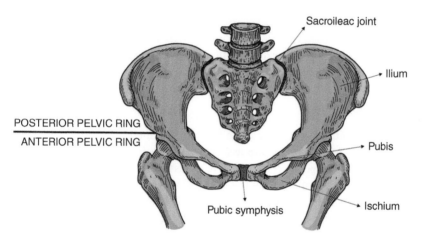

Sacroileac joint

Ilium

POSTERIOR PELVIC RING

ANTERIOR PELVIC RING

Pubis

Pubic symphysis

Ischium

Figure 9.8 Bony pelvis anatomy.

bulbomembranous junction [16]. This is important because the external sphincter complex is closely associated with the membranous urethra so the location and degree of the injury may jeopardize future continence (Figure 9.7). Interestingly, the proposed classification systems focus on the degree of the injury but not its location in relation to the sphincteric mechanism.

Fractures of the Bony Pelvis

The bony pelvis is made up of the paired iliac bones, which articulate posteriorly with the sacrum at the sacroiliac joints (forming the posterior arch) and are continued anteriorly with the ilio- and ischio-pubic rami which join at the midline in the pubic symphysis (forming the anterior arch). The integrity of the posterior arch is the most important for the stability of the pelvic ring (Figure 9.8).

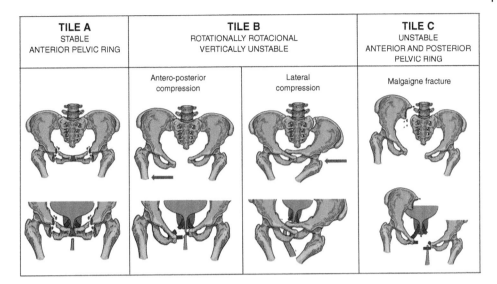

TILE A	TILE B		TILE C
STABLE	ROTATIONALLY ROTACIONAL		UNSTABLE
ANTERIOR PELVIC RING	VERTICALLY UNSTABLE		ANTERIOR AND POSTERIOR PELVIC RING
	Antero-posterior compression	Lateral compression	Malgaigne fracture

Figure 9.9 Initial options for management of urethral trauma.

The most commonly used classification for pelvic fractures is that of Tile, who divides them according to the rotational and vertical stability of the pelvis [17]. There are three types of fractures, with A being stable, B being partially stable, and C being unstable. The frequency and severity of the posterior urethral lesion is associated with the severity and stability of the pelvic fracture and within each type of fracture there are some that are more frequently associated with urethral injury (Figure 9.9) [18]:

- **Tile A fractures** only have involvement of the anterior arch; they are rotationally and vertically stable fractures. The ones most frequently associated with a urethral injury are those that affect the four pubic ramus, creating a bone segment "in butterfly wings" that may cause a shear between the prostate and the membranous urethra, injuring the urethra at this level.
- **Tile B fractures** have complete involvement of the anterior arch and partial damage of the posterior arch. They are partially stable fractures with rotational instability but vertically stable. Those that are most associated with urethral lesion are fractures in "open book," "closed book," or in "bucket handle." The open book fractures are usually produced by an anteroposterior compression of the pelvis causing rupture of the anterior arch and a corresponding sacroiliac subluxation, causing the hemipelvis to rotate externally and injure the urethra by avulsion. The closed book and the bucket handle injuries are produced by a lateral compression. In the closed book fracture, ipsilateral injuries such as sacroiliac subluxation and rupture of the pubic symphysis or pubic branches are found, and in the bucket handle fracture there is an ipsilateral sacroiliac injury and a contralateral rupture of the pubic branches. In both cases, the hemipelvis rotates internally and injure the urethra by a crush mechanism.
- **Tile C fractures** have a complete fracture-dislocation of the anterior and posterior arches and are unstable fractures rotationally and vertically. They are the fractures most

frequently associated with lesion of the posterior urethra, mainly the Malgaigne fracture (fracture of both pubic rami and fracture-dislocation of the sacroiliac or ipsilateral ilium) in which the urethra can suffer a rupture with dislocation of the ends.

Displacement of the fractured pelvis abruptly distracts the membranous urethra that is fixed by the pubo-prostatic ligaments and the urogenital diaphragm, producing different degrees of injury: contusion of the wall and urethral mucosa (25%), partial rupture (25%), or complete rupture (50%) [7, 19]. As expected, complete tears tend to be more frequent in unstable fractures [18]. Urethral injury can also be caused by the direct impact of a bone fragment ("spring knife" or "switchblade" effect). In more complex cases, the bladder, bladder neck, and/or rectum (and the vagina in women) can also be damaged.

Posterior urethral injuries in children are less frequent and are usually located in the bladder neck or prostatic urethra, because the prostate is still not developed and its fixations to the pelvis are more lax than in adults [20].

RUG, discussed above, provides the most important information about urethral injury; CT scan can provide additional information at the level of the posterior urethra such as darkening of the adipose plane of the urogenital diaphragm and bulbocavernosus muscle and hematoma of the ischiocavernosus and obturator internus muscles [21].

Management in the Acute Phase

Early diagnosis and appropriate acute injury management establish prompt urinary drainage and serve to reduce associated complications, such as urethral stenosis and urinary incontinence [7, 18]. In the acute setting, a prime objective is to establish prompt urinary drainage [4]. A gentle attempt to pass a soft 14–16 Fr catheter can be made, ideally by an experienced operator in the emergency room or under fluoroscopy at the time of the admission RUG. If there is any difficulty in passing the catheter, a suprapubic cystostomy should be placed, especially in unstable patients.

Initial management will depend on the type of urethral lesion (partial or complete) and the overall severity of injuries and hemodynamic status of the patient. The options are primary urethral realignment (simple urethral catheterization, endoscopic primary realignment, open primary realignment), or placement of suprapubic cystostomy for delayed reconstruction [1, 7, 22] (Figure 9.10).

- **Primary urethral realignment:**
- *Simple urethral catheterization*: Passage of a well-lubricated soft rubber Foley catheter can be attempted in cases of partial injury, under fluoroscopy by a trained operator at the time of admission RUG. If it is successful, the catheter is maintained for two to three weeks. Prior to removal, a peri-catheter urethrogram is performed. If extravasation persists, the catheter is maintained, and imaging is repeated at intervals until resolution [1].
- *Primary endoscopic or open realignment*: This is considered in patients in whom urethral catheterization could not be performed due to complete injury or other complicating factors. The objective is to intubate the rupture leaving a urethral catheter in place [23].
  - **Primary endoscopic realignment**: It can be performed with rigid or flexible cystoscope, or with combined technique in a retrograde and antegrade way through a suprapubic access. It must be done when the patient's situation allows it and up to

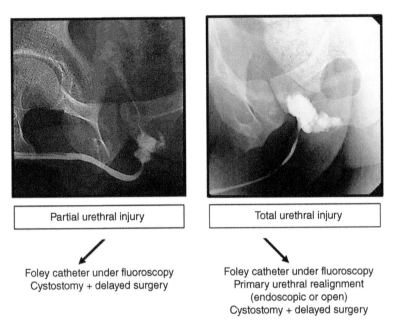

| Partial urethral injury | Total urethral injury |

Foley catheter under fluoroscopy
Cystostomy + delayed surgery

Foley catheter under fluoroscopy
Primary urethral realignment
(endoscopic or open)
Cystostomy + delayed surgery

Figure 9.10 Initial management of urethral trauma.

2 weeks post-trauma, but the ideal period is within the first 48 hours [24]. The goal is to pass a catheter across the injury to allow healing by second intention. Importantly, prolonged and obstinate attempts at endoscopic realignment should be avoided [4]. If successful, the catheter is maintained for three to eight weeks. Intubation has been reported as successful in 70–93% of attempts, but the main problem of realignment is the high rate of subsequent stenosis (up to 90%) that will require additional surgical procedures for resolution [25]. In addition, the time taken until the definitive solution of the urethral problem has been reported is much longer in cases of endoscopic realignment compared with cystostomy and delayed surgery (average 122 months vs. 7 months) [26]. For this reason, in front of a recurrence after realignment, the recommendation is urethroplasty [27]. In spite of this, there are groups that prefer endoscopic realignment as it is a minimally invasive, low morbidity procedure that allows to avoid a suprapubic cystostomy, which could mean a potential risk of infection of the osteosynthesis material, in case open reduction and internal fixation (ORIF) of the pelvic fracture is required [25]. Additionally, it has been suggested that if a stenosis occurs after primary realignment, it could be of less surgical complexity [24, 28].

- **Open primary realignment**: It is considered in patients who will undergo an exploratory laparotomy for other reasons and are stable enough for a realignment attempt. The bladder is accessed and opened longitudinally at the dome. Urethral intubation is performed using a combined technique (retrograde and antegrade). You actually have to get into the hematoma to connect the two catheter tips. This approach has the same drawbacks as the endoscopic technique. Excessive traction on the catheters during manipulation could potentially exacerbate injuries.

- **Suprapubic cystostomy and deferred urethroplasty**:
  - If any difficulty is found in simple urethral catheterization, the procedure should be suspended and a suprapubic cystostomy placed, percutaneously under ultrasonographic control or open by means of a laparotomy, always in the midline, two finger widths above the pubic symphysis and with a caliber of at least 14F. This will ensure adequate bladder drainage and has the benefit of facilitating future delayed urethroplasty [1, 22].

There are situations in which early realignment and other immediate surgical procedures are indicated [1, 7]:

- Complete disruption of the urethra with a large pelvic hematoma, rupture of the puboprostatic ligaments and cephalad displacement of the bladder ("pie in the sky bladder"), causing great distraction of the two urethral ends. This may make deferred urethroplasty difficult, indicating the need for primary realignment.
- Associated rectal or vaginal lesion, which must be repaired primarily to avoid pelvic sepsis.
- Injury of the bladder neck, which must be carefully repaired immediately as future urinary continence will depend on the normal functioning of the internal sphincter located at this level.
- In rare cases with injury to the sacral plexus, in which the bladder neck remains open by denervation. In this situation, extravasation of urine into the perivesical space can occur, despite having a suprapubic cystostomy. This indicates the need for primary realignment.

Very importantly, immediate retropubic urethroplasty is never indicated because it has been linked with an increased risk of stenosis, urinary incontinence, and erectile dysfunction [29].

Delayed Management

Lesions of the posterior urethra are repaired by excision and primary bulbo-prostatic anastomosis (end-to-end urethroplasty). Of utmost importance, endoscopic urethrotomy is not indicated in trauma cases due to the high risk of stricture recurrence.

The waiting time recommended in the literature for delayed urethroplasty is three to six months to allow resolution of the hematoma and post-traumatic inflammation. However, in some patients, the reconstruction could be carried out earlier. In our experience, a satisfactory reconstruction is possible as early as four to six weeks, as long as there is no induration of the perineum on rectal examination, the pelvic fracture is found to be stable enough to tolerate high lithotomy position, and that associated lesions are stabilized [30].

In the pre-operative study, urethral lesion, sphincter function, and erectile function should be evaluated.

The key elements for the success of this urethroplasty are a complete excision of the scar and pelvic fibrosis and a well-vascularized, spatulated tension-free mucosa to mucosa anastomosis. To achieve tension-free approximation of the urethral ends there are several sequential maneuvers, such as mobilization of the urethral bulb, distal urethral mobilization from the cavernous bodies, and splitting of the intercrural septum. In more complex cases, it may also be necessary to perform an inferior pubectomy and even a supracrural urethral re-routing [31]. In cases where, despite performing these maneuvers, good access is not achieved, an abdominal-perineal approach should be considered. Fortunately, these more complex maneuvers are very rarely necessary.

Following these recommendations and in the hands of an experienced surgeon, the long-term success rates of urethroplasty are 90–98% [3, 7].

Trauma to the Anterior Urethra

The most frequent injuries to the anterior urethra are those caused by iatrogenic injuries and also by blunt trauma by a direct blow to the perineum or straddle injuries. Other mechanisms are shown in Table 9.2 [32]. Regardless of the etiology, emergency management should include providing prompt urinary drainage.

The most characteristic sign is the presence of blood in the meatus. Others are the inability to urinate, perineal urinoma, or a butterfly-shaped perineal hematoma [4, 6].

In blunt trauma to the perineum, the bulb is crushed against the pubic symphysis, resulting in rupture of the urethra at the site of compression, causing a bulbar urethral injury.

Iatrogenic urethral injury can be caused by urethral catheterization (false passage, inflation of the catheter's balloon into the urethra, or removal of the catheter with a non-deflated balloon), instrumentation of the urethra (endoscopic procedures), or surgical complications (penile prosthesis implant, penile surgery). The most important measure to avoid iatrogenic urethral injury is to secure the proper training for each procedure [33].

Penetrating injuries are rare and are usually associated with genital injuries (penile and/or testicular) or pelvic injuries.

Penile fracture may be accompanied by a urethral injury (partial or complete) and usually occurs after blunt trauma with the erect penis, mainly during sexual activity. Overall incidence has been reported to be 10–20%. The patients report a "snapping" sound, followed by pain, penile detumescence, and penile deviation. A hematoma is formed that may be limited or extend to the perineum (in butterfly wings); this will depend on the fact that Buck's fascia is injured. If urethral injury occurs, blood at the meatus and difficulty to void are the rule. In these cases, early surgical treatment is mandatory [13].

Table 9.2 Mechanisms of anterior urethra injury.

Blunt Trauma	Direct blow Astride impact
Penetrating Trauma	Projectile
	Stab wound
	Impalement
	Bites
	Amputations
Constrictive Trauma	Condom catheter
	Psychiatric patients
Sex-related Trauma	Penile fracture
	Sexual devices
Internal Trauma	Foreign bodies
	Iatrogenic trauma

Minor perineal trauma may go unnoticed and subsequently be manifested as a urethral stricture.

Management in the Acute Phase

Management recommendations depend on the etiology and general condition of the patient [32, 34].

- *Urethral contusion*: A gentle attempt to urethral catheterization should be performed under fluoroscopy; if any difficulty is found, a suprapubic cystostomy is placed.
- *Partial or complete lesions*: It is difficult to establish strict recommendations due to the great variability in mechanism of injury and condition of the patient. The management strategies likewise vary, according to the general and local conditions, as well as the experience of the attending team. A gentle attempt at soft urethral catheterization under fluoroscopy is always an option; if successful, a peri-catheter urethrogram is performed at two to four weeks. Another alternative is endoscopic or open urethral realignment in patients in whom urethral catheterization was not successful and require surgery for other injuries. Patients treated by catheter realignment should be followed closely, since they have a high risk of stricture. As for iatrogenic lesions, most are resolved by catheter drainage for two weeks.

Immediate primary surgical repair can be considered for uncomplicated penetrating injuries. On the contrary, primary repair in blunt injuries is exceptional and the best option is a suprapubic cystostomy for delayed repair at four to six weeks.

In urethral injury related to penile fracture, early surgery must be performed. The recommended surgical technique includes penile degloving that provides excellent exposure of the urethra and corpus cavernosum. In addition to the repair of the lesion of the corpus cavernosum, if the associated urethral injury is partial, its repair is primary closure; however, complete urethral injury needs end-to-end urethroplasty. The most common complications are urethral strictures, urethra-cutaneous fistula, and penile deformity, so it is important to monitor the patient [13].

Delayed Management

Post-traumatic strictures usually occur at the bulbar urethra and are accompanied by moderate to severe fibrosis, so management with direct vision internal urethrotomy it is contraindicated. For defects up to 2.5–3 cm, the treatment of choice is excision of the scar and anastomotic urethroplasty. Longer defects may need the addition of a dorsal buccal mucosa graft as an augmented anastomotic urethroplasty. Due to fibrosis of the spongiosum, the use of grafts in the ventral position is not considered. In some rare occasions with very extensive defects, a mixed combined technique, with a dorsal graft and a ventral fascio-cutaneous flap, may be required [34, 35].

In addition to recurrent urethral stricture, patients with anterior urethral trauma may have long-term complications after treatment, such as erectile dysfunction or urinary incontinence. Therefore, it is recommended to monitor these patients for at least one year following urethral injury [4].

Conclusions

Urethral injuries do not constitute a life-threatening emergency by themselves, but early diagnosis and adequate acute management are crucial to avoid severe complications and long-term sequela. Prompt urinary drainage is mandatory, linked to a decision for immediate or delayed treatment commanded by the local and general conditions of each case. Available experience and resources are also determining factors, therefore judicious placement of a suprapubic cystostomy is always a recommendable temporizing option allowing time for transferral to a specialized center for specific treatment.

References

1 Velarde, L., Gómez, R., Campos, F., and Portillo, J.A. (2016). Lesiones traumáticas de la uretra posterior. *Actas Urol. Esp.* 40 (9): 539–548. https://doi.org/10.1016/j. acuro.2016.03.011.

2 Bjurlin, M.A., Fantus, R.J., Mellett, M.M., and Goble, S.M. (2009). Genitourinary injuries in pelvic fracture morbidity and mortality using the National Trauma Data Bank. *J. Trauma* 67 (5): 1033–1039. https://doi.org/10.1097/TA.0b013e3181bb8d6c.

3 Gómez, R., Mundy, T., Dubey, D. et al. (2013). SIU/ICUD consultation on urethral strictures: pelvic fracture urethral injuries. *Urology* 83 (3): S48–S58. https://doi.org/10.1016/j.urology. 2013.09.023.

4 Morey, A., Brandes, S., Dugi, D.D. et al. (2014). AUA guideline. *J. Urol.* 192 (2): 327–335.

5 Krishnan, V., Chawla, A., Sharbidre, K.G., and Peh, W. (2018). Currents techniques and clinical applications of computed tomography urography. *Curr. Probl. Diagn. Radiol.* 47: 245–256. https://doi.org/10.1067/j.cpradiol.2017.07.002.

6 Kitrey, N.D., Djakovic, N., Hallscheidt, P. et al. (2018). EAU guideline on urological trauma. EAU Guidelines Office, Arnhem, The Netherlands. http://uroweb.org/guidelines/ compilations-of-all-guidelines/.

7 Kulkarni, S., Joshi, P., and Ramírez Pérez, E.A. (2020). Surgical reconstruction of pelvic fracture urethral injury. In: *Textbook of Male Genitourethral Reconstruction*, vol. 21 (eds. F.E. Martins, S.B. Kulkarni and T. Kohler), 253–266.

8 Maciejewski, C. and Rourke, K. (2015). Imaging of urethral stricture disease. *Transl. Androl. Urol.* 4 (1): 2–9. https://doi.org/10.3978/j.issn.2223-4683.2015.02.03.

9 Furr, J. and Gelman, J. (2020). Functional anatomy of the male urethra for the reconstructive surgeon. In: *Textbook of Male Genitourethral Reconstruction*, vol. 2 (eds. F.E. Martins, S.B. Kulkarni and T. Kohler), 17–24.

10 Myers, R.P. (2001). The male striated urethral sphincter. In: *The Urinary Sphincter*, vol. 3 (eds. J. Corcos and E. Schick), 25–42.

11 Macura, K.J., Genadry, R., Borman, T. et al. (2004). Evaluation of the female urethra with intraurethral magnetic resonance imaging. *J. Magn. Reson. Imaging* 20: 153–159. https:// doi.org/10.1002/jmri.20058.

12 Latini, J.M., JW, M.A., Brandes, S.B. et al. (2014). SIU/ICUD Consultation on urethral strictures: Epidemiology, etiology, anatomy, and nomenclature of urethral stenoses, strictures, and pelvic fracture urethral disruption injuries. *Urology* 83 (Suppl): S1–S7. https://doi.org/10.1016/j.urology.2013.09.009.

13 Barros, R., Silva, M., Antonucci, V. et al. (2018). Primary urethral reconstruction results in penile fracture. *Ann. R. Coll. Surg. Engl.* 100 (1): 21–25. https://doi.org/10.1308/rcsann.2017.0098.

14 Rosenberg, S., Joshi, P., Laerence, A. et al. (2014). Management of female urethral trauma. *J. Urol.* 191 (suppl 4): 129.

15 Black, P.C., Miller, E.A., Porter, J.R., and Wessells, H. (2006). Urethral and bladder neck injury associated with pelvic fracture in 25 female patients. *J. Urol.* 175 (6): 2140–2144; discussion 2144. doi:https://doi.org/10.1016/S0022-5347(06)00309-0.

16 Mouraviev, V.B. and Santucci, R.A. (2005). Cadaveric anatomy of pelvic fracture urethral distraction injury: most injuries are distal to the external urinary sphincter. *J. Urol.* 173: 869–872. https://doi.org/10.1097/01.ju.0000152252.48176.69.

17 Tile, M. (1988). Pelvic ring fractures: should they be fixed? *J. Bone Joint Surg. Br.* 70: 1–12. PMID: 3276697.

18 Andrich, D.E., Day, A., and Mundy, A.R. (2007). Proposed mechanisms of lower urinary tract injury in fractures of the pelvic ring. *BJU Int.* 100: 567–573. https://doi.org/10.1111/j.1464-410X.2007.07020.x.

19 Ríos, E., Martínez-Piñeiro, L., and Álvarez-Maestro, M. (2014). Reparación de la estenosis de uretra posterior tras traumatismo y fractura pélvica. Monográfico de cirugía uretral. *Arch. Esp. Urol.* 67 (1): 68–76.

20 Pichler, R., Fritsch, H., Skradski, V. et al. (2012). Diagnosis and management of pediatric urethral injuries. *Urol. Int.* 89: 136–142. https://doi.org/10.1159/000336291.

21 Ali, M., Safriel, Y., Sclafani, S.J., and Schulza, R. (2003). CT signs of urethral injury. *Radiographics* 23: 951–963. https://doi.org/10.1148/rg.234025097.

22 Gelman, J. and Wisenbaugh, E.S. (2015). Posterior urethral strictures. *Adv. Urol.* 2015: 628107. https://doi.org/10.1155/2015/628107.

23 Olapade-Olaopa, E.O., Atalabi, O.M., Adekanye, A.O. et al. (2010). Early endoscopic realignment of traumatic anterior and posterior urethral disruptions under caudal anaesthesia – a 5-year review. *Int. J. Clin. Pract.* 64: 6–12. https://doi.org/10.1111/j.1742-1241.2007.01481.x.

24 Stein, D.M. and Santucci, R.A. (2015). Pro: endoscopic realignment for pelvic fracture urethral injuries. *Transl. Androl. Urol.* 4 (1): 72–78. https://doi.org/10.3978/j.issn.2223-4683.2015.01.11.

25 Chung, P.H., Wessells, H., and Voelzke, B.B. (2017). Updated outcomes of early endoscopic realignment for pelvic fracture urethral injuries at a level 1 trauma center. *Urology* 112: 191–197. https://doi.org/10.1016/j.urology.2017.09.032.

26 Johnsen, N.V., Dmochowski, R.R., Mock, S. et al. (2015). Primary endoscopic realignment of urethral disruption injuries. A double-edged sword? *J. Urol.* 194 (4): 1022–1026. https://doi.org/10.1016/j.juro.2015.03.112.

27 Gómez, R., Storme, O., Velarde, L., and Finsterbusch, C. (2013). Catheter realignment versus suprapubic cystostomy + delayed urethroplasty for pelvic fracture urethral injuries: a goal-oriented retrospective comparison. *Urology* 189 (4S): e4. https://doi.org/10.1016/j.juro.2013.02.1384.

28 Koraitim, M.M. (2012). Effect of early realignment on length and delayed repair of postpelvic fracture urethral injury. *Urology* 79: 912–915. https://doi.org/10.1016/j.urology.2011.11.054.

29 Morehouse, D.D., Belitsky, P., and Mackinnon, K. (1972). Rupture of the posterior urethra. *J. Urol.* 107 (2): 255–258. https://doi.org/10.1016/s0022-5347(17)60996-0.

30 Scarberry, K., Bonomo, J., and Gómez, R. (2018). Delayed posterior urethroplasty following pelvic fracture urethral injury: do we have to wait 3 months? *Urology* 116: 193–197. https://doi.org/10.1016/j.urology.2018.01.018.

31 Webster, G.D. and Ramon, J. (1991). Repair of pelvic fracture posterior urethral defects using an elaborated perineal approach: experience with 74 cases. *J. Urol.* 145: 744–748. https://doi.org/10.1016/s0022-5347(17)38442-2.

32 Morey, A.F. and Tausch, T. (2018). Management of complications related to traumatic injuries. *Complications Urol. Surg.* 15: 169–176.e5.

33 Summerton, D.J., Kitrey, N.D., Lumen, N. et al. (2012). EAU guidelines on iatrogenic trauma. *Eur. Urol.* 62 (4): 628–639. https://doi.org/10.1016/j.eururo.2012.05.058.

34 Dobrowolski, Z.F., Weglarz, W., Jakubik, P. et al. (2002). Treatment of posterior and anterior urethral trauma. *BJU Int.* 89 (7): 752–754. https://doi.org/10.1046/j.1464-410X.2002.02719.x.

35 Biserte, J. and Nivet, J. (2006). Trauma to the anterior urethra: diagnosis and management. *Ann. Urol.* 40 (4): 220–232. https://doi.org/10.1016/j.anuro.2006.05.002.

36 Moore, E.E., Cogbill, T.H., Malangoni, M.A. et al. (1995). Organ Injury Scaling. Surg Clin North Am. 75 (2): 293–303.

10

Acute Management of Urethral Stricture

Akio Horiguchi

Department of Urology, National Defense Medical College, Tokorozawa, Japan

Introduction

Urethral stricture is a relatively common urologic problem caused by fibrosis or inflammation of the epithelial tissue and corpus spongiosum that results in stenosis of the urethral lumen. Most urethral strictures occur in males; as a result of the rarity of female urethral strictures, this review limits its focus to urethral stricture management in men. Urethral stricture not only adversely impacts patient-reported quality of life but also overall health status, and urologists and other healthcare professionals need to know the appropriate immediate and longer-term management of urethral strictures.

Etiology of Urethral Stricture

The male urethra is traditionally divided into the anterior urethra, which is surrounded by the corpus spongiosum, and posterior urethra, which is surrounded by the sphincter mechanisms and prostate. Most strictures are in the anterior urethra and half of such strictures are located in the bulbar urethra [1–3]. A recent meta-analysis of the literature has shown that most anterior urethral strictures in patients in developed countries are iatrogenic, idiopathic, and, to a lesser extent, traumatic and inflammatory [1–3]. Iatrogenic urethral strictures are caused by improper or prolonged catheterization and by transurethral procedures, especially transurethral resection of the prostate. Iatrogenic strictures are typically found at the junction of the bulbar and penile urethra, or in the proximal bulbar urethra [4, 5]. Traumatic anterior urethral strictures are caused by blunt or penetrating trauma. A typical injury of the bulbar urethra causing a stricture is a straddle injury, which crushes the bulbar urethra against the underside of the pubic symphysis [6, 7]. So-called idiopathic strictures are probably caused by unrecognized childhood perineal trauma [8]. One of the most important etiologies in inflammatory urethral strictures is lichen sclerosus (LS), which is a chronic inflammatory, hypomelanotic, lymphocyte-mediated skin disorder with

A Clinical Guide to Urologic Emergencies, First Edition. Edited by Hunter Wessells, Shigeo Horie, and Reynaldo G. Gómez.
© 2021 John Wiley & Sons Ltd. Published 2021 by John Wiley & Sons Ltd.
Companion website: www.wiley.com/go/wessells/urologic

a progressive sclerosing process that can involve the penile shaft skin, glans, meatus, and finally extend into the anterior urethra [9]. While recurrent gonococcal urethritis remains a main cause of anterior urethral stricture in low and middle-income countries, it has become uncommon in developed countries due to the advent of effective antibiotic treatment [10]. Surgery for hypospadias is another important cause of anterior urethral strictures [11, 12]. On the other hand, posterior urethral stricture commonly occurs due to iatrogenic etiology including instrumentation of the urethra, transurethral resection of prostate surgery, and various types of prostate cancer treatment [13]. Posterior urethral stricture, other than iatrogenic stricture, is uncommon and most commonly caused by pelvic fracture urethral injury (PFUI) [14].

It is important to note that urethral stricture is not a disease of the elderly but affects all ages [2, 3]. Urethral stricture patients were found to have predominantly idiopathic causes in men younger than 45 years, with iatrogenic causes (specifically, previous transurethral resection of the prostate) found most commonly in men older than 45 years [2].

Patient History and Physical Examination

Many patients with urethral strictures present initially with lower urinary tract symptoms such as weak urinary stream, straining to void, urinary hesitancy, incomplete emptying, nocturia, frequency, and urinary retention [15]. Patients may also present with symptoms other than lower urinary tract symptoms including gross hematuria, urinary tract infection, genitourinary pain, incontinence, and sexual dysfunction, and may suffer from life-threatening conditions including renal insufficiency or necrotizing fasciitis [15].

The patient should be asked about a history of difficult urethral catheterization, urinary tract infection, and previous trauma to the penis or perineum. History of prior treatment, such as urethral dilation and surgical procedures for urethral stricture, should be gathered in patients with previous diagnosis of urethral stricture. Physical examination of the abdomen in a patient with urethral stricture may identify chronic urinary retention and a palpably distended bladder. Examination of the penile skin may reveal the presence of LS, an important cause of inflammatory urethral strictures. Examination of the urethral meatus may reveal stenosis or sequela of hypospadias. Palpation of the urethra often reveals thickening and/or induration which, when present, correlates with the severity of periurethral fibrosis identified intra-operatively. Some patients with stricture after PFUI are unable to flex their hips due to dissociation of the pelvic ring; it is therefore important to check whether the lithotomy position can be used to gain access to the perineum. A urethral fistula may be detected in some cases, particularly in patients who have undergone previous urethral surgery.

Evaluation of Urethral Stricture

Clinicians planning elective intervention for stricture should determine the characteristics of the urethral stricture in advance [16]. It is important to know the number of strictures, location and length of each stricture, degree of spongiofibrosis, and lumen diameter of each stricture, in order to formulate a proper management plan. At the time of evaluation,

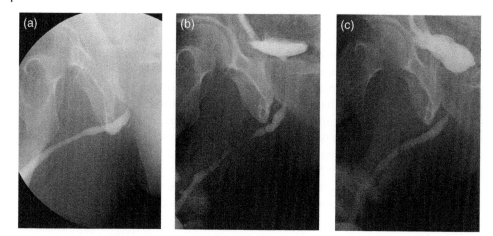

Figure 10.1 (a) RUG immediately after catheter removal in patient after failed multiple transurethral procedures for penobulbar strictures. (b) RUG three months after suprapubic tube placement, clearly delineating stricture. (c) RUG from same patient after substitution urethroplasty, showing a widely patent urethral lumen.

the patient's stricture should be stable and no longer contracting for accurate staging. Men presenting with an indwelling catheter or following recent urethral manipulation will have unstable stricture anatomy. In these patients, "urethral rest" should be accomplished by removal of the indwelling catheter and cessation of intermittent self-catheterization, and if necessary, suprapubic tube placement. The urethra should not be instrumented for at least three months for stricture maturation [17]. Urethral rest promotes identification of severe fibrotic segments, enabling proper selection of a surgical procedure and a more successful reconstruction (Figure 10.1) [17].

Voiding Symptoms and Uroflowmetry

Symptomatic assessment is best formulized using American Urological Association Symptom Score (AUA-SS) [18] or a specifically designed patient reported outcome measurement (PROM), such as one developed in the UK [19]. A urinary flow rate showing the long slow protracted flow pattern with the appearance of a plateau is typical in patients with urethral stricture. For accurate readings, a voided volume of at least 150 ml is preferred. If the voided volume and flow rate suggest a urethral stricture, urethro-cystoscopy, retrograde urethrography (RUG), voiding cystourethrography (VCUG), or ultrasound urethrography are the next steps to make a definitive diagnosis of a stricture [16].

Urethrography

The most common methods for imaging the male urethra are RUG and VCUG. RUG is the gold standard for evaluation of anterior urethral strictures. Oblique positioning of the patient (45°) is a critically important step, and the downward obturator fossa should be completely closed on the scout film (see Figure 10.1) to confirm appropriate positioning, in order to position the urethra as parallel as possible to the film [20]. RUG should ideally be conducted (or directly supervised) and interpreted by the treating urologists, because in many centers independently reported retrograde urethrographies will not be as accurate as specialty physician-reported RUG [21]. It is important to note that the posterior urethra is not open physiologically during RUG and will not be distended. Moreover, in cases of severe or complete urethral occlusion, retrograde assessment of the proximal to the obstruction is often impossible. VCUG is typically most useful for visualizing the posterior urethra and segment of the urethra proximal to a urethral stricture.

Ultrasound Urethrography

Although urethrography is the cornerstone assessment method of urethral stricture, it has several drawbacks. First, it can over- and under-estimate stricture length; second, it is sometimes difficult to assess associated periurethral problems such as the degree of spongiofibrosis [22]. To overcome the limitation of urethrography, ultrasound urethrography was introduced for evaluation of urethral stricture and has been refined [20]. The utility of ultrasound urethrography is, however, limited by stricture location, with this modality being more sensitive to identify strictures located in the penile urethra compared to the bulbar portion [23]. Strictures in the more proximal bulbar urethra are difficult to assess using ultrasound urethrography, because the bulbar urethra curves into the pelvis away from the skin and from the ultrasound probe [24]. In selected cases, ultrasound urethrography may be more sensitive than RUG in the assessment of stricture length and degree of spongiofibrosis: however, ultrasound urethrography is not necessary in most stricture patients, and the clinical relevance of these findings remains uncertain [25].

Urethro-Cystoscopy

Flexible cystoscopy is an excellent modality for determining the presence or absence of a urethral stricture. Cystoscopy is also useful for visualizing the fibrosis of urethral mucosa that cannot be seen on a urethrogram, which is particularly important in patients with previous history of urethrotomy or dilation. However, cystoscopy alone does not show the stricture length or state of the urethra proximal to the stricture, and its use in combination with urethrography is necessary. In patients with complete urethral disruption, antegrade flexible cystoscopy through the suprapubic catheter tract may be used to evaluate the proximal stump in conjunction with RUG to accurately delineate the urethral gap. Moreover, cystoscopy via the suprapubic tract also allows the assessment of bladder neck competence in patients with PFUI, which is important information for post-operative urinary continence [26].

MRI

Magnetic resonance imaging (MRI) is a non-invasive imaging modality, has multiplanar capabilities, does not subject patients to ionizing radiation, and provides detailed information regarding periurethral tissues and pathology. MRI is especially useful in the evaluation of the tunica albuginea disruption in traumatic bulbar urethral strictures [27] and prostatic displacement or concomitant rectal injury in PFUI [28, 29], providing information that conventional urethrography may not capture. MRI correctly estimates the length of urethral defects in 85% of cases, displacement of the prostate apex in 90% of PFUI cases, precisely delineates the site and density of scar tissue, and surgical approach in 26% changed based on MRI findings [28, 30]. Despite its high resolution, the cost of MRI is about 5 times that of urethrography and the appropriate indication and cost-effectiveness of MRI should be confirmed in future studies [22].

Emergency Management of Urinary Retention and Unexpected Urethral Stricture

Patients may not notice the presence of urethral stricture until going into urinary retention or unsuccessful attempts at urinary catheterization on the operating table [15]. In such situations, clinicians may utilize transurethral management to place a urethral catheter after confirming the characteristics of the stricture by urethro-cystoscopy and/or RUG [16]. If the stricture is flimsy, clinicians might dilate only enough to allow passage of a catheter over a guide wire by dilators such as filiforms and followers, balloon dilators, or sounds [16] (Figure 10.2). If the stricture is dense, direct vision internal urethrotomy (DVIU) may be performed instead of dilation [16]. Unless the catheterization is complex, the urethral catheter can be safely removed after 24–72 hours [16]. Suprapubic tube placement is recommended when urethral catheterization fails, the urethra is traumatized by improper catheterization, or severe complication such as massive extravasation or periurethral abscess is encountered. Afterward, the status of the stricture should be evaluated and be treated as described below. If a stricture patient awaiting elective management goes into urinary retention or requires frequent intermittent self-catheterization, placement of a suprapubic tube instead of ongoing DVIU/dilation is necessary to provide a period of urethral rest.

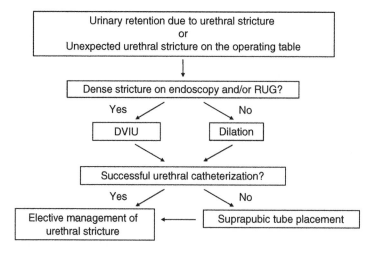

Figure 10.2 A flow chart of emergent urethral stricture management.

Elective Management of Urethral Stricture

There are a variety of options in elective management of urethral strictures, which are mainly categorized into two groups: one is transurethral procedures including dilation, DVIU, and urethral stents, and the other is open surgical management (formal urethroplasty). The advantages of transurethral procedures are that they can be conducted under local anesthesia in an outpatient setting with a low complication rate and virtually no risk of mortality, but the success rate is generally low [31, 32]. On the other hand, the success rate of urethroplasty is excellent, but it is technically more demanding than transurethral procedures [33, 34]. There is some evidence that transurethral procedures are being used excessively and inappropriately because of their simplicity and ease of repetition and because there is a lack of familiarity with urethroplasty [35, 36]. The characteristics of urethral strictures differ among patients, and it is important to select an appropriate management plan for each patient. The flow chart of management plans of urethral strictures is shown in Figure 10.3.

Transurethral Procedures

DVIU and Dilation

DVIU and dilation are minimally invasive interventions most often used for treating urethral strictures, and their effectiveness is equal for the initial treatment of strictures [35–37]. Primary DVIU and dilation are best suited as first-line therapies for strictures with favorable characteristics that fulfill all the following characteristics: short (within 1–2 cm), single, non-traumatic, bulbar urethral strictures (Figure 10.3). A stricture-free rate for patients with these favorable characteristics may be up to 50–70% [35]. On the other hand, DVIU and dilation are futile for long, multiple, obliterative, traumatic, penile, or penobulbar strictures, and they should be treated with formal urethroplasty as a primary management plan, unless patient preference dictates a less effective management strategy [35]. Urethral strictures that recur within six months after DVIU/dilation or are refractory to a second DVIU/dilation should also be treated with formal urethoplasty, unless the patient has co-morbidities or agrees to be palliated by repeated DVIU/dilation [16]. Successive urethral dilation and urethrotomy are not cost-effective [38–40] and may make eventual urethroplasty more difficult [41, 42] with lower than predicted long-term success [43–46].

Figure 10.3 A flow chart of elective urethral stricture management.

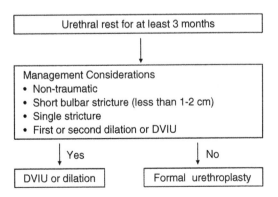

Urethral Stents

A permanent metallic urethral stent, Urolume*, which is incorporated into the urethral wall, has been used to maintain urethral patency following DVIU or dilation in the management of recurrent urethral strictures [47]. Despite initial enthusiasm, tissue ingrowth and granulation through the permanent stent occur and the long-term outcome revealed a high failure rate [48, 49]. Permanent urethral stenting is not recommended for patients with strictures who are considered to be candidates for urethroplasty and might be considered only for patients with short, recurrent bulbar strictures who are medically unfit for urethroplasty and cannot tolerate intermittent-self catheterization [31]. A temporary urethral stent, Memokath*, is a thermos-expansible urethral stent designed for easy deployment and removal. The aim of temporary urethral stenting is to maintain urethral patency without the risk of permanent implantation after urethral dilation or DVIU [50]. Jordan and associates reported that patients with recurrent bulbar urethral strictures treated with Memokath insertion for 12 months following dilation or DVIU maintained significantly longer urethral patency than those treated with dilation or DVIU alone [50]. Wong also reported a series of 22 patients with recurrent bulbar urethral strictures with mean stricture length of 2.4 cm who underwent DVIU or dilation [51]. Memokath was indwelled for three months, and 78% of patients remained stricture-free at a mean follow-up of 23 months [51]. However, the stricture-free rate was much lower than that of urethroplasty [52, 53]. Moreover, urethral stenting using Memokath is the transurethral procedure with the highest risk of increasing stricture complexity and necessitating the use of a complex repair procedure [42]. The appropriate circumstances for temporary urethral stenting have not been determined, and although the device has been approved in several countries, the procedure remains largely experimental [31].

Urethroplasty

For most patients for whom DVIU or dilation are inappropriate, or in whom it has failed, urethroplasty is usually the only curative option. The procedures of urethroplasty can be categorized into anastomotic urethroplasty (excision and primary anastomosis, EPA) and substitution urethroplasty. The length and location of stricture, etiology, and history of previous urethral surgery or instrumentation help one to decide which urethroplasty method to use. Before undertaking urethroplasty, the urologist must be familiar with the use of numerous reconstructive surgical techniques, because it is unpredictable what kind of technique will be required during surgery and the pre-operative surgical plan needs to be modified intra-operatively when faced with unexpected findings [54]. A flow chart of the surgical steps in urethroplasty is shown in Figure 10.4.

EPA

The principal of EPA consists of resecting all fibrosis and approximating both urethral ends, without tension, to bridge the gap using fine interrupted absorbable sutures. EPA is the preferred method of urethral reconstruction whenever possible, because of the high success rate and durability compared to substitution urethroplasty [52, 53, 55]. It is best suited for traumatic or other short strictures of the bulbar or membranous urethra with excellent long-term success rate [52, 53, 56–58]. The factors limiting the potential for using

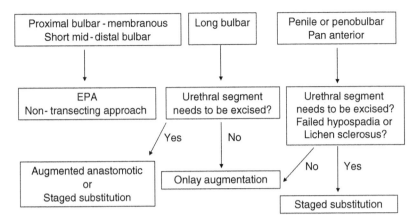

Figure 10.4 Surgical steps in urethroplasty according to stricture location.

EPA are the length and location of the stricture [34, 57, 59]. When the stricture is in the proximal bulbar urethra or membranous urethra, longer strictures can be bridged because the bulbar urethra can be fully elongated by mobilization; separating the corpora and/or inferior pubectomy can straighten the natural curve of the bulbar urethra and shorten its course [57]. However, the more distal the stricture is in the bulbar urethra, the shorter the gap that can be bridged due to the limited length of the mobilized bulbar urethra. For a mid-bulbar urethral stricture, anastomotic urethroplasty is applicable only for short (probably within 1 cm) strictures where tension-free anastomosis is achievable. It is very uncommon to be able to perform EPA for long strictures in the bulbar urethra or any more distal stricture in the penile urethra because of the potential risk for causing chordee. Recently, the non-transecting approach has emerged as an alternative management of short and proximal bulbar strictures with minimal spongiofibrosis, which enables preserving the blood supply with equivalent outcome, but EPA remains appropriate for strictures with full-thickness spongiofibrosis developing after perineal trauma [60, 61].

Substitution Urethroplasty
Substitution urethroplasty is the procedure of choice for urethral strictures that are too long to be excised and re-anastomosed. In contemporary practice, penile skin and oral mucosa are most commonly used as urethral substitutes. Barbagli recently reported the long-term success rate of anterior substitution urethroplasty, and oral mucosa showed a greater failure-free survival rate than penile skin [62]. Currently, buccal mucosa is most widely used as a urethral substitute; lingual mucosa has emerged as an alternative substitution with equivalent urethroplasty outcome (Figure 10.5) [63, 64].

Substitution urethroplasty is categorized into one-stage or staged urethral reconstruction. One-stage substitution urethroplasty is divided into augmented anastomotic (to excise the stricture and restore a roof strip of the native urethra augmented by a patch), onlay augmentation (to incise the stricture and carry out a patch augmentation), and tube augmentation (to excise the stricture and put in a circumferential patch) procedures [33]. Strictures that have tight segments to be excised and that are too long to be managed

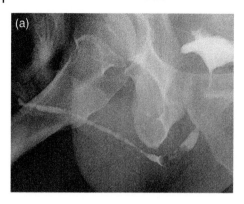
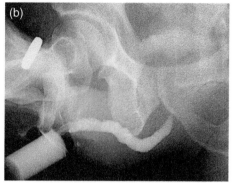

Figure 10.5 RUG showing pan-anterior urethral stricture secondary to lichen sclerosus (a). Stricture was successfully reconstructed by buccal mucosal substitution urethroplasty (b).

through EPA, are indication of the augmented anastomotic procedure [65]. The tight segment of a stricture is excised after which the urethral ends are anastomosed as a roof or floor strip, augmented in a ventral or dorsal onlay fashion respectively [65]. The one-stage tube augmentation procedure is associated with high failure rate and should be avoided [66, 67]. Regarding onlay augmentation, location of the graft (ventral or dorsal) has been debated, but the different graft positions have shown no difference in success rate in bulbar urethroplasty [68, 69]. The advantages of the ventral onlay procedure include limited urethral mobilization with preservation of perforating arteries and shorter operative time compared to the dorsal onlay procedure, while the advantages of the dorsal onlay procedure include a more stable and reliably well-vascularized graft bed and less possibility of sacculation [69]. The choice of location of grafting depends largely on the surgeon's preference. For patients with proximal bulbar stricture or obese patients, dorsal graft placements are typically more difficult to sew in a deep and proximal wound. In patients who have undergone repeated DVIUs or urethroplasty, the urethral lumen may be adherent and firmly fixed to the tunica albuginea, and urethral mobilization from the corpora cavernosa is difficult. In these situations, we prefer to use the ventral onlay procedure. On the other hand, we prefer to use the dorsal onlay procedure in the distal bulbar urethra, because application of the graft to the tunica albuginea of the corpora cavernosa in the distal bulbar urethra is easier than that in the proximal bulbar urethra. In the penile urethra, corpus spongiosum is too small to cover the ventrally applied graft, and mobilization of the penile urethra for a dorsal onlay graft may compromise critical blood supply from the circumferential arteries. Thus, the dorsal inlay technique described by Asopa with a ventral sagittal urethrotomy transluminal approach without urethral mobilization is well-suited for penile urethral strictures [70, 71]. Urethroplasty can be difficult in men with strictures associated with failed hypospadias repair or LS, in which the penis is fully involved in the disease and requiring a staged approach. The use of oral mucosa is mandatory in patients with genital LS, because any skin that is used as graft material already is or may become diseased (Figure 10.5) [72]. Staged procedures involve excision of the stricture and abnormal urethral and reconstruction of a roof strip, which is allowed to heal prior to final tubularization [33].

Post-operative Follow-Up

Post Transurethral Procedures

There is no evidence that leaving the urethral catheter longer than 72 hours after DVIU/ dilation improves safety or outcome, and catheters may be removed after 24–72 hours [16]. Because recurrent stricture is common after transurethral procedures, clinicians should carefully follow the patient. Intermittent self-catheterization after transurethral procedures may be recommended to patients who are not candidates for urethroplasty, to maintain temporary urethral patency and to reduce stricture recurrence rate [16]. However, urethro-plasty should be offered to patients who hope to cure urethral stricture instead of repeated transurethral procedures and physicians who are not familiar with urethroplasty should consider referral to expert reconstructive urologists [16].

Post Urethroplasty

A 14–16 Fr urethral catheter is placed after urethroplasty and pericatheter RUG is per-formed after two to three weeks. If extravasation was absent, the urethral catheter can be removed and the patient can start voiding thereafter. There is no established regimen for post-operative follow-up. In our practice, patients are followed up at 3, 6, and 12 months and annually thereafter by uroflowmetry and questionnaires using validated PROM. Flexible cystoscopy is done when a recurrent stricture is suspected on uroflowmetry or from a PROM.

Conclusion

Male urethral stricture is a relatively common disease that causes problems including not only lower urinary tract symptoms but also urinary tract infection or renal insufficiency in severe cases. Clinicians encountering patients going into urinary retention or having diffi-cult catheterization due to urethral stricture may proceed with transurethral procedures such as DVIU and dilation or suprapubic tube placement. However, transurethral proce-dures are not optimal as elective managements in most urethral stricture patients and ure-throplasty is the gold standard management. EPA is the most durable surgical treatment for short bulbar urethral strictures and substitution urethroplasty using buccal mucosa graft is the procedure of choice for a long stricture in the proximal bulbar urethra and strictures of any length located anywhere from the distal bulbar urethra to the penile urethra. Because urethral stricture recurrence following elective management can occur at any time in the post-operative period [16], clinicians should follow stricture patients carefully.

References

1 Fenton, A.S., Morey, A.F., Aviles, R. et al. (2005). Anterior urethral strictures: etiology and characteristics. *Urology* 65: 1055.
2 Lumen, N., Hoebeke, P., Willemsen, P. et al. (2009). Etiology of urethral stricture disease in the 21st century. *J. Urol.* 182: 983.

3 Palminteri, E., Berdondini, E., Verze, P. et al. (2013). Contemporary urethral stricture characteristics in the developed world. *Urology* 81: 191.

4 Edwards, L.E., Lock, R., Powell, C. et al. (1983). Post-catheterisation urethral strictures. A clinical and experimental study. *Br. J. Urol.* 55: 53.

5 Nielsen, K.K. and Nordling, J. (1990). Urethral stricture following transurethral prostatectomy. *Urology* 35: 18.

6 Mundy, A.R. and Andrich, D.E. (2011). Urethral trauma. Part II: types of injury and their management. *BJU Int.* 108: 630.

7 Mundy, A.R. and Andrich, D.E. (2011). Urethral trauma. Part I: introduction, history, anatomy, pathology, assessment and emergency management. *BJU Int.* 108: 310.

8 Viers, B.R., Pagliara, T.J., Rew, C.A. et al. (2017). Characteristics of idiopathic urethral strictures: a link to remote perineal trauma? *Urology* 110: 228.

9 Stewart, L., McCammon, K., Metro, M. et al. (2014). SIU/ICUD consultation on urethral strictures: anterior urethra-lichen sclerosus. *Urology* 83: S27.

10 Latini, J.M., McAninch, J.W., Brandes, S.B. et al. (2014). SIU/ICUD consultation on urethral strictures: epidemiology, etiology, anatomy, and nomenclature of urethral stenoses, strictures, and pelvic fracture urethral disruption injuries. *Urology* 83: S1.

11 Amukele, S.A., Stock, J.A., and Hanna, M.K. (2005). Management and outcome of complex hypospadias repairs. *J. Urol.* 174: 1540.

12 Myers, J.B., McAninch, J.W., Erickson, B.A. et al. (2012). Treatment of adults with complications from previous hypospadias surgery. *J. Urol.* 188: 459.

13 Herschorn, S., Elliott, S., Coburn, M. et al. (2014). SIU/ICUD consultation on urethral strictures: posterior urethral stenosis after treatment of prostate cancer. *Urology* 83: S59.

14 Gomez, R.G., Mundy, T., Dubey, D. et al. (2014). SIU/ICUD consultation on urethral strictures: pelvic fracture urethral injuries. *Urology* 83: S48.

15 Rourke, K. and Hickle, J. (2012). The clinical spectrum of the presenting signs and symptoms of anterior urethral stricture: detailed analysis of a single institutional cohort. *Urology* 79: 1163.

16 Wessells, H., Angermeier, K.W., Elliott, S. et al. (2016). Male urethral stricture: AUA guideline. *J. Urol.* 197: 182.

17 Terlecki, R.P., Steele, M.C., Valadez, C. et al. (2011). Urethral rest: role and rationale in preparation for anterior urethroplasty. *Urology* 77: 1477.

18 Morey, A.F., McAninch, J.W., Duckett, C.P. et al. (1998). American Urological Association symptom index in the assessment of urethroplasty outcomes. *J. Urol.* 159: 1192.

19 Jackson, M.J., Sciberras, J., Mangera, A. et al. (2011). Defining a patient-reported outcome measure for urethral stricture surgery. *Eur. Urol.* 60: 60.

20 Gallentine, M.L. and Morey, A.F. (2002). Imaging of the male urethra for stricture disease. *Urol. Clin. North Am.* 29: 361.

21 Bach, P. and Rourke, K. (2014). Independently interpreted retrograde urethrography does not accurately diagnose and stage anterior urethral stricture: the importance of urologist-performed urethrography. *Urology* 83: 1190.

22 Theisen, K.M., Kadow, B.T., and Rusilko, P.J. (2016). Three-dimensional imaging of urethral stricture disease and urethral pathology for operative planning. *Curr. Urol. Rep.* 17: 54.

23 Nash, P.A., McAninch, J.W., Bruce, J.E. et al. (1995). Sono-urethrography in the evaluation of anterior urethral strictures. *J. Urol.* 154: 72.

24 Mundy, A.R. and Andrich, D.E. (2011). Urethral strictures. *BJU Int.* 107: 6.

25 Angermeier, K.W., Rourke, K.F., Dubey, D. et al. (2014). SIU/ICUD consultation on urethral strictures: evaluation and follow-up. *Urology* 83: S8.

26 Iselin, C.E. and Webster, G.D. (1999). The significance of the open bladder neck associated with pelvic fracture urethral distraction defects. *J. Urol.* 162: 347.

27 Horiguchi, A., Edo, H., Soga, S. et al. (2019). Magnetic resonance imaging findings of traumatic bulbar urethral stricture help estimate repair complexity. *Urology* 135: 146–153.

28 Koraitim, M.M. and Reda, I.S. (2007). Role of magnetic resonance imaging in assessment of posterior urethral distraction defects. *Urology* 70: 403.

29 Horiguchi, A., Edo, H., Soga, S. et al. (2017). Pubourethral stump angle measured on preoperative magnetic resonance imaging predicts urethroplasty type for pelvic fracture urethral injury repair. *Urology* 112: 198–204.

30 Narumi, Y., Hricak, H., Armenakas, N.A. et al. (1993). MR imaging of traumatic posterior urethral injury. *Radiology* 188: 439.

31 Buckley, J.C., Heyns, C., Gilling, P. et al. (2014). SIU/ICUD consultation on urethral strictures: dilation, internal urethrotomy, and stenting of male anterior urethral strictures. *Urology* 83: S18.

32 Santucci, R. and Eisenberg, L. (2010). Urethrotomy has a much lower success rate than previously reported. *J. Urol.* 183: 1859.

33 Chapple, C., Andrich, D., Atala, A. et al. (2014). SIU/ICUD consultation on urethral strictures: the management of anterior urethral stricture disease using substitution urethroplasty. *Urology* 83: S31.

34 Morey, A.F., Watkin, N., Shenfeld, O. et al. (2014). SIU/ICUD consultation on urethral strictures: anterior urethra – primary anastomosis. *Urology* 83: S23.

35 Bullock, T.L. and Brandes, S.B. (2007). Adult anterior urethral strictures: a national practice patterns survey of board certified urologists in the United States. *J. Urol.* 177: 685.

36 van Leeuwen, M.A., Brandenburg, J.J., Kok, E.T. et al. (2011). Management of adult anterior urethral stricture disease: nationwide survey among urologists in The Netherlands. *Eur. Urol.* 60: 159.

37 Steenkamp, J.W., Heyns, C.F., and de Kock, M.L. (1997). Internal urethrotomy versus dilation as treatment for male urethral strictures: a prospective, randomized comparison. *J. Urol.* 157: 98.

38 Wright, J.L., Wessells, H., Nathens, A.B. et al. (2006). What is the most cost-effective treatment for 1 to 2-cm bulbar urethral strictures: societal approach using decision analysis. *Urology* 67: 889.

39 Rourke, K. and Jordan, G. (2005). Primary urethral reconstruction: the cost minimized approach to the bulbous urethral stricture. *J. Urol.* 173: 1206.

40 Greenwell, T., Castle, C., Andrich, D. et al. (2004). Repeat urethrotomy and dilation for the treatment of urethral stricture are neither clinically effective nor cost-effective. *J. Urol.* 172: 275.

41 Hudak, S.J., Atkinson, T.H., and Morey, A.F. (2012). Repeat transurethral manipulation of bulbar urethral strictures is associated with increased stricture complexity and prolonged disease duration. *J. Urol.* 187: 1691.

42 Horiguchi, A., Shinchi, M., Masunaga, A. et al. (2018). Do transurethral treatments increase the complexity of urethral strictures? *J. Urol.* 199: 508.

43 Singh, B.P., Andankar, M.G., Swain, S.K. et al. (2010). Impact of prior urethral manipulation on outcome of anastomotic urethroplasty for post-traumatic urethral stricture. *Urology* 75: 179.

44 Lumen, N., Hoebeke, P., Troyer, B.D. et al. (2009). Perineal anastomotic urethroplasty for posttraumatic urethral stricture with or without previous urethral manipulations: a review of 61 cases with long-term Followup. *J. Urol.* 181: 1196.

45 Culty, T. and Boccon-Gibod, L. (2007). Anastomotic urethroplasty for posttraumatic urethral stricture: previous urethral manipulation has a negative impact on the final outcome. *J. Urol.* 177: 1374.

46 Breyer, B.N., McAninch, J.W., Whitson, J.M. et al. (2010). Multivariate analysis of risk factors for long-term urethroplasty outcome. *J. Urol.* 183: 613.

47 Shah, D.K., Paul, E.M., and Badlani, G.H. (2003). 11-year outcome analysis of endourethral prosthesis for the treatment of recurrent bulbar urethral stricture. *J. Urol.* 170: 1255.

48 Hussain, M., Greenwell, T.J., Shah, J. et al. (2004). Long-term results of a self-expanding wallstent in the treatment of urethral stricture. *BJU Int.* 94: 1037.

49 De Vocht, T.F., van Venrooij, G.E., and Boon, T.A. (2003). Self-expanding stent insertion for urethral strictures: a 10-year follow-up. *BJU Int.* 91: 627.

50 Jordan, G.H., Wessells, H., Secrest, C. et al. (2013). Effect of a temporary thermo-expandable stent on urethral patency after dilation or internal urethrotomy for recurrent bulbar urethral stricture: results from a 1-year randomized trial. *J. Urol.* 190: 130.

51 Wong, E., Tse, V., and Wong, J. (2014). Durability of Memokath urethral stent for stabilisation of recurrent bulbar urethral strictures – medium-term results. *BJU Int.* 113 (Suppl 2): 35.

52 Santucci, R.A., Mario, L.A., and McAninch, J.W. (2002). Anastomotic urethroplasty for bulbar urethral stricture: analysis of 168 patients. *J. Urol.* 167: 1715.

53 Eltahawy, E.A., Virasoro, R., Schlossberg, S.M. et al. (2007). Long-term followup for excision and primary anastomosis for anterior urethral strictures. *J. Urol.* 177: 1803.

54 Andrich, D.E., O'Malley, K.J., Summerton, D.J. et al. (2003). The type of urethroplasty for a pelvic fracture urethral distraction defect cannot be predicted preoperatively. *J. Urol.* 170: 464.

55 Andrich, D.E., Dunglison, N., Greenwell, T.J. et al. (2003). The long-term results of urethroplasty. *J. Urol.* 170: 90.

56 Park, S. and McAninch, J.W. (2004). Straddle injuries to the bulbar urethra: management and outcomes in 78 patients. *J. Urol.* 171: 722.

57 Mundy, A.R. (2005). Anastomotic urethroplasty. *BJU Int.* 96: 921.

58 Koraitim, M.M. (2005). On the art of anastomotic posterior urethroplasty: a 27-year experience. *J. Urol.* 173: 135.

59 Morey, A.F. and Kizer, W.S. (2006). Proximal bulbar urethroplasty via extended anastomotic approach – what are the limits? *J. Urol.* 175: 2145.

60 Andrich, D.E. and Mundy, A.R. (2012). Non-transecting anastomotic bulbar urethroplasty: a preliminary report. *BJU Int.* 109: 1090.

61 Ivaz, S., Bugeja, S., Frost, A. et al. (2017). The nontransecting approach to bulbar urethroplasty. *Urol. Clin. North Am.* 44: 57.

62 Barbagli, G., Kulkarni, S.B., Fossati, N. et al. (2014). Long-term followup and deterioration rate of anterior substitution urethroplasty. *J. Urol.* 192: 808.

63 Simonato, A., Gregori, A., Ambruosi, C. et al. (2008). Lingual mucosal graft urethroplasty for anterior urethral reconstruction. *Eur. Urol.* 54: 79.

64 Barbagli, G., De Angelis, M., Romano, G. et al. (2008). The use of lingual mucosal graft in adult anterior urethroplasty: surgical steps and short-term outcome. *Eur. Urol.* 54: 671.

65 Guralnick, M.L. and Webster, G.D. (2001). The augmented anastomotic urethroplasty: indications and outcome in 29 patients. *J. Urol.* 165: 1496.

66 Patterson, J.M. and Chapple, C.R. (2008). Surgical techniques in substitution urethroplasty using buccal mucosa for the treatment of anterior urethral strictures. *Eur. Urol.* 53: 1162.

67 Greenwell, T.J., Venn, S.N., and Mundy, A.R. (1999). Changing practice in anterior urethroplasty. *BJU Int.* 83: 631.

68 Vasudeva, P., Nanda, B., Kumar, A. et al. (2015). Dorsal versus ventral onlay buccal mucosal graft urethroplasty for long-segment bulbar urethral stricture: a prospective randomized study. *Int. J. Urol.* 22: 967.

69 Figler, B.D., Malaeb, B.S., Dy, G.W. et al. (2013). Impact of graft position on failure of single-stage bulbar urethroplasties with buccal mucosa graft. *Urology* 82: 1166.

70 Pisapati, V.L., Paturi, S., Bethu, S. et al. (2009). Dorsal buccal mucosal graft urethroplasty for anterior urethral stricture by Asopa technique. *Eur. Urol.* 56: 201.

71 Asopa, H.S., Garg, M., Singhal, G.G. et al. (2001). Dorsal free graft urethroplasty for urethral stricture by ventral sagittal urethrotomy approach. *Urology* 58: 657.

72 Barbagli, G. (2007). Interview with Dr Guido Barbagli. Substitution urethroplasty: which tissues and techniques are optimal for urethral replaceåment? *Eur. Urol.* 52: 602.

11

Prostatitis and Prostatic Abscess

Hunter Wessells

Department of Urology, University of Washington School of Medicine, Seattle, WA, USA

Introduction

The advent of highly effective antimicrobial agents and improvement in diagnosis have transformed the management of prostatic infections. Acute prostatitis remains a rare genitourinary infection with risk of systemic response and progression to abscess formation. Appropriate antimicrobial therapy and surgical drainage in selected cases can prevent septic shock in all but the most compromised and high-risk patients. This chapter restricts its content to acute bacterial infections of the prostate and indications for imaging and surgical intervention.

Classification

The National Institute of Diabetes and Digestive and Kidney Diseases classification system for prostatitis syndromes designates acute infection of the prostate as distinct from other chronic bacterial, chronic nonbacterial, and asymptomatic prostatitis and accounts for <5% of all prostatitis syndromes [1]. Reflecting the etiology and treatment needs of acute prostatic infection, prostatitis uniformly falls under the "Complicated urinary tract infection (UTI)" nomenclature of the Infectious Diseases Society of America (IDSA) [2]. A more comprehensive approach to classification has been proposed, acknowledging the diversity of presentation of infections of the male accessory glands, severity and specificity of symptoms, patterns of infection, urological factors, and pathogens [3].

Presentation

Acute prostatitis may begin insidiously. Vague discomfort in the lower abdomen, perineum, and rectum rapidly progresses to the onset of fever, chills, and symptoms of lower urinary tract obstruction (decreased force of stream, incomplete emptying, urinary

A Clinical Guide to Urologic Emergencies, First Edition. Edited by Hunter Wessells, Shigeo Horie, and Reynaldo G. Gómez.
© 2021 John Wiley & Sons Ltd. Published 2021 by John Wiley & Sons Ltd.
Companion website: www.wiley.com/go/wessells/urologic

retention) or overactivity (frequency, urgency) [4]. Pain in the low back, suprapubic, perineal, and rectal areas characterize acute prostatic infection. Associated malaise, arthralgia, and myalgia reflect systemic manifestations. The history of present illness should describe recent or past history of urinary tract infection, indwelling or intermittent urethral catheterization, urethral instrumentation, prostate biopsy, as well as traditional risk factors and immunocompromised states including diabetes, Human Immunodeficiency Virus (HIV), and chronic kidney disease (CKD). Past antibiotic exposure and duration will also inform decision-making and antibiotic selection and must be recorded.

Vital signs may reveal elevation in temperature, respiratory rate, heartrate, and low blood pressure. Affected men appear ill. Physical examination should assess for signs of systemic toxicity, bladder distension, and any associated urethral discharge or testicular enlargement. A rectal exam must be performed because an exquisitely tender swollen prostate gland on examination is pathognomonic. The consistency of the gland can vary from boggy and irregular to firm, and may be warm to the touch. Extensive manipulation is discouraged to reduce the likelihood of severe pain and/or bacteremia [5].

Ultrasonographic post void residual (US PVR) urine volume should be measured to ensure complete bladder emptying. If retention is suspected, and US PVR is not available, urethral straight catheterization is appropriate to ensure emptying and collect urine for culture.

Urinalysis will demonstrate bacteriuria, pyuria, and hematuria. Midstream or catheterized urine should be collected for culture and antibiotic sensitivity. Other laboratory studies should include complete blood count with differential, blood cultures, and chemistry studies. In men with risk factors for sexually transmitted infection, urine nucleic acid amplification testing is mandatory to identify chlamydial and gonococcal infection.

Pathogens associated with acute prostatic infection include the entire range of urinary microbiota including *Escherichia coli* most commonly [6], followed by other *Enterobacteriaciae, Staphylococcus, Enterococcus, Neisseria gonorrhea*, and *Chlamydia trachomatis* [7]. In immunocompromised men, a broader differential diagnosis is required.

Management

Acute bacterial prostatitis requires prompt initiation of empiric oral or intravenous antimicrobial therapy. The route of administration (intravenous vs. oral) should be chosen based on overall acuity of infection. Practitioners should use local antibiograms and resistance patterns to guide antibiotic selection, with consideration for prior exposure to agents that may lead to multidrug resistance. Concerns about antibiotic penetration of prostatic tissue are of limited relevance in acute prostatic infection, and fluoroquinolones, cephalosporins, and sulfonamides will generally achieve effective intraprostatic levels of drug. Supportive measures should include hydration, analgesics, antipyretics, and bed rest [8]. Acute urinary retention due to acute prostatitis (or prostatic abscess) can be managed with transurethral catheterization without increasing risk of exacerbating the response to infection. Suprapubic cystostomy should be reserved for cases in which anatomical abnormalities preclude urethral catheter use.

Table 11.1 Empirical antibiotic choices for acute prostatitis.

Clinical Scenario	First Line	Alternative
STI-related prostatitis	Ceftriaxone (Rocephin), 250 mg (intramuscular) IM *then* Doxycycline, 100 mg po BID for 10 days	Erythromycin base 500 mg orally four times a day for 7 days *or* Erythromycin ethylsuccinate 800 mg orally four times a day for 7 days *or* Levofloxacin 500 mg orally once daily for 7 days
Low risk of systemic infection (outpatient)	Ciprofloxacin 500 mg BID *or* Levofloxacin 500 mg daily	Trimethoprim/ sulfamethoxazole 160/800 mg po BID
High risk of systemic infection	Piperacillin/tazobactam, 3.375 g IV every 6 hours *plus* aminoglycoside *or* Cefotaxime (Claforan), 2 g IV every 4 hours *plus* aminoglycosides *or* Ceftazidime (Fortaz), 2 g IV every 8 hours *plus* aminoglycosides	
High risk of antibiotic resistance	Parenteral antibiotics as described for high risk of systemic infection	

STI: sexually transmitted infections.
Source: adapted from Ref. [4] and Center for Disease Control and, Prevention Sexually Transmitted Diseases Treatment Guidelines. 2015. Available from: http://www.cdc.gov/std/tg2015/epididymitis.htm.

Temperature, vital signs, white blood cell count, serum measures of renal function, and general appearance of the patient indicate whether outpatient management is appropriate or there is a need for hospitalization and potential ICU (intensive care unit) admission. Contemporary antibiotic regimens are listed in Table 11.1. Imaging is not required at presentation.

Urine culture and sensitivity testing dictates whether antimicrobial coverage can be narrowed and transitioned to oral agents. Incomplete patient response may indicate the need to alter antibiotic therapy, perform imaging (see below) to identify the presence of prostatic abscess or anatomical abnormalities, as well as investigate other complicating factors (incomplete bladder emptying, immunocompromised state). Therapy should be continued for a total of four weeks after the diagnosis of acute prostatitis to prevent the development of chronic bacterial prostatitis [8].

Prostatic abscess occurs in a subset of patients with acute prostatitis, with estimates ranging from 2.7 [9] to 21% [6]. Variation in rates may reflect different definitions of abscess and frequency of imaging. Compared to patients without prostatic abscess, those with abscess present with a longer duration of symptoms (7.8 vs. 3.0 days), higher percentage with diabetes (52 vs. 27%), and objective evidence of urinary obstruction (e.g. peak uroflometry <5 cc/s or elevated PVR (post void residual), 50 vs. 14%) [6].

Diagnostic Imaging

In cases of urinary retention, persistent fever and/or hemodynamic instability despite appropriate antimicrobial therapy, the presence of prostatic abscess, urinary stone disease, or upper urinary tract conditions should be investigated with cross-sectional imaging. Computed tomography (CT) of the abdomen and pelvic with intravenous contrast represents the best study (Figures 11.1 and 11.2), because in addition to excellent visualization of the prostate, it provides high resolution imaging of other organ systems susceptible to abscess formation including the kidneys, liver, and spleen. Abdominal ultrasonography lacks sensitivity and specificity for prostatic abscess, although it may successfully detect large abscesses. Magnetic resonance imaging (MRI) has been used extensively for prostate imaging, but surprisingly little literature exists on features of acute bacterial infection of the prostate. Transrectal ultrasonography will identify prostatic abscess accurately, but is operator dependent and may not be available in the emergency setting.

Prostatic Abscess

The decision to proceed with drainage of a prostatic abscess should take into consideration ongoing evidence of systemic infection, abscess size, suitability for drainage, and other patient factors. Small abscesses, <2 cm in size, may respond to antibiotic therapy alone [6].

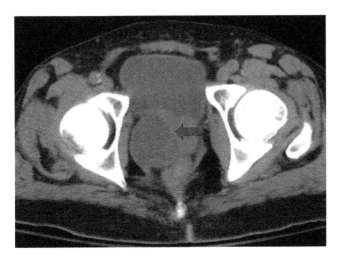

Figure 11.1 Axial image from contrast enhanced pelvic CT scan demonstrating large low-density collection (arrow) within right side of the prostate. This patient required drainage transurethrally (see Figure 11.3).

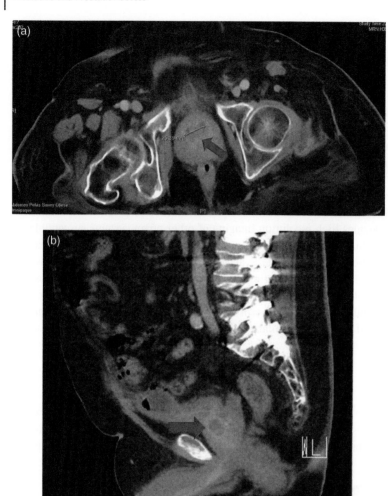

Figure 11.2 Axial (a) and saggital (b) image from contrast enhanced pelvic CT scan demonstrating 2.5 cm low-density collection (arrow) within right side of the prostate.

An abscess that fails to respond to antibiotics is optimally drained by the transurethral route. In a large contemporary cases series, 45% of prostatic abscesses, all >2 cm in size, underwent a transurethral drainage procedure. Prompt drainage, in combination with appropriate antimicrobial therapy, resolves most abscesses. Transurethral, perineal, and transrectal drainage of prostatic abscesses have been described [10]. Ultrasound guided transurethral incision or resection of the prostate is now the most common treatment strategy for prostatic abscess [11, 12]. It is important to resect deeply enough into the respective prostatic lobe to widely unroof the abscess and allow free drainage of the purulent material (Figure 11.3). Nickel makes the caveat that when the abscess has penetrated beyond the prostatic capsule or penetrated through the levator ani muscle, a transperineal approach may be necessary [13].

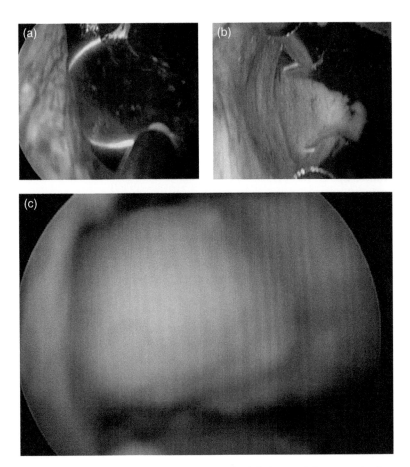

Figure 11.3 Endoscopic images of transurethral drainage of the prostatic abscess shown in Figure 11.1. (a) Right lobe of prostate before drainage. (b) Transurethral resection of portion of right lobe, before unroofing. (c) Purulent drainage into the prostatic fossa. See related video for complete resection. (*Source:* courtesy of B. Figler, MD, FACS)

Conclusions

The diagnosis of acute prostatitis relies on history, physical examination, and urinalysis. Identification of urinary retention should prompt catheterization after which immediate empiric broad-spectrum antimicrobial therapy can be started. A long course of culture specific therapy is critical in order to ensure complete eradication and avoid bacterial resistance. Use of cross-sectional imaging allows identification of abscess and other complicating factors, and helps determine whether surgical intervention is required.

References

1 Krieger, J.N., Nyberg, L. Jr., and Nickel, J.C. (1999). NIH consensus definition and classification of prostatitis. *JAMA* 282: 236–237.
2 Gupta, K., Hooton, T.M., Naber, K.G. et al. (2011). International clinical practice guidelines for the treatment of acute uncomplicated cystitis and pyelonephritis in women: a 2010

update by the Infectious Diseases Society of America and the European Society for Microbiology and Infectious Diseases. *Clin. Infect. Dis.* 52 (5): e103–e120. https://doi.org/10.1093/cid/ciq257.

3 Johansen, T.E., Botto, H., Cek, M. et al. (2011). Critical review of current definitions of urinary tract infections and proposal of an EAU/ESIU classification system. *Int. J. Antimicrob. Agents* 38 (Suppl): 64–70. https://doi.org/10.1016/j.ijantimicag.2011.09.009.

4 Coker, T.J. and Dierfeldt, D.M. (2016). Acute bacterial prostatitis: diagnosis and management. *Am. Fam. Physician* 93 (2): 114–120.

5 Krieger, J.N. (1984). Prostatitis syndromes: pathophysiology, differential diagnosis, and treatment. *Sex. Transm. Dis.* 11: 100–112.

6 Lee, D.S., Choe, H.S., Kim, H.Y. et al. (2016). Acute bacterial prostatitis and abscess formation. *BMC Urol.* 16 (1): 38. Published 2016 Jul 7. doi:https://doi.org/10.1186/s12894-016-0153-7.

7 Roberts, R.O., Lieber, M.M., Bostwick, D.G., and Jacobsen, S.J. (1997). A review of clinical and pathological prostatitis syndromes. *Urology* 49: 809–821.

8 Meares, E.M. Jr. (1980). Prostatitis syndromes: new perspectives about old woes. *J. Urol.* 123: 141–147.

9 Millán-Rodríguez, F., Palou, J., Bujons-Tur, A. et al. (2006). Acute bacterial prostatitis: two different sub-categories according to a previous manipulation of the lower urinary tract. *World J. Urol.* 24 (1): 45–50. https://doi.org/10.1007/s00345-005-0040-4.

10 Barozzi, L., Pavlica, P., Menchi, I. et al. (1998). Prostatic abscess: diagnosis and treatment. *AJR Am. J. Roentgenol.* 170: 753–757.

11 Meares, E.M. Jr. (1986). Prostatic abscess. *J. Urol.* 136: 1281–1282.

12 Trauzzi, S.J., Kay, C.J., Kaufman, D.G., and Lowe, F.C. (1994). Management of prostatic abscess in patients with human immunodeficiency syndrome. *Urology* 43 (5): 629–633. https://doi.org/10.1016/0090-4295(94)90176-7.

13 Nickel, J.C. (2016). Inflammatory and pain conditions of the male genitourinary tract: prostatitis and related pain conditions, orchitis, and epididymitis. In: Campbell-Walsh Urology, (eds. A.J. Wein, L.R. Kavoussi, A.W. Partin and C.A. Peters), 304–333.11th Edition. Philadelphia, PA: Elsevier.

Section III

External Genitalia

12

Fournier's Gangrene

Kosuke Kitamura and Shigeo Horie

Department of Urology, Juntendo University Graduate School of Medicine, Tokyo, Japan

Introduction

Fournier's gangrene (FG) is a fulminant form of infective fasciitis that necrotizes the perineal, genital, and perianal regions. FG commonly afflicts men, but women and children can contract FG as well. It was first reported in the late 1800s by Jean Alfred Fournier [1–3]. Anaerobic bacteria proliferate in a hypoxic environment, produce gas, and subsequently accumulate in the soft tissue spaces [4]. The prevalence of the disease is relatively low, but the mortality rate still remains high without appropriate intensive care and rapid surgical intervention. External wounds such as hemorrhoids or anorectal abscess, complex urethral stricture disease, combined with conditions like diabetes mellitus and other immunocompromised states, predispose an individual to FG. Irrespective of causative microorganisms, its consensus treatment includes emergent removal of necrotic tissues, treatment of sepsis-induced hemodynamic disturbances, and intravenous administration of broad-spectrum antibiotics [5].

Epidemiology

The overall incidence rate of FG is 1.6 cases per 100 000 males per year. FG is diagnosed more frequently among males. FG is rare in pediatric patients, with the rate rising with age to reach its peak at the age of 50. Incidence remains steady afterwards with 3.3 cases per 100 000 males [6–8]. By contrast, prevalence of FG is low among women and children. Sorensen et al. identified only 39 women who met their diagnosis criteria for FG, while they identified 1641 male patients in the same cohort [6]. Eke et al. reviewed 1762 cases of FG in total and reported that male patients far outnumber female patients, in a ratio of 10:1 [9].

Traditionally reported mortality rates range from 3.6 to 40%, with even higher rates reported; recent National Surgical Quality Improvement Program data suggest a modern

A Clinical Guide to Urologic Emergencies, First Edition. Edited by Hunter Wessells, Shigeo Horie, and Reynaldo G. Gómez.
© 2021 John Wiley & Sons Ltd. Published 2021 by John Wiley & Sons Ltd.
Companion website: www.wiley.com/go/wessells/urologic

mortality of about 10% [10–13]. Advanced age and complications are associated with augmented mortality. FG patients were at elevated risk of death when they required the following procedures during admission: colostomy, penectomy, mechanical ventilation, and dialysis [14, 15]. FG patients often have physiological or surgical comorbidities, which predispose them to the condition, as well as a subsequent more severe or fatal outcome.

Etiology

The etiology of FG is a polymicrobial infection induced by both anaerobic and aerobic bacteria [16]. FG can occur from surgical wounds, skin abscess, pressure sores, anorectal infection, ischiorectal abscesses, and colon perforations. Other less frequent causes include a urethral stricture and a trauma from an indwelling Foley catheter. In female patients, it has commonly been ascribed to Bartholin abscesses or vulvar skin infections [4].

Focal infections of the urinary tract, skin, or rectal anus spread to fascia subcutaneously (Colles fascia, Scarpa's fascia, Buck's fascia, and Dartos fascia). Anatomically, subcutaneous tissues of the scrotum and the perineum have an insufficient blood flow, making them a hotbed for bacterial proliferation (Figure 12.1). In FG, suppurative bacterial infection results in microthrombosis of the small subcutaneous vessels leading to the development of gangrene of the overlying skin [2, 9]. The combination of edema, inflammation, and infection in an enclosed space further impairs the blood supply; the resulting hypoxia promotes the growth of anaerobic bacteria [18]. Predisposing factors for all-cause FG are poor perfusion (peripheral vascular disease), hypertension, renal insufficiency,

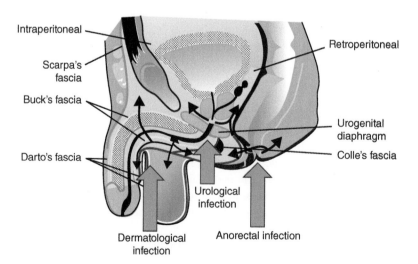

Figure 12.1 The spreading infectious process may arise from local skin, urinary tract, and colorectal regions (arrows). Infection in FG tends to spread along the fascial planes, as subcutaneous tissue of the scrotum and the perineum has poor blood supply [17].

trauma, diabetes mellitus, malnutrition, smoking, obesity, immunocompromised status, intravenous drug abuse, malignancy, and spinal cord injury [13]. The underlying principle of all these conditions is compromised host immunity creating a favorable environment to establish infection. Malnutrition and lower socio-economic status have also been shown to be associated with the development of FG [19]. Alcoholism and diabetes mellitus are the most common in Western countries, with rates of 25–50% and 10–60%, respectively [20, 21]. An evaluation of cases of FG in diabetics patients has shown that this co-morbid condition has an impact on the clinical course of the soft-tissue infection. Primarily, the patient profile tends to be of a younger age and wound cultures reveal different bacterial colonies [19]. SGLT2 inhibitors such as empagliflozin have recently been linked with an increase in the risk of developing Fournier's gangrene in diabetic patients, prompting issuance of an FDA black box safety warning for these medications [22]. This class of medications promote urinary glucose excretion, and episodes of euglycemic diabetic ketoacidosis may underlie the increased risk unique to the genitalia, although the precise causal mechanism remains unclear. While SGLT inhibitor-related Fournier's still predominantly affects males, between one-quarter to one-third of these rare cases occur in females [23].

FG is a devastating condition that affects mostly patients whose immunity has been reduced. There is evidence for increasing incidence of the disease in those with Human Immunodeficiency Virus (HIV) disease. HIV has been reported as a comorbidity in 4% of patients with FG. Various studies have documented a significant rise in the prevalence of cases of FG since the advent of the HIV epidemic [24–26].

Patients with poor general health are particularly prone to FG. This includes malnutrition or obesity, chronic renal failure, chronic liver disease, malignancies, and other conditions causing immunosuppression [3, 10]. Additional predisposing conditions include paralysis/neurological deficit, debility, advanced age, and anorectal diseases [3, 27]. Perforation of rectum after neoadjuvant or therapeutic chemoradiotherapy can cause FG [20].

Bacteriology

FG is typically caused by a polymicrobial infection, with an average of 3 bacteria cultured from each diagnosed patient [16]. Bacteria isolated from FG patients usually derive from the normal flora of the urogenital or anorectal region, such as enteric Gram-negative rods (*Escherichia coli*, *Klebsiella* spp., *Proteus* spp.), Gram-positive cocci (staphylococci, streptococci, enterococci) and obligate anaerobic bacteria (*Clostridium* spp., *Bacteroides* spp., *Fusobacterium* spp., *Peptococcus* spp., *Peptostreptococcus* spp.) [3, 9, 16, 28]. The most commonly detected bacteria are *Bacteroides fragilis*, while *Staphylococcus aureus* or *Streptococci* are frequently identified in patients with diabetes mellitus [21, 29, 30]. Among them, *E. coli* has been reported to be the most common bacteria isolated from the infected lesion, presumably due to its commensal nature in the perineal region. Anaerobes are less frequently isolated than expected, which could be attributable to technical laboratory difficulties. Rare reports of other causative organisms include *Candida albicans* and *Lactobacillus gasseri* [2].

Clinical Symptoms and Imaging

The typical clinical symptoms of FG are a sudden acute pain in the scrotum, prostration, pallor, and fever. When the disease progresses slowly, patients are often unable to remember a specific date of symptom onset or sometimes report a date more recent than the actual date. Physical examination shows intense inflammation in the perineal region with strong erythema and edema that extend progressively beyond the genitals. Signs of suppuration are purulent exudate, and crepitation upon palpation. In addition, violet coloring of the area indicates hypoxia/ischemia and is often followed by the blackish color of necrosis (Figure 12.2) [31, 32]. Intense pain accompanies the condition [33]. It begins with a prodromal period of genital discomfort and pruritus followed by sudden onset of perianal or perineal pain out of proportion to the physical findings [13].

Plain radiographs and ultrasound can demonstrate gas accumulation in soft tissue (Figure 12.3a and b). Gas production under fascia is rarely seen. Compared to radiographs and ultrasound, computed tomography (CT) has a higher specificity for the detection of FG [34]. Although the diagnosis of FG is most commonly made clinically, CT can be an instrumental diagnostic tool to detect early stage disease or patients with indistinctive symptoms. There are few studies that report imaging findings associated with FG [35]. The characteristic features of FG obtained by CT include soft tissue thickening and inflammation. Signature findings by CT comprise asymmetric fascial thickening, concurrent fluid collection or abscess, fat stranding around the infected tissues, and subcutaneous emphysema secondary to proliferation of gas-forming bacteria (Figure 12.4) [36]. Accurate risk estimation for mortality is important to determine appropriate treatment strategy. To this end, several methods of mortality prediction have been implemented, as exemplified by Fournier's Gangrene Severity Index (FGSI), which is the most commonly-used traditional scoring system (Table 12.1) [5, 13]. Others, such as the Uludag Fournier's Gangrene Severity Index (UFGSI) and the Age Adjusted Charlson Comorbidity Index (ACCI), are among the most commonly-used scoring systems to determine FG prognosis and mortality [38, 39]. Specifically, the mean FGSI score at the time of admission was 5.04 ± 2.49 (standard deviation: SD) for survivors, as

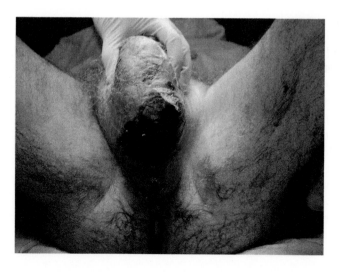

Figure 12.2 Photograph of patient with violet/black color scrotal skin indicative of necrosis *Source:* courtesy of Hunter Wessells, MD.

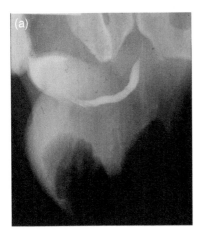
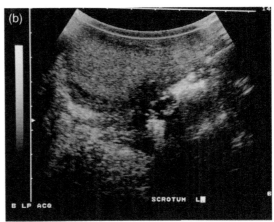

Figure 12.3 CT demonstrating gas in scrotum and posterior tracking into perineum. (a) Retrograde urethrogram demonstrating plain x-ray finding of gas in scrotum and normal anterior urethra. (b) Sonographic appearance of gas in scrotal wall. Note highly echogenic focus.

Figure 12.4 CT demonstrating gas in the scrotal wall consistent with subcutaneous emphysema.

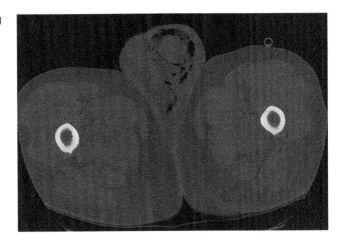

compared to 13.6 ± 4.61 (SD) for non-survivors [13, 27]. The FGSI can predict mortality with a probability of 75% and survival with a probability of 78% for patients with FG [40]. Roghmann et al. compared several published scoring systems for predicting results (FGSI, UFGSI, ACCI, etc.) [41]. All scores are useful to predict mortality. Despite including more variables, the UFGSI does not seem to be more powerful than the FGSI. Thus, the FGSI allows us to evaluate severity of the condition and predict the outcome with a high degree of certainty in this complex patient population [18].

Treatment

FG remains a urological emergency. The mainstay of its treatment is early radical debridement of necrotic tissues, drainage, and antimicrobial therapy (see below), as well as hemodynamic stabilization of the patient. Of note, the time required for the

Table 12.1 Fournier's Gangrene Severity Index (FGSI).

Variable	High Abnormal Values				Normal	Low Abnormal Values			
	+4	+3	+2	+1	0	+1	+2	+3	+4
Temperature (°C)	>41	39–40.9	–	38.5–389	36–38.4	34–35.9	32–33.9	30–31.9	<29.9
Heart rate (bpm)	>180	140–179	110–139	–	70–109	–	55–69	40–54	
Respiration rate	>50	35–49	–	25–34	12–24	10–11	6–9	–	<5
Serum sodium (mmol/l)	>180	160–179	155–159	150–154	130–149	–	120–129	111–119	<110
Serum K^{2+} (mmol/l)	>7	6–6.9	–	5.5–5.9	3.5–5.4	3–3.4	2.5–2.9	–	<2.5
Serum creatinine (mg/100 ml)*	>3.5	2–3.4	1.5–1.9	–	0.6–1.4	–	<0.6	–	–
Hematocrit (%)	>60	–	50–59.9	46–49.4	30–45.9	–	20–29.9	–	<20
White blood cell count (total/mm^3 × 1000)	>40	–	20–39.9	15–19.9	3–14.9	–	1–2.9	–	<1
Serum bicarbonate venous (mmol/l)	>50	41–15.9	–	32–40.9	22–31.9		18–21.9	15–17.9	<15

The FGSI is a numeric score obtained from a combination of admission physiological parameters, including temperature, heart and respiration rates, sodium, potassium, creatinine, white blood cell count, hematocrit, and sodium bicarbonate [13, 18, 37].

initiation of surgical debridement after admission was not statistically different between survivors and non-survivors.

Many studies have pointed out that timing and the extent of the first debridement are the most important prognosis-determining factors regarding mortality rate [42]. The extent of surgical debridement was probably the most clinically significant parameter between survivors and non-survivors (Figure 12.5) [43]. Early surgical intervention (within two days of admission) significantly reduced FG case fatality as compared with delayed intervention (within three to five days of admission) [44]. Surgical reexamination of the infected area and removal of necrotic tissue is advocated within 24 hours and should be carried out repeatedly. After initial surgical debridement, occasionally a series of debridement is required. In all-cause FG, an average of 3.5 procedures is required [12]. Planning initial debridement with an eye toward subsequent reconstruction has been demonstrated to limit the need for skin grafting or other complex wound closures after necrotizing soft tissue infection in other body regions [45, 46]. There may be limitations in application of these techniques to the external genitalia due to differences in baseline patient disease (chronic underlying microvascular disease limiting perfusion of raised skin flaps) and anatomy (thin superficial soft tissue over the penile shaft), but this technique could prove useful with infections involving the scrotum and perineum and warrants further investigation.

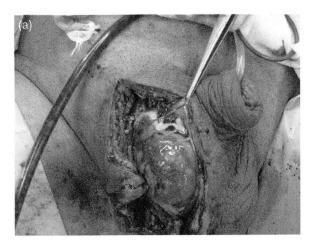 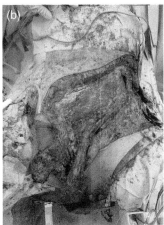

Figure 12.5 Appearance of genitalia after surgical debridement for Fournier's Gangrene (FG) (a) FG involving right hemi-scrotum and inguinal area (b) Debridement of perineum and lower abdominal wall in another patient to remove necrotic tissue and prevent spread of infection. Note absence of left hemi-scrotum and exposed testis within the tunica vaginalis.

An effective dressing is also important. In recent years, it has been reported that the method called negative-pressure wound therapy (NPWT) is useful for wound healing of FG [47, 48]. Extensive debridement, including a slim window of healthy adjacent tissue, has been advocated in the literature. Close observation of the wound and repeated debridement are necessary measures to control the infection [19]. Patients should be returned to the operating room within the next 24 hours for evaluation of the wound. Another debridement will be performed if the necrosis seems to continue, followed by a wound dressing [48]. Understanding the somatic clues of skin and soft tissue viability is essential in consummating its preservation. Meticulous serial surgical debridement coupled with NPWT may contribute to fostering the development of healthy skin and soft tissue granulation suitable for staged complex closures [49, 50].

Regarding surgical intervention, cystostomy, colostomy, and orchiectomy did not significantly affect mortality. As to whether stoma formation reduces the FG case fatality, it is rather controversial. Some earlier studies maintain that an increased mortality was seen among FG patients who underwent stoma formation; however, it can be ascribable to selection bias in which patients with advanced disease were selected for stoma formation [44]. Colostomy has been used for fecal diversion in cases of severe perineal involvement in all-cause FG with anal sphincter involvement; fecal incontinence; and continuous fecal contamination of the wound margins [20]. Rectal diversion decreases the number of germs in the perineal region and improves wound healing. The primary colostomy rate is 16–17%, whereas the secondary colostomy rate is 35–40% [51, 52].

The surgical wounds are usually left for secondary healing or delayed primary wound closure; patients with large tissue defects become candidates for reconstructive surgery with local skin flaps or skin grafts [53]. When additional necrotic lesions were identified after the first debridement, repeating debridement, and the placement of ostomy would be required [54].

Antibiotic regimens vary depending on center and resistance to specific antibiotics in the geographical area where certain microorganisms are isolated. Recent studies recommend the initiation of empirical antibiotic therapy with third-generation cephalosporins for Gram-negative bacteria and metronidazole for anaerobes bacteria, with the arbitrary addition of aminoglycosides [55]. Coverage for anaerobes bacteria requires careful consideration; metronidazole, clindamycin, or carbapenems are considered to be effective.

Excellent wound care is critical to the successful management of FG patients after debridement. The standard care has been saline wet-to-dry dressings changed twice daily or more often as needed. Vacuum-assisted closure (VAC) therapy has been applied to FG wounds with the aim to clean and decontaminate (Figure 12.6). A recent prospective, comparative study showed that patients treated with a VAC device had a significantly lower mortality than historical controls treated only with daily antiseptic dressings [56, 57]. Hyperbaric oxygen therapy is believed to be an effective adjunctive therapy in the treatment of FG, even though conclusive evidence regarding its effectiveness is lacking. In hyperbaric oxygen therapy, patients are placed in an environment of increased ambient pressure while inhaling 100% oxygen, resulting in elevated oxygenation of the arterial

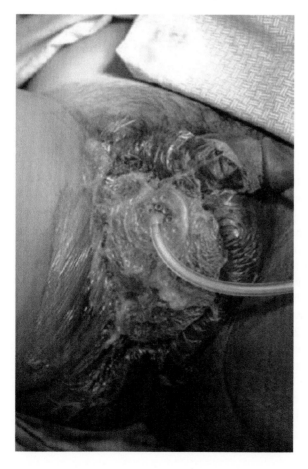

Figure 12.6 Vacuum assisted closure device applied to large scrotal wound. Foley catheter in urethra not visible.

blood and tissues. The indications for adjunctive hyperbaric oxygen therapy in FG still remain controversial, although several groups have reported optimistic results [58].

Perineoscrotal defects should be reconstructed using well-vascularized flaps to avoid complications that include impairment of bladder function, bowel function, and hip joint movement [59]. Perforator flaps, when appropriate, are a minimally invasive alternative, because they do not require sacrificing muscles, and they utilize a reliable blood supply with a wide vascular territory [60, 61]. Split thickness skin grafts remain the mainstay of coverage for larger defects and when the necrotizing soft tissue infection (NSTI) compromises available skin for flap reconstruction [62].

Conclusions

Fournier's Gangrene is a gas-forming, necrotizing soft tissue infection affecting the perineum. It spreads rapidly along the deep fascial planes and is associated with a high mortality rate. The mainstay of treatment is early radical debridement of necrotic tissues, drainage, and antibiotic treatment, as well as hemodynamic stabilization of the patient. NPWT in addition to traditional dressings helps to promote wound healing and to reduce the extent of reconstructive surgery required for ultimate coverage.

References

1 Smith, G.L., Bunker, C.B., and Dinneen, M.D. (1998). Fournier's gangrene. *Br. J. Urol.* 81 (3): 347–355.

2 Thwaini, A., Khan, A., Malik, A. et al. (2006). Fournier's gangrene and its emergency management. *Postgrad. Med. J.* 82 (970): 516–519.

3 Aridogan, I.A., Izol, V., Abat, D. et al. (2012). Epidemiological characteristics of Fournier's gangrene: a report of 71 patients. *Urol. Int.* 89 (4): 457–461.

4 Misiakos, E.P., Bagias, G., Patapia, P. et al. (2014). Current concepts in the management of necrotizing fasciitis. *Front. Surg.* 1: 36.

5 Yilmazlar, T., Işık, Ö., Öztürk, E. et al. (2014). Fournier's gangrene: review of 120 patients and predictors of mortality. *Ulus Travma Acil Cerrahi Derg* 20 (5): 333–337.

6 Sorensen, M.D., Krieger, J.N., Rivara, F.P. et al. (2009). Fournier's Gangrene: population-based epidemiology and outcomes. *J. Urol.* 181 (5): 2120–2126.

7 Korkut, M., Içöz, G., Dayangaç, M. et al. (2003). Outcome analysis in patients with Fournier's gangrene: report of 45 cases. *Dis. Colon Rectum* 46 (5): 649–652.

8 Norton, K.S., Johnson, L.W., Perry, T. et al. (2002). Management of Fournier's gangrene: an eleven year retrospective analysis of early recognition, diagnosis, and treatment. *Am. Surg.* 68 (8): 709–713.

9 Eke, N. (2000). Fournier's gangrene: a review of 1726 cases. *Br. J. Surg.* 87 (6): 718–728.

10 Hakkarainen, Kopari, Pham, T.W., N.M., T.N. et al. (2014). Necrotizing soft tissue infections: review and current concepts in treatment, systems of care, and outcomes. *Curr. Probl. Surg.* 51 (8): 344–362.

11 Mills, M.K., Faraklas, I., Davis, C. et al. (2010). Outcomes from treatment of necrotizing soft-tissue infections: results from the National Surgical Quality Improvement Program database. *Am. J. Surg.* 200 (6): 790–796; discussion 796-7.

12 Chawla, S.N., Gallop, C., and Mydlo, J.H. (2003). Fournier's gangrene: an analysis of repeated surgical debridement. *Eur. Urol.* 43 (5): 572–575.

13 Yeniyol, C.O., Suelozgen, T., Arslan, M. et al. (2004). Fournier's gangrene: experience with 25 patients and use of Fournier's gangrene severity index score. *Urology* 64 (2): 218–222.

14 Sorensen, M.D., Krieger, J.N., Rivara, F.P. et al. (2009). Fournier's gangrene: management and mortality predictors in a population-based study. *J. Urol.* 182 (6): 2742–2747.

15 Yaghan, R.J., Al-Jaberi, T.M., and Bani-Hani, I. (2000). Fournier's gangrene: changing face of the disease. *Dis. Colon Rectum* 43 (9): 1300–1308.

16 Bjurlin, M.A., O'Grady, T., Kim, D.Y. et al. (2013). Causative pathogens, antibiotic sensitivity, resistance patterns, and severity in a contemporary series of Fournier's gangrene. *Urology* 81 (4): 752–758.

17 Rajan, D.K. and Scharer, K.A. (1998). Radiology of Fournier's gangrene. *AJR Am. J. Roentgenol.* 170 (1): 163–168.

18 Corcoran, A.T., Smaldone, M.C., Gibbons, E.P. et al. (2008). Validation of the Fournier's gangrene severity index in a large contemporary series. *J. Urol.* 180 (3): 944–948.

19 Singh, A., Ahmed, K., Aydin, A. et al. (2016). Fournier's gangrene. A clinical review. *Arch. Ital. Urol. Androl.* 88 (3): 157–164.

20 Bruketa, T., Majerovic, M., and Augustin, G. (2015). Rectal cancer and Fournier's gangrene – current knowledge and therapeutic options. *World J. Gastroenterol.* 21 (30): 9002–9020.

21 Nisbet, A.A. and Thompson, I.M. (2002). Impact of diabetes mellitus on the presentation and outcomes of Fournier's gangrene. *Urology* 60 (5): 775–779.

22 https://www.fda.gov/drugs/drug-safety-and-availability/fda-warns-about-rare-occurrences-serious-infection-genital-area-sglt2-inhibitors-diabetes. Accessioned 10/15/2020.

23 Hu, Y., Bai, Z., Tang, Y. et al. (2020). Fournier Gangrene associated with sodium-glucose cotransporter-2 Inhibitors: A pharmacovigilance study with data from the U.S. FDA Adverse Event Reporting System. *J. Diabetes Res.* https://doi.org/10.1155/2020/3695101.

24 Ngugi, P., Magoha, G., and Nyaga, P. (2014). Fournier's ganrene in the HIV era. *Afr. Health Sci.* 14 (4): 1063–1068.

25 Elem, B. and Ranjan, P. (1995). Impact of immunodeficiency virus (HIV) on Fournier's gangrene: observations in Zambia. *Ann. R. Coll. Surg. Engl.* 77 (4): 283–286.

26 Chazan, B., Chen, Y., Raz, R. et al. (2007). Fournier's gangrene as the initial presentation of HIV infection. *Int. J. Infect. Dis.* 11 (2): 184–185.

27 Ulug, M., Gedik, E., Girgin, S. et al. (2009). The evaluation of microbiology and Fournier's gangrene severity index in 27 patients. *Int. J. Infect. Dis.* 13 (6): e424–e430.

28 Kalorin, C.M. and Tobin, E.H. (2007). Community associated methicillin resistant *Staphylococcus aureus* causing Fournier's gangrene and genital infections. *J. Urol.* 177 (3): 967–971.

29 Paty, R. and Smith, A.D. (1992). Gangrene and Fournier's gangrene. *Urol. Clin. North Am.* 19 (1): 149–162.

30 Efem, S.E. (1993). Recent advances in the management of Fournier's gangrene: preliminary observations. *Surgery* 113 (2): 200–204.

31 Tehrani, M.A. and Ledingham, I.M. (1977). Necrotizing fasciitis. *Postgrad. Med. J.* 53 (619): 237–242.

32 Scott, S.D., Dawes, R.F., Tate, J.J. et al. (1988). The practical management of Fournier's gangrene. *Ann. R. Coll. Surg. Engl.* 70 (1): 16–20.

33 Rubegni, P., Lamberti, A., Natalini, Y. et al. (2014). Treatment of two cases of Fournier's gangrene and review of the literature. *J. Dermatolog. Treat.* 25 (2): 189–192.

34 Wong, C.H., Khin, L.W., Heng, K.S. et al. (2004). The LRINEC (Laboratory Risk Indicator for Necrotizing Fasciitis) score: a tool for distinguishing necrotizing fasciitis from other soft tissue infections. *Crit. Care Med.* 32 (7): 1535–1541.

35 Ballard, D.H., Raptis, C.A., Guerra, J. et al. (2018). Preoperative CT findings and interobserver reliability of Fournier gangrene. *AJR Am. J. Roentgenol.* 211 (5): 1051–1057.

36 Levenson, R.B., Singh, A.K., and Novelline, R.A. (2008). Fournier gangrene: role of imaging. *Radiographics* 28 (2): 519–528.

37 Erol, B., Tuncel, A., Hanci, V. et al. (2010). Fournier's gangrene: overview of prognostic factors and definition of new prognostic parameter. *Urology* 75 (5): 1193–1198.

38 Ureyen, O., Acer, A., Gökçelli, U. et al. (2017). Usefulness of FGSI and UFGSI scoring systems for predicting mortality in patients with Fournier's gangrene: a multicenter study. *Ulus. Travma Acil Cerrahi Derg.* 23 (5): 389–394.

39 St-Louis, E., Iqbal, S., Feldmen, L.S. et al. (2015). Using the age-adjusted Charlson comorbidity index to predict outcomes in emergency general surgery. *J. Trauma Acute Care Surg.* 78 (2): 318–323.

40 Yilmazlar, T., Ozturk, E., Ozguc, H. et al. (2010). Fournier's gangrene: an analysis of 80 patients and a novel scoring system. *Tech. Coloproctol.* 14 (3): 217–223.

41 Roghmann, F., von Bodman, C., Löppenberg, B. et al. (2012). Is there a need for the Fournier's gangrene severity index? Comparison of scoring systems for outcome prediction in patients with Fournier's gangrene. *BJU Int.* 110 (9): 1359–1365.

42 Morpurgo, E. and Galandiuk, S. (2002). Fournier's gangrene. *Surg. Clin. North Am.* 82 (6): 1213–1224.

43 McCormack, M., Valiquette, A.S., and Ismail, S. (2015). Fournier's gangrene: a retrospective analysis of 26 cases in a Canadian hospital and literature review. *Can. Urol. Assoc. J.* 9 (5–6): E407–E410.

44 Sugihara, T., Yasunaga, H., Horiguchi, H. et al. (2012). Impact of surgical intervention timing on the case fatality rate for Fournier's gangrene: an analysis of 379 cases. *BJU Int.* 110 (11 Pt C): E1096–E1100.

45 Rüfenacht, M.S., Montaruli, E., Chappuis, E. et al. (2016). Skin-sparing débridement for necrotizing fasciitis in children. *Plast Reconstr Surg.* 138 (3): 489e–497e. https://doi.org/10.1097/PRS.0000000000002478. PMID: 27556624.

46 Tom, L.K., Maine, R.G., Wang, C.S. et al. (2020). Comparison of traditional and skin-sparing approaches for surgical treatment of necrotizing soft-tissue infections. *Surg. Infect. (Larchmt.)* 21 (4): 363–369. https://doi.org/10.1089/sur.2019.263. Epub 2019 Dec 3. PMID: 31800370.

47 Chang, F.S., Chou, C., Hu, C.Y. et al. (2018). Suture technique to prevent air leakage during negative-pressure wound therapy in Fournier gangrene. *Plast. Reconstr. Surg. Glob. Open* 6 (1): e1650.

48 Ozkan, O.F., Koksal, N., Altinli, E. et al. (2016). Fournier's gangrene current approaches. *Int. Wound J.* 13 (5): 713–716.

49 Perry, T.L., Kraker, L.M., Mobley, E.E. et al. (2018). Outcomes in Fournier's gangrene using skin and soft tissue sparing flap preservation surgery for wound closure: an alternative approach to wide radical debridement. *Wounds* 30 (10): 290–299.

50 Verbelen, J., Hoeksema, H., Heyneman, A. et al. (2011). Treatment of Fournier's gangrene with a novel negative pressure wound therapy system. *Wounds* 23 (11): 342–349.

51 Corman, J.M., Moody, J.A., and Aronson, W.J. (1999). Fournier's gangrene in a modern surgical setting: improved survival with aggressive management. *BJU Int.* 84 (1): 85–88.

52 Chen, C.S., Liu, K.L., Chen, H.W. et al. (1999). Prognostic factors and strategy of treatment in Fournier's gangrene: a 12-year retrospective study. *Changgeng Yi Xue Za Zhi* 22 (1): 31–36.

53 Sroczynski, M., Sebastian, M., Rudnicki, J. et al. (2013). A complex approach to the treatment of Fournier's gangrene. *Adv. Clin. Exp. Med.* 22 (1): 131–135.

54 Hong, K.S., Yi, H.J., Lee, R.A. et al. (2017). Prognostic factors and treatment outcomes for patients with Fournier's gangrene: a retrospective study. *Int. Wound J.* 14 (6): 1352–1358.

55 Jimenez-Pacheco, A., Arrabal-Polo, M.Á., Arias-Santiago, S. et al. (2012). Fournier gangrene: description of 37 cases and analysis of associated health care costs. *Actas Dermosifiliogr.* 103 (1): 29–35.

56 Zagli, G., Cianchui, G., Degl'innocenti, S. et al. (2011). Treatment of Fournier's gangrene with combination of vacuum-assisted closure therapy, hyperbaric oxygen therapy, and protective colostomy. *Case. Rep. Anesthesiol.* 2011: 430983.

57 Czymek, R., Schmidt, A., Eckmann, C. et al. (2009). Fournier's gangrene: vacuum-assisted closure versus conventional dressings. *Am. J. Surg.* 197 (2): 168–176.

58 Li, C., Zhou, X., Liu, L.F. et al. (2015). Hyperbaric oxygen therapy as an adjuvant therapy for comprehensive treatment of Fournier's gangrene. *Urol. Int.* 94 (4): 453–458.

59 Hong, J.P., Kim, C.G., Suh, H.S. et al. (2017). Perineal reconstruction with multiple perforator flaps based on anatomical divisions. *Microsurgery* 37 (5): 394–401.

60 Koshima, I. and Soeda, S. (1989). Inferior epigastric artery skin flaps without rectus abdominis muscle. *Br. J. Plast. Surg.* 42 (6): 645–648.

61 Kadota, H., Momii, K., Hanada, M. et al. (2019). Simultaneous deep inferior epigastric and bilateral anterolateral thigh perforator flap reconstruction of an extended perineoscrotal defect in Fournier's gangrene: a case report. *Microsurgery* 39 (3): 263–266.

62 Wessells, H. (1999). Genital skin loss: unified reconstructive approach to a heterogeneous entity. *World J. Urol.* 17 (2): 107–114.

13

Traumatic Penile Injuries

Ariel Fredrick[1] and Alex J. Vanni[2]

[1] Lahey Hospital and Medical Center, Lahey Institute of Urology at Portsmouth and Rochester, Portsmouth and Rochester, NH, USA
[2] Center for Reconstructive Urologic Surgery, Lahey Hospital and Medical Center, Burlington, MA, USA

Introduction

Penile trauma is uncommon, accounting for only 10–16% of all genitourinary traumatic injuries (Table 13.1) [1]. While traumatic penile injury is uncommon, the mechanism of injury has an important impact on subsequent treatment. Approximately 45% of injuries to the external genitalia result from penetrating injury, 45% from blunt injury, while 10% are due to burns and industrial accidents [2]. Traumatic injury to the flaccid penis is rare, usually resulting from penetrating trauma or machinery accidents [1, 3, 4]. Although civilian penile trauma is a rare event, battlefield penile injuries occur more frequently due to the use of improvised explosive devices (IED). Fortunately, improvements in protective armor have limited battlefield penile injury to 6% of all genitourinary trauma [5, 6]. Prompt diagnosis and treatment are required to avoid potentially devastating long-term physical, psychological, and functional sequel of traumatic penile injuries. Rapid treatment of most penile injuries will prevent the development of permanent sexual dysfunction. Lastly, recent publication, and update of the American Urological Association (AUA) Urotrauma Guideline, provide clinicians with a systematic review of the literature with evidence-based guidelines in the appropriate methods of evaluation and management of traumatic penile injuries [7]. In this chapter, we will reference the guidelines to highlight the relevant information as it pertains to a given topic.

Pathophysiology of Traumatic Penile Injury

Blunt Penile Injury (Penile Fracture)

Penile fracture is an injury of the tunica albuginea that occurs only with full penile rigidity. Penile fracture typically involves men between the ages of 30 and 40, happens most frequently on the weekends and during the summer, and most commonly occurs during sexual intercourse as a result of missed intromission, masturbation, rolling over in bed, and

A Clinical Guide to Urologic Emergencies, First Edition. Edited by Hunter Wessells, Shigeo Horie, and Reynaldo G. Gómez.
© 2021 John Wiley & Sons Ltd. Published 2021 by John Wiley & Sons Ltd.
Companion website: www.wiley.com/go/wessells/urologic

Table 13.1   American Association for the Surgery of Trauma (AAST Penis Injury Scale).

Grade[a]	Description of injury
I	Cutaneous laceration/contusion
II	Bucks' fascia (cavernosum) laceration without tissue loss
III	Cutaneous avulsion/laceration through glans/meatus/cavernosal or urethral defect <2 cm
IV	Cavernosal or urethral defect >3 cm/partial penectomy
V	Total penectomy

[a] Advance one grade for multiple injuries up to grade III. Advance one grade for bilateral lesions up to grade V. Source Mohr et al [3].

kneading the penis to achieve detumescence [8–14]. The largest series of cases has been reported in the Middle East and North Africa, suggesting a higher frequency in these areas compared to North America [8–10]. This is thought to be due to the practice of Taqaandan, which involves bending the distal end of the erect penis while holding the base of the penis in place. Blunt trauma to the flaccid penis requires extensive force because the tunica albuginea can undergo significant degrees of bending without damage. During erection, the tunica albuginea thins to approximately 0.25 mm, making subsequent injury more likely [15]. A penile fracture occurs when a sudden rise in intracorporeal pressure associated with bending compromises the integrity of the tunica albuginea, causing a tunical tear [11, 16]. Tears in the tunica albuginea tend to be unilateral and transverse, but are bilateral in 5–14% of cases. "False" penile fracture is indistinguishable from a true penile fracture in most cases. It can be the result of rupture of a superficial dorsal vein, a deep dorsal vein, a dorsal artery, or nonspecific dartos bleeding [17]. The absence of immediate detumescence may alert the provider to this diagnosis [18].

Bending injuries to the penis can result in significant penile sequela. Injuries in either the flaccid or erect state, are thought to play a role in the development of Peyronie's disease. In addition to penile fracture, sexual activity with a partial erection due to erectile dysfunction (ED) may also be a risk facture for the development of Peyronie's disease. Twenty-one to forty percent of men with Peyronie's disease report trauma to the penis in either the flaccid state or during intercourse [19, 20].

Penetrating Penile Injury

Gunshot Wounds

Gunshot wounds (GSW) to the penis are rare due to the anatomical location, size, and mobility of the flaccid penis. Due to the rarity of this injury, most series have been reported in large metropolitan areas or after wars [1, 21, 22]. Up to 80% of patients with penetrating penile injuries have other associated injuries [4]. The degree of tissue destruction is highly dependent on the caliber of weapon and velocity of missile. Military injuries differ from civilian injuries because they are generally caused by high-velocity projectiles, produce greater tissue loss, and often require urinary diversion with staged repair. In the modern era, IEDs account for the vast majority of projectile penetrating injury. Improved body armor in modern warfare has decreased the incidence of penile injuries. Only 6% of genitourinary injuries affected the penis in Operation Iraqi Freedom compared to 16–40% in the Vietnam War era [6, 21, 23].

Stab Wounds/Amputation

Penile stab wounds or amputations are devastating injuries that occur as a result of assault or are self-inflicted. Self-inflicted penile amputation is a result of a psychotic event in 87% of patients, with schizophrenia (51%) and depression (19%) the most common causes. Amputations have also been reported in transgender patients [24]. The largest series of penile amputations was reported in Thailand in the 1980s. In this series of approximately 100 cases, most amputations were carried out by disgruntled wives of philandering husbands [25].

Avulsion/Bites

Historically, avulsion injuries to the penis most frequently occurred as a result of power machinery accidents when clothing became entrapped in the moving machinery parts. Fortunately, the incidence has decreased with improved safety measures. Today, most genital skin avulsion injury results from motorcycle or bicycle collisions [26].

Bites to the penis are exceedingly rare and can result in skin loss, infection, injury to the urethra, and partial or complete loss of the organ. Bites are most frequently caused by canine attack and most frequently occur in children [27]. Human bites are even more rare and usually present in a delayed fashion due to embarrassment or fear of retribution.

Burns

Isolated penile burns are extremely rare, and are usually part of a larger surface area burn, occurring in 5–13% of burn cases [28]. Burns can be thermal, chemical, or electrical in nature. They require immediate referral to a burn center and demonstrate an average total body surface area of 21–56% for patients with perineal burns [28–30]. Patients with genital burns have been found to have a greater than average total burn surface area and higher mortality [31].

Initial Evaluation

Penile Fracture

"Clinicians must suspect penile fracture when a patient presents with penile ecchymosis, swelling, pain cracking or snapping sound during intercourse or manipulation and immediate detumescence" [7]. Most frequently this occurs during intercourse as the erect penis slips out of the vagina and strikes against the pubic bone or perineum. A classic "eggplant deformity" is present when Buck's fascia remains intact and hematoma is confined to the penis (Figure 13.1a). The ecchymosis will spread to the scrotum and perineum if Buck's fascia is disrupted. Diagnosis can reliably be made based on history and physical examination. "Clinicians may perform ultrasound in patients with equivocal signs and symptoms of penile fracture" [7]. Ultrasonography is inexpensive, non-invasive, and helps with diagnosis in uncertain cases. If diagnosis remains equivocal after ultrasonography, surgical exploration should be performed [7]. Magnetic Resonance Imaging (MRI) can accurately demonstrate the presence, location, and extent of a tunical tear [32], but its use in the acute setting is not recommended because it is costly, time-consuming, and can delay prompt surgical intervention [33]. Cavernosography to evaluate for extravasation involves (a)　　　　　　　　　　　　　　(b)

(c)

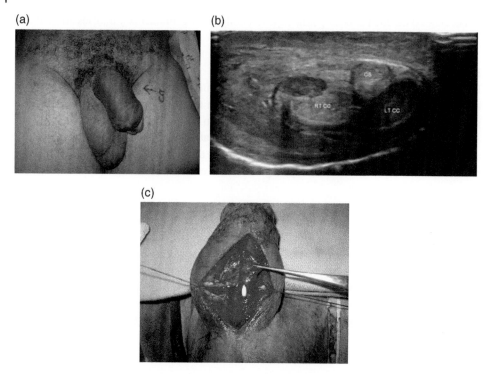

Figure 13.1 Penile fracture: (a) Ecchymosis and eggplant deformity. (b) Ultrasound of penile fracture. Note hypoechoic focus of hematoma arising out of the right corpus cavernosum (RT CC) and intact corpus spongiosum (CS) and left corpus cavernosum (LT CC). (c)Ventral tunica rupture in a different patient crossing midline with associated urethral injury exposing urethral catheter. *Source:* courtesy Alex J. Vanni, MD, FACS.

intracorporal injection of contrast medium followed by fluoroscopy. This has limited sensitivity and specificity for the diagnosis of penile fracture and can easily be misinterpreted by urologists and radiologists due to lack of familiarity with the technique [34].

Tears in the tunica albuginea may extend to affect the corpus spongiosum and urethra in 6–22% of cases [2]. "Clinicians must perform evaluation for concomitant urethral injury in patients with penile fracture or penetrating trauma who present with blood at the urethral meatus, gross hematuria, or inability to void (Guideline 29: Standard; Evidence Strength: Grade B) [7]. These patients must undergo evaluation for urethral injury with retrograde urethrography (RUG) or flexible cystoscopy [13, 35]. Associated urethral injury has been shown to be more common in coital-related injuries, whereas urethral injury rarely occurs (1.6%) when the fracture has a non-coital etiology [8].

Penetrating Injury

The initial evaluation of any penetrating injury should include careful search for associated injuries. Civilian GSWs in general have associated injuries in 80–90% cases, most commonly the thigh (69–75%) and scrotum (56–56%) [1, 4, 36]. Some studies have suggested that RUG be performed in all patients with gunshot injury to the penis, given that up to half of patients may have an associated urethral injury [1]. However, other studies have shown only a 6–24% rate of associated urethral injury, suggesting that RUG may be performed on a case-by-case basis [1, 4, 36]. In general, all patients with penetrating injury to the penis should undergo surgical exploration, with concomitant evaluation for urethral injury. For patients with lacerations or bites to the penis that are obviously superficial to Buck's fascia, a conservative approach may be warranted.

Amputation

Initial evaluation should focus on stabilization of the patient, both medically and psychologically. "Surgeons should perform prompt penile replantation in patients with traumatic penile amputation, with the amputated appendage wrapped in saline-soaked gauze, in a plastic bag and placed on ice during transport" (Guideline 32: Clinical Principle) [7]. If feasible, the patient should be transferred to a center with expertise in microvascular surgery. Evaluation of both the penile stump and amputated organ are undertaken to determine the feasibility of replantation. An attempt to salvage the organ and perform replantation should be made within 24 hours, as success has been reported after 18 hours of warm ischemia and up to 24 hours of cold ischemia time [37–39]. Prior to operative intervention, patients need to be kept well-hydrated and kept warm to maximally dilate the peripheral vasculature. The penile stump may bleed significantly, and thus manual compression may be required to prevent ongoing blood loss until definitive surgical management of the penile stump and appendage can be performed. Additionally, managing the bladder until definitive surgery will depend on multiple factors including the time to definitive surgery, degree of ongoing penile stump bleeding, and nature of the penile injury. If feasible, a urethral catheter may be placed, otherwise suprapubic tube drainage should be performed.

Management

Penile Fracture

"Surgeons should perform prompt surgical exploration and repair in patients with acute signs and symptoms of penile fracture" (Guideline 27: Standard; Evidence Strength: Grade B) [7]. Conservative management alone has a high risk of long-term ED and penile angulation [16, 40, 41]. Up to 50% of patients managed conservatively will have either ED or penile deviation [40, 42]. Despite the emergent nature of the injury, studies have shown that delayed repair up to seven days does not result in any significant long-term serious deformities or erectile function [43, 44]. The injured corpus cavernosum can be exposed through either a circumferential subcoronal degloving incision, ventral midline incision, or longitudinal incision directly over the tunica tear. One of the disadvantages of a longitudinal incision directly over the tear is the risk of missing a bilateral rupture. A ventral midline incision can provide exposure as good as degloving, as the penis can be inverted through the ventral midline incision and may be preferred in patients with a delayed presentation when the hematoma is more organized and degloving more challenging. Once the incision is made the hematoma is evacuated and tunica repaired with absorbable sutures. In the event that the tunica rupture extends behind the corpus spongiosum, the urethra is mobilized to allow adequate visualization of the injury (Figure 13.1b). Similarly, if the rupture occurs on the dorsal aspect of the penis, the neurovascular bundle should be elevated over the tear to minimize injury to the neurovascular bundle during repair. The corpus spongiosum must be inspected at the time of exploration, given the approximate 20% rate of associated urethral injury and the possibility of a falsely negative retrograde urethrogram or cystourethroscopy. If urethral injury is present, the urethra is repaired primarily in two layers over a urethral catheter, taking care to avoid narrowing the urethral lumen. The urethral catheter should be left in place for approximately two to three weeks with a pericatheter retrograde urethrogram performed prior to catheter removal to evaluate for urethral healing.

Penetrating GSW and Stab Wounds

Surgical exploration must be performed in all cases of penetrating penile injury, except in superficial, tangential injuries that clearly do not involve structures deep to the dartos [4]. Mainstays of treatment are debridement of devitalized tissues, copious irrigation with saline, and assessment of associated injuries. When possible, immediate reconstruction should be attempted. However, more extensive injuries may require urinary diversion and delayed reconstruction. The caliber and velocity of weapon in patients with GSWs has a significant impact on the extent of injury. Low-velocity GSWs usually do not have damage outside the path of projectile. Higher velocity missiles carry the risk of damage outside the path of fire [45]. Patients with higher velocity injury or injury from an IED should have management strategies that first prevent further damage to local tissues and prevent sepsis. Major debridement is deferred until local tissue viability has declared itself. Subsequent surgical management is then performed in which debridement, primary closure, or delayed primary closure and/or split thickness skin grafting is performed, depending on the local tissue viability [46].

Amputation

The penile stump with Microvascular reattachment has shown superior outcomes with decreased skin necrosis, improved sensation, and superior function compared to macrovascular technique, in which only the corpora and urethra are reattached [47, 48]. The urethra is spatulated and repaired in a two-layer fashion with slowly absorbable sutures (Figure 13.2). A urethral catheter is placed to stabilize the penis. Next, the tunica albuginea of the corpora cavernosa are anastomosed with slowly absorbable sutures. Sutures may be

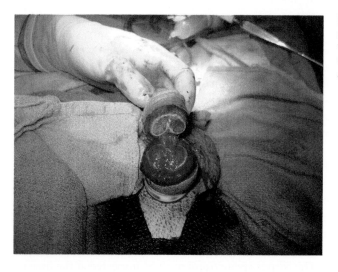

Figure 13.2 Penile amputation reattachment with urethra anastomosis complete. *Source:* courtesy Alex J. Vanni, MD, FACS.

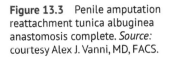

Figure 13.3 Penile amputation reattachment tunica albuginea anastomosis complete. *Source:* courtesy Alex J. Vanni, MD, FACS.

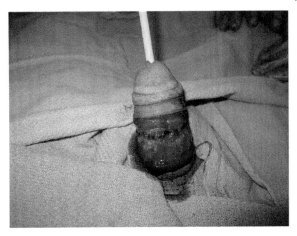

placed in the septum to provide additional stability to the penis (Figure 13.3). This restores blood flow to the shaft of the penis. Lastly, microsurgical anastomosis of dorsal arteries, dorsal vein, and dorsal nerves is performed with fine nonabsorbable sutures. The skin is loosely approximated to allow for post-operative edema. Post-operatively, the patient is kept in a warm room on bed rest to maximize arterial blood flow. Serial vascular checks on the glans are performed with a Doppler. In the event of vascular congestion of the distal penile flap, leech therapy may be initiated.

If the patient presents without the amputated penis, the amputated organ is not salvageable, or if the graft bed is not compatible with replantation, reconstructing the penile stump or total phallic replacement with a free flap are the remaining options. The penile stump is initially managed by over-sewing the corpora and the urethra brought out to the skin and marsupialized as distally as possible. A perineal urethrostomy should be avoided if possible, to allow for the possibility of free flap phalloplasty in the future. Additionally, a split thickness skin graft may be required, depending on whether the native skin is salvageable.

Abrasions/Lacerations/Avulsion

Degloving injuries or lacerations to the penis can be closed primarily when the injury does not put the closure on tension. Split-thickness skin grafting can be performed if the injury is not possible without tension or if there is full thickness circumferential penile skin injury precluding closure. When the mechanism is due to the shear forces of a motor vehicle collision, the injury may be suitable for cleansing and immediate split-thickness skin grafting. However, in cases of a rotating machinery injury, the wound should be initially managed with wet-to-dry dressings to allow for demarcation of viable tissue.

Bites

Infection is one of the most devastating complications of penile bites and can occur in up to 30% of wounds. Immediate irrigation and debridement, along with broad-spectrum antibiotic prophylaxis and tetanus/rabies immunizations (when appropriate) are the mainstays of therapy followed by primary wound closure whenever possible. More extensive injuries may require mobilization of a local skin flap or skin grafting [34]. The wound must be free of infection with clean skin edges prior to reconstruction.

Burns

Initial management involves removal of clothing, aggressive fluid replacement, and Foley or suprapubic tube placement to measure urine output. Burns are stratified into three categories. First-degree burns involve only the epidermis and appear pink with significant pain. Second-degree burns involve the epidermis and papillary demise, and appear as pink, moist, tender skin with thin-walled blisters. First- and second-degree burns can be treated without debridement with 1% silver sulfadiazine. Third-degree burns are full-thickness, painless lesions that appear white or brown and firm. Third-degree burns require debridement of all nonviable tissue, as delay in surgical intervention leads to an increased incidence of infection, longer hospital stays, and risk of burn scar contracture [26]. Third-degree thermal burns should be immediately skin grafted. Electrical burns require careful evaluation of the depth and degree of the burn and should initially be managed conservatively to characterize the full extent of involvement. Often, they require serial debridement and extensive skin grafting.

Conclusions

Prompt diagnosis and treatment are required to avoid potentially devastating long-term physical, psychological, and functional sequel of traumatic penile injuries. Rapid treatment of most penile injuries will prevent the development of permanent sexual dysfunction. "Clinicians should initiate ancillary psychological, interpersonal, and/or reproductive counseling and therapy for patients with genital trauma when loss of sexual, urinary, and/or reproductive function is anticipated" (Guideline 33: Expert Opinion) [7].

References

1 Cerwinka, W.H. and Block, N.L. (2009). Civilian gunshot injuries of the penis: the Miami experience. *Urology* 73 (4): 877–880.

2 Brandes, S.B. and McAninch, J.W. External genital trauma: amputation, degloving, and burns. *Atlas Urol. Clin. N. Am.* 6 (2): 127–142.

3 Mohr, A.M., Pham, A.M., Lavery, R.F. et al. (2003). Management of trauma to the male external genitalia: the usefulness of American Association for the Surgery of Trauma organ injury scales. *J. Urol.* 170 (6 Pt 1): 2311–2315.

4 Phonsombat, S., Master, V.A., and McAninch, J.W. (2008). Penetrating external genital trauma: a 30-year single institution experience. *J. Urol.* 180 (1): 192–195; discussion 5–6.

5 Waxman, S., Beekley, A., Morey, A., and Soderdahl, D. (2009). Penetrating trauma to the external genitalia in Operation Iraqi Freedom. *Int. J. Impot. Res.* 21 (2): 145–148.

6 Paquette, E.L. (2007). Genitourinary trauma at a combat support hospital during Operation Iraqi Freedom: the impact of body armor. *J. Urol.* 177 (6): 2196–2199; discussion 9.

7 Morey, A.F., Brandes, S., Dugi, D.D. 3rd et al. (2014). Urotrauma: AUA guideline. *J. Urol.* 192 (2): 327–335.

8 El Atat, R., Sfaxi, M., Benslama, M.R. et al. (2008). Fracture of the penis: management and long-term results of surgical treatment. Experience in 300 cases. *J. Trauma* 64 (1): 121–125.

9 El-Assmy, A., El-Tholoth, H.S., Mohsen, T., and el Ibrahiem, H.I. (2010). Long-term outcome of surgical treatment of penile fracture complicated by urethral rupture. *J. Sex. Med.* 7 (11): 3784–3788.

10 Zargooshi, J. (2002). Penile fracture in Kermanshah, Iran: the long-term results of surgical treatment. *BJU Int.* 89 (9): 890–894.

11 Eke, N. (2002). Fracture of the penis. *Br. J. Surg.* 89 (5): 555–565.

12 El-Sherif, A.E., Dauleh, M., Allowneh, N., and Vijayan, P. (1991). Management of fracture of the penis in Qatar. *Br. J. Urol.* 68 (6): 622–625.

13 Koifman, L., Barros, R., Junior, R.A. et al. (2010). Penile fracture: diagnosis, treatment and outcomes of 150 patients. *Urology* 76 (6): 1488–1492.

14 Pariser, J.J., Pearce, S.M., Patel, S.G., and Bales, G.T. (2015). National patterns of urethral evaluation and risk factors for urethral injury in patients with penile fracture. *Urology* 86 (1): 181–186.

15 Cendron, M., Whitmore, K.E., Carpiniello, V. et al. (1990). Traumatic rupture of the corpus cavernosum: evaluation and management. *J. Urol.* 144 (4): 987–991.

16 Orvis, B.R. and McAninch, J.W. (1989). Penile rupture. *Urol. Clin. North Am.* 16 (2): 369–375.

17 El-Assmy, A., El-Tholoth, H.S., Abou-El-Ghar, M.E. et al. (2010). False penile fracture: value of different diagnostic approaches and long-term outcome of conservative and surgical management. *Urology* 75 (6): 1353–1356.

18 Ruckle, H.C., Hadley, H.R., and Lui, P.D. (1992). Fracture of penis: diagnosis and management. *Urology* 40 (1): 33–35.

19 Chilton, C.P., Castle, W.M., Westwood, C.A., and Pryor, J.P. (1982). Factors associated in the aetiology of Peyronie's disease. *Br. J. Urol.* 54: 748–750.

20 Jarow, J.P. and Lowe, F.C. (1997). Penile trauma: an etiologic factor in Peyronie's disease and erectile dysfunction. *J. Urol.* 158: 1388–1390.

21 Salvatierra, O. Jr., Rigdon, W.O., Norris, D.M., and Brady, T.W. (1969). Vietnam experience with 252 urological war injuries. *J. Urol.* 101 (4): 615–620.

22 Hudolin, T. and Hudolin, I. (2003). Surgical management of urogenital injuries at a war hospital in Bosnia-Hrzegovina, 1992 to 1995. *J. Urol.* 169 (4): 1357–1359.

23 Selikowitz, S.M. (1977). Penetrating high-velocity genitourinary injuries. Part II: ureteral, lower tract, and genital wounds. *Urology* 9 (5): 493–499.

24 Baltieri, D.A. and de Andrade, A.G. (2005). Transsexual genital self-mutilation. *Am. J. Forensic Med. Pathol.* 26 (3): 268–270.

25 Bhanganada, K., Chayavatana, T., Pongnumkul, C. et al. (1983). Surgical management of an epidemic of penile amputations in Siam. *Am. J. Surg.* 146 (3): 376–382.

26 Chang, A.J. and Brandes, S.B. Advances in diagnosis and Management of Genital Injuries. *Urol. Clin.* 40 (3): 427–438.

27 Gomes CM, Ribeiro-Filho L, Giron AM et al. Genital trauma due to animal bites. *J. Urol.* 165(1):80–3.

28 Michielsen, D., Van Hee, R., Neetens, C. et al. (1998). Burns to the genitalia and the perineum. *J. Urol.* 159 (2): 418–419.

29 McDougal, W.S., Peterson, H.D., Pruitt, B.A., and Persky, L. (1979). The thermally injured perineum. *J. Urol.* 121 (3): 320–323.

30 Peck, M.D., Boileau, M.A., Grube, B.J., and Heimbach, D.M. (1990). The management of burns to the perineum and genitals. *J. Burn Care Rehabil.* 11 (1): 54–56.

31 Harpole, B.G., Wibbenmeyer, L.A., and Erickson, B.A. (2014). Genital burns in the national burn repository: incidence, etiology, and impact on morbidity and mortality. *Urology* 83 (2): 298–302.

32 Choi, M.H., Kim, B., Ryu, J.A. et al. (2000). MR imaging of acute penile fracture. *Radiographics* 20 (5): 1397–1405.

33 Muglia V, Tucci S, Jr., Elias J, Jr et al. Magnetic resonance imaging of scrotal diseases: when it makes the difference. *Urology* 2002;59(3):419–23.

34 Morey, A.F., Metro, M.J., Carney, K.J. et al. (2004). Consensus on genitourinary trauma: external genitalia. *BJU Int.* 94 (4): 507–515.

35 Ghilan, A.M., Al-Asbahi, W.A., Ghafour, M.A. et al. (2008). Management of penile fractures. *Saudi Med. J.* 29 (10): 1443–1447.

36 Kunkle, D.A., Lebed, B.D., Mydlo, J.H., and Pontari, M.A. (2008). Evaluation and management of gunshot wounds of the penis: 20-year experience at an urban trauma center. *J. Trauma* 64 (4): 1038–1042.

37 Wei, F.C., McKee, N.H., Huerta, F.J., and Robinette, M.A. (1983). Microsurgical replantation of a completely amputated penis. *Ann. Plast. Surg.* 10 (4): 317–321.

38 Hayhurst, J.W., O'Brien, B.M., Ishida, H., and Baxter, T.J. (1974). Experimental digital replantation after prolonged cooling. *Hand* 6 (2): 134–141.

39 Ching, W.C., Liao, H.T., Ulusal, B.G. et al. (2010). Salvage of a complicated penis replantation using bipedicled scrotal flap following a prolonged ischaemia time. *J. Plast. Reconstr. Aesthet. Surg.* 63 (8): e639–e643.

40 Gamal WM, Osman MM, Hammady A et al. Penile fracture: long-term results of surgical and conservative management. *J. Trauma* 2011;71(2):491–3.

41 Yapanoglu, T., Aksoy, Y., Adanur, S. et al. (2009). Seventeen years' experience of penile fracture: conservative vs. surgical treatment. *J. Sex. Med.* 6 (7): 2058–2063.

42 Yamaçake, K.G.R., Tavares, A., Padovani, G.P. et al. (2013). Long-term treatment outcomes between surgical correction and conservative management for Penile fracture: retrospective analysis. *Korean J. Urol.* 54 (7): 472–476.

43 Kozacioglu, Z., Degirmenci, T., Arslan, M. et al. (2011). Long-term significance of the number of hours until surgical repair of penile fractures. *Urol. Int.* 87 (1): 75–79.

44 El-Assmy, A., El-Tholoth, H.S., Mohsen, T., and el Ibrahiem, H.I. (2011). Does timing of presentation of penile fracture affect outcome of surgical intervention? *Urology* 77 (6): 1388–1391.

45 Jolly, B.B., Sharma, S.K., Vaidyanathan, S., and Mandal, A.K. (1994). Gunshot wounds of the male external genitalia. *Urol. Int.* 53 (2): 92–96.

46 Banti, M., Walter, J., Hudak, S., and Soderdahl, D.J. (2016 Jan). Improvised explosive device-related lower genitourinary trauma in current overseas combat operations. *J. Trauma Acute Care Surg.* 80 (1): 131–134.

47 Biswas, G. (2013). Technical considerations and outcomes in penile replantation. *Semin Plast. Surg.* 27 (4): 205–210.

48 Roche, N.A., Vermeulen, B.T., Blondeel, P.N., and Stillaert, F.B. (2012). Technical recommendations for penile replantation based on lessons learned from penile reconstruction. *J. Reconstr. Microsurg.* 28 (4): 247–250.

14

Priapism

Akash A. Kapadia, Kevin Ostrowski, and Thomas J. Walsh

Department of Urology, University of Washington School of Medicine, Seattle, WA, USA

Introduction

Callaway first described priapism in the medical literature in 1824 where he referred to an erection that "occurred during but was not diminished by repeat connexion" [1]. The term priapism comes from Priapus, the Greek god of seduction, fertility, and sexuality, who was well-known for his large phallus. The natural history of untreated priapism was detailed by Frank Hinman, Sr. in 1914 [2], and since then multiple other sources have confirmed the severe consequences of untreated prolonged erections.

The American Urological Association (AUA) defines priapism as a persistent penile erection that continues hours beyond, or is unrelated to, sexual stimulation [3]. Three common types of priapism are described: ischemic (low-flow, veno-occlusive), non-ischemic (high-flow, arterial), and stuttering (intermittent, recurrent) priapism. This chapter aims to discuss the epidemiology, etiology, pathophysiology, and treatment for all types of priapism in a clinically oriented and practical manner.

Epidemiology

There is limited data evaluating the prevalence and incidence of priapism. The incidence in the general population is estimated as between 0.3 and 1.1 cases per 100 000 person-years in Europe [4, 5]. The expected prevalence is higher in the United States (U.S.), Latin America, and Africa, due to the higher incidence of hemoglobinopathies, especially sickle cell disease (SCD).

Multiple studies have tried to identify the incidence of ischemic priapism in patients with SCD, and have found the lifetime probability to be between 29 and 42% [4, 6]. A case series by Nelson and Winter found 23% of adult cases and 63% of pediatric cases of ischemic priapism to be related to SCD [7]. An international multi-center observation study of 130 men with SCD found a mean age of priapism onset at 11 years old with 25% presenting

A Clinical Guide to Urologic Emergencies, First Edition. Edited by Hunter Wessells, Shigeo Horie, and Reynaldo G. Gómez.
© 2021 John Wiley & Sons Ltd. Published 2021 by John Wiley & Sons Ltd.
Companion website: www.wiley.com/go/wessells/urologic

during pre-pubertal years [6]. Aliyu et al. estimated the prevalence of SCD in 2008 based upon data from the World Health Organization. According to the study, 20–25 million individuals worldwide have homozygous SCD: 12–15 M in sub-Saharan Africa, 5–10 M in India, and 3 M in other regions. As many as 70 000 patients with SCD live in the US [8]. As such, SCD-related priapism is estimated to affect six million individuals worldwide, assuming a 30% lifetime probability.

Information on non-ischemic priapism is exclusively based on reports from case series of patients with blunt perineal trauma [9].

Pathophysiology and Causes

Ischemic

Ischemic priapism is a penile compartment syndrome characterized by hypoxia, hypercapnia, and acidosis within the corpora cavernosa (Table 14.1). Smooth muscle exposure to this environment for a prolonged time can cause irreversible erectile damage from necrosis, inflammation, and eventual corporal fibrosis. Hypoxia in any area of the body activates endothelial cells which leads to a cascade of reactions characterized by increased neutrophil adhesion, decreased mitochondrial chain activity, and increased intracellular calcium. After re-establishing blood flow there is also reperfusion of ischemic tissues, which initiates the production of reactive oxygen species, leading to further cellular damage.

The majority of episodes of ischemic priapism are idiopathic; however, a detailed evaluation is required to exclude potential inciting events or influences. Causes of ischemic priapism include medications, illicit drug use, parenteral nutrition, hematologic/metabolic/neurologic diseases, and neoplasms (Table 14.2).

Drugs (prescription and recreational) are responsible for approximately 30% of ischemic priapism cases [11]. Intracavernosal injection of vasoactive drugs for the treatment of erectile dysfunction (ED) remains a major cause of priapism. The clinical trials of the Alprostadil Study Group found prolonged erection (4–6 hours) in 5% of subjects, with priapism (>6 hours) occurring in 1% of subjects [12]. Very few cases of ischemic priapism have been reported with PDE-5 inhibitors; the majority of these cases occur in men with increased risk for priapism [13].

Table 14.1 Blood gas findings in priapism.

	PO$_2$ (mmHg)	PCO$_2$ (mmHg)	pH
Normal arterial blood	>90	<40	7.40
Mixed venous blood	40	50	7.35
Ischemic priapism	<30	>60	<7.25
Nonischemic priapism	>90	<40	7.4

Adapted from Ref. [3].

Table 14.2 Etiology of ischemic priapism.

Medications	
Intracavernosal agents	Papaverine, prostaglandin 1, phenoxybenzamine, phentolamine
Central nervous system (CNS) agents	Trazodone, benzodiazepines, phenothiazines
PDE-5 inhibitors	Sildenafil, tadalafil, vardenafil
Anti-hypertensives	Prazosin, phenoxybenzamine, calcium channel blockers, beta blockers, hydralazine
Anti-coagulants	Heparin, warfarin
Hormones	Testosterone, gonadotropin releasing hormone, antiestrogens (tamoxifen)
Illicit Drugs	Cocaine, marijuana
Parenteral nutrition	High concentration lipid infusions
Hematologic Disorders:	
Hyperviscous and hyper-coagulable states	Polycythemia vera, Protein C deficiency, Protein S deficiency
Hemoglobinopathies	Sickle cell disease, thalassemias
Immunologic diseases	Lupus, protein C deficiencies
Metabolic diseases:	Gout, diabetes, nephrotic syndrome, renal failure, amyloidosis, Fabry's disease, hypertriglyceridemia
Neurologic diseases:	Spinal cord injuries, autonomic neuropathy, spinal stenosis
Neoplastic disorders:	Leukemia, multiple myeloma, prostate/bladder/ rectosigmoid/kidney cancers
Idiopathic	

Source: adapted from Ref. [3, 10].

Cocaine is an increasingly common cause of ischemic priapism. The mechanism is complex because it is both a norepinephrine re-uptake inhibitor (preventing detumescence) and serotonin re-uptake inhibitor (central nervous system [CNS] stimulation and peripheral vasodilation) [14, 15]. In addition to cocaine, marijuana has been associated with priapism.

Some anti-hypertensive drugs can cause priapism through alpha-adrenergic antagonism, which prevents, or delays physiologic detumescence [16]. This same mechanism is thought to underlie the risk of priapism resulting from use of psychotropic drugs such as tricyclic antidepressants and trazodone [11, 17].

Heparin and warfarin have been associated with ischemic priapism through a poorly understood mechanism. Singhal et al. found 17 of 3337 hemodialysis patients who received heparin experienced an acute episode of priapism [18]. The episode of priapism may be due to a relative hypercoagulable state after heparin therapy but more studies are needed [19]. The same mechanism is proposed in cases of priapism following parenteral nutrition. [20]

The most commonly known intrinsic causes of ischemic priapism are hematologic disorders. The prevalence of SCD in African Americans is 8%, with a significant number experiencing priapism both in pre-pubertal and post-pubertal years [21–23]. During penile erection, the deoxygenated hemoglobin S (HbS) polymerizes, injuring the sickled erythrocyte. This activates the cascade of hemolysis and vaso-occlusion. The damaged erythrocytes release free hemoglobin into the plasma, causing it to react with nitric oxide to produce methemoglobin and nitrate. This causes functional nitric oxide deficiency and contributes to the development of vasculopathy. In addition, as the ischemic corporal tissue is re-perfused, there is oxidative damage and free radical generation. All of these steps cause obstruction from venous outflow altering natural detumescence [24]. More recent animal studies have confirmed decreased nitric oxide and phosphodiesterase-5 (PDE-5) activity along with increased reactive oxygen species in penile tissue from transgenic sickle cell mice [25].

Malignant priapism is rare; however, most of the cancers associated with priapism are urological in nature (bladder 30%, prostate 30%, rectosigmoid colon 16%, kidney 11%). This is most likely due to venous obstruction in a pro-coagulant state. Direct occlusion of the corporal outflow by malignant infiltration is also possible [26].

Non-ischemic

Non-ischemic priapism is a result of unregulated increased cavernous arterial inflow causing penile tumescence [10]. In most cases a ruptured artery allows unregulated inflow of oxygenated blood to fill the sinusoids and results in penile erection of varying degrees. Venous drainage from the corpora cavernosa continues unabated, preventing stasis of blood flow and therefore tissue ischemia. This phenomenon explains why pain is not often a presenting symptom. Blunt or penetrating trauma resulting in laceration of the cavernous artery or one of its branches within the corpora is the most common cause. This causes an arterial-lacunar fistula leading to the unregulated release of endothelial nitric oxide. Nitric oxide is a potent vasodilator and prevents penile detumescence as well as clotting of the fistula [10].

Stuttering

Stuttering priapism is characterized by a pattern of recurrent ischemic priapism. This was first described by Hinman Sr. [2] and then further elucidated by Emond et al. with homozygous SCD patients in Jamaica [4]. They found a 42% prevalence rate with median age of onset of 21 years. They identified two predominant patterns: (i) short episodes lasting <3 hours with normal sexual function afterwards; and (ii) prolonged erections (normally >24 hours) commonly followed by ED [4]. A multicenter study of 130 patients with SCD found that 35% (46 pts) had a history of priapism with 75% occurring before the age of 20. Of these patients, 72% (33 pts) had stuttering priapism [6].

Evaluation and Diagnostic Workup

The AUA Guideline on the Management of Priapism from 2003 (updated in 2010) serve as the basis of evaluation and treatment for priapism [3]. The evaluation of patient with priapism includes a combination of detailed history, physical exam, laboratory work, and/or

Table 14.3 Clinical findings in priapism.

	Ischemic Priapism	Non-ischemic Priapism
Fully rigid corpora cavernosa	Usually	Rarely
Penile pain	Usually	Rarely
Abnormal penile blood gas	Usually	Rarely
Blood abnormalities and hematologic malignancy	Sometimes	Rarely
Recent intracavernous vasoactive drug injection	Sometimes	Rarely
Chronic, well tolerated tumescence without full rigidity	Rarely	Usually
Perineal Trauma	Rarely	Sometimes

Source: adapted from Ref. [3].

radiographic studies. A thorough history can help differentiate between an ischemic or non-ischemic condition, and must include specific information, such as duration of erection, degree of pain, use of medications or illicit drugs, history of blood dyscrasias, and history of pelvic or genital traumas. On physical exam, the corpora cavernosa are completely rigid and tender to palpation during ischemic priapism. During a non-ischemic event, however, the corpora cavernosa may be tumescent without complete rigidity and tenderness on examination (see Table 14.3).

Recommended laboratory studies include complete blood count (CBC) with differential, toxicology screening if clinical suspicion is present, and penile blood gas testing. A CBC can help rule out acute infections or dyscrasias, such as leukemia or platelet abnormalities. In cases with high index of suspicion, hemoglobin electrophoresis may help identify previously unknown hemoglobinopathies such as thalassemias in men of African, Mediterranean, or Southeast Asian descent. Other rare hematological disorders can be investigated on a case-by-case basis including Protein C and S deficiency; Factor V Leiden deficiency; Antithrombin III deficiency; Prothrombin gene mutation; and anti-phospholipid antibody.

Penile blood gas testing is essential in differentiating ischemic and non-ischemic priapism. Cavernosal blood in men with ischemic priapism typically appears dark due to severe hypoxia. A typical pattern of blood gas levels in ischemic priapism is as follows: PO_2 (partial pressure of oxygen) < 30, PCO_2 (partial pressure of carbon dioxide) > 60, and pH < 7.25. In contrast, aspirated blood in non-ischemic priapism is bright red due to adequate oxygenation. Expectedly, the blood gas pattern is as follows: $PO_2 > 90$, $PCO_2 < 40$, and pH ~ 7.4 (Table 14.1).

Color duplex ultrasonography can be performed as an alternative or an adjunct to penile blood gas study in order to differentiate the two etiologies. Ultrasonography can be particularly helpful when assessing the patient who may have undergone an intervention or shunt procedure. In ischemic priapism, cavernosal arteries typically demonstrate absent or significantly compromised blood flow velocities (Figure 14.1a); whereas, in non-ischemic priapism, blood velocities are much higher, normal or close to normal for a penile erection (Figure 14.1b). Further imaging studies, such as penile arteriography, can be performed with the intent of treatment with embolization if there is a high suspicion for cavernous artery fistula (Figure 14.1c).

(a)

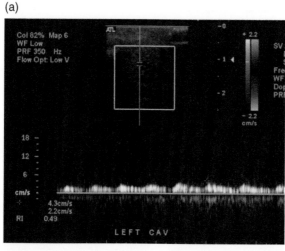

(b)   (c)

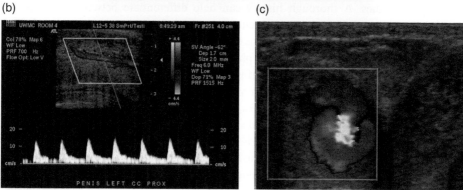

Figure 14.1   Penile ultrasonography of patients with priapism. (a) Color duplex Doppler ultrasound study of the left cavernosal artery demonstrating severely diminished peak systolic velocity (PSV) confirming ischemic priapism. (b) Color duplex Doppler ultrasound study demonstrating low-normal PSV suggestive of non-ischemic priapism. (c) Color Doppler ultrasound study of the corpora cavernosa demonstrating significant color flow on the right side, consistent with non-ischemic priapism due to a large anterio-venous fistula. *Source:* courtesy of H. Wessells, MD.

Treatment

Treatment for priapism is also directed by the AUA Guideline, and is based upon the type of priapism identified on evaluation. In the treatment of ischemic priapism, a step-wise approach is recommended as outlined in the algorithm in Figure 14.2. A penile block with or without systemic analgesia is initiated followed by aspiration/irrigation treatment. Data from Ateyah et al. [28] shows that a combination of aspiration with cold saline irrigation resolved 66 versus 24% with aspiration alone; however, irrigation is optional per the AUA Guideline [3].

Next, use of a sympathomimetic agent (phenylephrine) intracavernosally ranging from 100 to 500 μg/ml every three to five minutes for up to one hour is recommended. Notably, lower doses should be used in pediatric patients or patients with severe cardiovascular risk

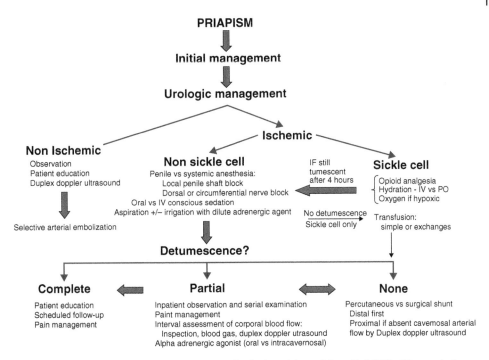

Figure 14.2 Algorithm for the management of priapism. Adapted from Ref. [27] with permission.

factors. Cardiovascular monitoring is also recommended (side effects of systemic phenylephrine include hypertensive crisis, reflex bradycardia, headache, and palpitations). If there is a failure of aspiration and repeated injections of a sympathomimetic agent, consideration of surgical intervention via shunt procedures should be made.

The type of surgical shunt procedure is chosen based upon the surgeon's experience; however, a corporoglanular (distal) shunt should be performed first, due to relative technical ease and fewer complications. Types of distal shunts are highlighted in Figure 14.3 and 14.4. As a general principle, less invasive distal shunts are recommended prior to more invasive proximal shunts, and success rates range from 66 to 74%. Of the distal shunts, the Al-Ghorab shunt (Figure 14.5) is the most effective, and can still be utilized after failure of other distal shunts. If distal shunts are unsuccessful, proximal shunts can be created between the corpus cavernosum and spongiosum (Quackels, Figure 14.6) or between corpus cavernosum and the saphenous vein (Grayhack). Proximal shunts are associated with higher rates of ED, but are effective in up to 77% of cases.

In non-ischemic priapism, observation is the initial form of management along with treatment of underlying conditions responsible for priapism. In selected cases, and after a detailed discussion, more invasive treatments can be considered. Androgen blockade is an effective treatment thought to be due to limiting nocturnal penile blood flow possibly causing spontaneous closure of the cavernous artery fistula [30]. Embolization using absorbable material is the first-line invasive treatment option. Surgical management with fistula ligation is a last resort. Selective arterial embolization offers a 90% success rate; however, 7–27% of temporary arterial embolization may recur. There has been a gradual

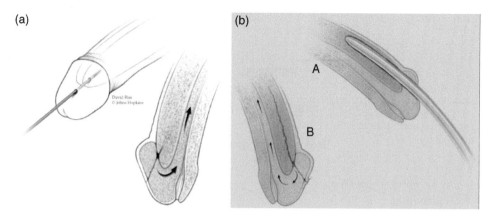

Figure 14.3 Conceptual basis for distal shunts for ischemic priapism. Note the larger connection created using the T shunt with "Snake" procedure (b) versus Winter shunt (a). Taken from Ref. [10] with permission.

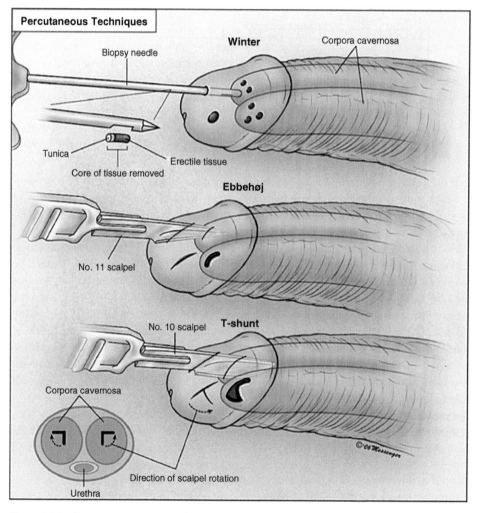

Figure 14.4 Percutaneous cavernosal spongiosal shunts. Top: Winter shunt with percutaneous needle perforation of distal tunica albuginea creating small opening(s) between cavernosum and spongiosum. Middle: Ebbehoj shunt in which scalpel is used to make opening in tunica. Bottom: T shunt with larger opening in tunica, through which one can perform "Snake" procedure (see Figure 14.3). Taken from Ref. [40] with permission.

Figure 14.5 Al-Ghorab distal shunt in which a transverse incision in the glans allows access to the tip of each corpus cavernosum, from which a small circle of tunica albuginea is excised to create a large bore shunt. Taken from Ref. [29] with permission.

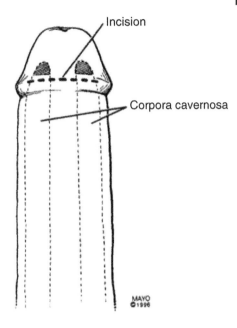

Incision

Corpora cavernosa

MAYO
©1996

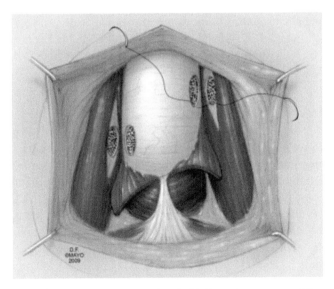

D.F.
©MAYO
2009

Figure 14.6 Proximal shunt (Quackel's). Note the shunts are bilateral in this depiction, offset in the proximal-distal axis so that the corpus spongiosum can be effectively approximated to the respective corpus cavernosum. Taken from Ref. [10] with permission.

evolution of treatment over the years, and there still remains a great paucity in the literature with a little over 100 reported cases. In a case series of 15 patients, approximately 20% of patients noticed a decrease in erectile quality and mean post-procedure International Index of Erectile Function (IIEF) score of 26.3 [31, 32].

In stuttering priapism, the goal is to prevent future episodes while management of each episode should follow the ischemic priapism management pathway (see above).

Table 14.4 Treatment options for stuttering priapism.

Medication	Administration	Side Effects
Antiandrogens	Oral	Gynecomastia, peripheral edema, anemia, hepatotoxicity, vasomotor effects
GNRH agonists or antagonists	Intramuscular	Gynecomastia, vasomotor effects, fatigue, osteoporosis, depression, etc.
Baclofen	Oral	Sedition, dizziness, fatigue, confusion, visual problems, etc.
Digoxin	Oral	Cardiac, gastrointestinal, gynecomastia, dizziness, visual problems
Alpha adrenergic agonists	Intracavernosal or Oral	Hypertension, bradycardia, headaches, palpitations
Gabapentin	Oral	Leukopenia, dizziness, fatigue, ataxia, weight gain, vision problems
Ketoconazole	Oral	Hepatotoxicity, gastrointestinal weakness, etc.

Adapted from Ref.[33].

Anti-androgens or agonists of gonadotropin-releasing hormones are an option in post-pubertal males. Self-administered phenylephrine intracavernosally should be discussed in patients not responding or not interested in systemic treatment. PDE-5 inhibitors have shown inconsistent results but may help some patients with stuttering priapism. Table 14.4 shows additional options of treatment for stuttering priapism.

Effects of Priapism on Erectile Function

The duration of priapism is the most important predictor of erectile function recovery after treatment. Bennett et al. reported on 39 SCD patients with priapism and found that all patients with priapism of more than 12 hours noted a decrease in penile rigidity. Return of spontaneous functional erections with or without sildenafil was: 100% (<12 hours), 78% (12–14 hours), 44% (24–36 hours), and 0% (>36 hours) [34]. Prolonged episodes of priapism can cause severe corporeal fibrosis that makes placement of a penile prosthesis technically difficult. This is associated with use of smaller-sized penile implants and a higher rate of complications compared to standard inflatable penile prosthesis placement [35]. Tausch et al. described placement of a malleable prosthesis as a treatment for refractory ischemic priapism [36, 37]. There is increasing evidence that early insertion of a semi-rigid device for refractory ischemic priapism is easier, more cost-effective, with lower complication rates, and allows for upsizing to a larger inflatable penile prosthesis at a later time [38, 39]

Summary

Prolonged erection persisting or unrelated to sexual stimulation requires emergency evaluation and determination of ischemic versus non-ischemic priapism. Ischemic priapism is a medical emergency and must be managed in a methodical fashion with early evaluation and intervention providing the best erectile function outcomes. Non-ischemic priapism is often caused by an arterial-lacunar fistula after perineal trauma and is not a medical emergency. Stuttering priapism, often seen in SCD, can be difficult to treat and each episode should be treated like ischemic priapism with multiple pharmacological prevention strategies available.

References

1 Callaway, T. (1824). Unusual case of priapism. *London Med. Rep.* 1: 286–287.

2 Hinman, F. (1914). Priapism: report of cases and clinical study of the literature with reference to its pathogenesis and surgical treatment. *Ann. Surg.* 60 (6): 689–716.

3 Montague, D., Jarow, J., Broderick, G. et al. (2003). American Urological Association guideline on the management of priapism. *J. Urol.* 170 (4): 1318–1324.

4 Emond, A., Holman, R., Hayes, R. et al. (1980). Priapism and impotence in homozygous sickle cell disease. *Arch. Intern. Med.* 140 (11): 1434–1437.

5 Kulmala, R., Lehtonen, T., and Tammela, T. (1995). Priapism, its incidence and seasonal distribution in Finland. *Scand. J. Urol. Nephrol.* 29 (1): 93–96.

6 Adeyoju, A., Olujohungbe, A., Morris, J. et al. (2002). Priapism in sickle-cell disease; incidence, risk factors and complications – an international multicentre study. *BJU Int.* 90 (9): 898–902.

7 Nelson, J. and Winter, C. (1977). Priapism: evolution of management in 48 patients in a 22-year series. *J. Urol.* 117 (4): 455–458.

8 Aliyu, Z., Kato, G., Taylor, J. et al. (2008). Sickle cell disease and pulmonary hypertension in Africa: a global perspective and review of epidemiology, pathophysiology, and management. *Am. J. Hematol.* 83 (1): 63–70.

9 Salonia, A., Eardley, I., Giuliano, F. et al. (2014). European Association of Urology guidelines on priapism. *Eur. Urol.* 65 (2): 480–489.

10 Broderick, G. (2021). Priapism. In: *Campbell-Walsh-Wein Urology* (ed. P.D.K. Peters) Chapter 27, 1539–1563. Elsevier.

11 Baños, J., Bosch, F., and Farré, M. (1989). Drug-induced priapism. Its aetiology, incidence and treatment. *Med. Toxicol. Adverse Drug Exp.* 4 (1): 46–58.

12 Porst, H. (1996). The rationale for prostaglandin E1 in erectile failure: a survey of worldwide experience. *J. Urol.* 155 (3): 802–815.

13 Broderick, G., Kadioglu, A., Bivalacqua, T. et al. (2010). Priapism: pathogenesis, epidemiology, and management. *J. Sex. Med.* 7 (1): 476–500.

14 Cocores, J., Dackis, C., and Gold, M. (1986). Sexual dysfunction secondary to cocaine abuse in two patients. *J. Clin. Psychiatry* 47 (7): 384–385.

15 Lakoski, J. and Cunningham, K. (1988). Cocaine interaction with central monoaminergic systems: electrophysiological approaches. *Trends Pharmacol. Sci.* 9 (5): 177–180.

16 Rubin, S. (1968). Priapism as a probable sequel to medication. *Scand. J. Urol. Nephrol.* 2 (2): 81–85.

17 Hanno, P., Lopez, R., and Wein, A. (1988). Trazodone-induced priapism. *Br. J. Urol.* 61 (1): 94.

18 Singhal, P., Lynn, R., and Scharschmidt, L. (1986). Priapism and dialysis. *Am. J. Neprol.* 6 (5): 358–361.

19 Burke, B., Scott, G., Smith, P. et al. (1983). Heparin-associated priapism. *Postgrad. Med. J.* 59 (691): 332–333.

20 Klein, E., Montague, D., and Steiger, E. (1985). Priapism associated with the use of intravenous fat emulsion: case reports and postulated pathogenesis. *J. Urol.* 133 (5): 857–859.

21 Fowler, J., Koshy, M., Strub, M. et al. (1991). Priapism associated with the sickle cell hemoglobinopathies: prevalence, natural history and sequelae. *J. Urol.* 145 (1): 65–68.

22 Hamre, M., Harmon, E., Kirkpatrick, D. et al. (1991). Priapism as a complication of sickle cell disease. *J. Urol.* 145 (1): 1–5.

23 Winter, C. and McDowell, G. (1988). Experience with 105 patients with priapism: update review of all aspects. *J. Urol.* 140 (5): 980–983.

24 Kato, G., Gladwin, M., and Steinberg, M. (2007). Deconstructing sickle cell disease: reappraisal of the role of hemolysis in the development of clinical subphenotypes. *Blood Rev.* 21 (1): 37–47.

25 Sopko, N., Matsui, H., Hannan, J. et al. (2015). Subacute hemolysis in sickle cell mice causes priapism secondary to NO imbalance and PDE5 dysregulation. *J. Sex. Med.* 12 (9): 1878–1885.

26 Huang, Y.C., Harraz, A., Shindel, A. et al. (2009). Evaluation and management of priapism: 2009 update. *Nat. Rev. Urol.* 6 (5): 262–271.

27 Berger, R., Billups, K., Brock, G. et al. (2001). Thought Leader Panel on Evaluation and Treatment of Priapism. Report of the American Foundation for Urologic Disease (AFUD). *Int J Impot Res.* 13 (suppl 5): S39–S43.

28 Ateyah, A., Rahman El-Nashar, A., Zohdy, A. et al. (2005). Intracavernosal irrigation by cold saline as a simple method of treating iatrogenic prolonged erection. *J. Sex. Med.* 2 (2): 248–253.

29 Harmon, W.J. and Nehra, A. (1997). Priapism: diagnosis and management. *Mayo Clin Proc.* 72 (4): 350–355.

30 Mwamukonda, K., Chi, T., Shindel, A. et al. (2010). Androgen blockade for treatment of high-flow priapism. *J. Sex. Med.* 7 (7): 2532–2537.

31 Kuefer, R., Bartsch, G., Herkommer, K. et al. (2005). Changing diagnostic and therapeutic concepts in high-flow priapism. *Int. J. Impot. Res.* 17 (2): 109–113.

32 Savoca, G., Pietropaolo, F., Scieri, F. et al. (2004). Sexual function after highly selective embolization of cavernous artery in patients with high flow priapism: long-term followup. *J. Urol.* 172 (2): 644–647.

33 O'Brien, K. and Munnariz, R. (2013). Priapism. In: *Urological Emergencies: A Practical Guide*, 2e (ed. H. Wessells). New York: Springer.

34 Bennett, N. and Mulhall, J. (2008). Sickle cell disease status and outcomes of African-American men presenting with priapism. *J. Sex. Med.* 5 (5): 1244–1250.

35 Trost, L., Patil, M., and Kramer, A. (2015). Critical appraisal and review of management strategies for severe fibrosis during penile implant surgery. *J. Sex. Med.* 12 (7): 439–447.

36 Tausch, T., Evans, A., and Morey, A. (2007). Immediate insertion of a semirigid penile prosthesis for refractor ischemic priapism. *Mil. Med.* 172 (11): 1211–1212.

37 Tausch, T., Zhao, L., and Morey, A. (2015). Malleable penile prosthesis is a cost-effective treatment for refractory ischemic priapism. *J. Sex. Med.* 12 (3): 824–826.

38 Zacharakis, E., Garaffa, G., Raheem, A. et al. (2014). Penile prosthesis insertion in patients with refractor ischaemic priapism: early vs delayed implantation. *BJU Int.* 114 (4): 576–581.

39 Zacharakis, E., De Luca, F., Raheem, A. et al. (2015). Early insertion of a malleable penile prosthesis in ischaemic priapism allows later upsizing of the cylinders. *Scan. J. Urol.* 49 (6): 468–471.

40 Burnett, A.L. and Sharlip, I.D. (2013). Standard operating procedures for priapism. *J Sex Med.* 10 (1): 180–194. (Wiley on line library).

15

Traumatic Scrotal and Testicular Injuries

Marios Hadjipavlou[1] and Davendra Sharma[2]

[1] Guy's Hospital, London, UK
[2] St George's Hospital, London, UK

Introduction

Traumatic injury of the scrotum and its contents is uncommon. The structures are relatively protected by the dependent and mobile nature of their anatomy. However, severe testicular trauma resulting in organ loss can affect fertility, contribute to hypogonadism, and affect social confidence and psychological well-being [1]. Prompt assessment and operative intervention, when required, is important to preserve normal testicular function.

Blunt scrotal trauma can cause scrotal skin ecchymosis, testicular hematoma, hematocele, testicular rupture, or dislocation. Blunt injuries account for 75–85% of cases, the majority of which are sustained during assault or sporting injury [2–5]. Less common mechanisms of injury are occupational accidents or motor vehicle collisions [5].

External genital injuries form up to 40–60% of all penetrating genitourinary trauma [4, 6]. While bilateral testicular injury is very rare in blunt trauma, it may be present in up to 30% of all penetrating scrotal injuries [5–8]. The most common causes for penetrating scrotal injuries in civilian series are gunshot wounds (55–95%), stab wounds (5–42%), and animal bites [6, 9]. Legal intoxication is often present in patients with penetrating external genital trauma [10].

External genital injuries have increased in the modern battlefield due to blast injuries from fragmentation devices and the lack of protective armor for the genital area [11]. These devastating injuries are associated with lower limb injury, pelvic fracture, and a high mortality [12]. Progress has been made with the development of protective equipment, survival (via advanced combat casualty care), and acute sperm retrieval [12–15].

The American Association for the Surgery of Trauma (AAST) produced a five grade scale system for scrotal (Table 15.1) and testicular (Table 15.2) injuries.

A Clinical Guide to Urologic Emergencies, First Edition. Edited by Hunter Wessells, Shigeo Horie, and Reynaldo G. Gómez.
© 2021 John Wiley & Sons Ltd. Published 2021 by John Wiley & Sons Ltd.
Companion website: www.wiley.com/go/wessells/urologic

Table 15.1 AAST scrotal injury scale [16].

Scrotum Injury Scale	
Grade	**Description of Injury**
I	Contusion
II	Laceration <25% of scrotal diameter
III	Laceration ≥25% of scrotal diameter
IV	Avulsion <50%
V	Avulsion ≥50%

Table 15.2 AAST testicular injury scale [16].

Testis Injury Scale	
Grade[a]	**Description of Injury**
I	Contusion/hematoma
II	Subclinical laceration of tunica albuginea
III	Laceration of tunica albuginea with <50% parenchymal loss
IV	Major laceration of tunica albuginea with ≥50% parenchymal loss
V	Total testicular destruction or avulsion

[a]Advance one grade for bilateral lesions up to grade V.

General Evaluation

The history should include the mechanism of injury, symptoms, and previous scrotal pathology or surgery. On physical examination, the injured scrotum is often difficult to palpate due to swelling and marked tenderness, making it challenging to assess the integrity of the testes. The degree of scrotal ecchymosis, swelling, and hematoma may not correlate with the severity of testicular injury, while lack of these signs does not always rule out testicular rupture [17]. An empty ecchymotic hemiscrotum should raise suspicion of testicular dislocation. A scrotal injury in the presence of blood at the urethral meatus and inability to void should raise the suspicion of associated urethral injury, particularly with penetrating mechanisms. Visible or microscopic haematuria should prompt the clinician to consider concomitant urinary tract injuries.

Imaging

Over the past 30 years, ultrasonography has proven a useful adjunct to clinical examination and forms the preferred non-invasive imaging modality in scrotal trauma. High-frequency real-time ultrasound using a linear transducer (>7.5 MHz) and grayscale, color, and Doppler flow technique in experienced hands is the modality of choice [18].

Testicular rupture may appear as a discontinuity of the tunica albuginea with an associated contour abnormality due to protrusion of the testicular parenchyma [18]. Heterogeneous echogenicity within the testis is considered a pathognomonic sign of rupture (Figure 15.1). Fracture of the tunica albuginea alone was used as the criterion for diagnosing testicular rupture; however, this has since been shown to have poor sensitivity [19–21]. Scrotal ultrasonography can be up to 100% sensitive in diagnosing testicular rupture and should prompt urgent surgical exploration [22].

Disruption of the tunica vasculosa, the layer underlying tunica albuginea comprising of internal capsular vessels, may result in loss of vascularity in a testicular segment [21]. Contusions, hematoceles, testicular dislocations, intratesticular hematomas, and testicular ruptures can also be visualized (Figure 15.2) [1].

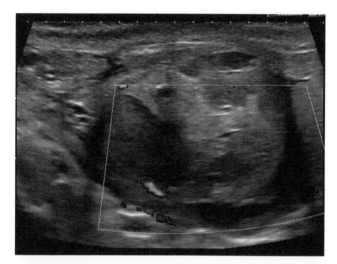

Figure 15.1 Ultrasonography demonstrating irregular hypoechoic regions with absent Doppler flow and increased peripheral flow. Surrounding fluid is evident. Although tunica albuginea appears intact, the features are highly suspicious of testicular rupture and emergency surgical exploration is indicated. *Source:* courtesy of Davendra Sharma, OBE, FRCS.

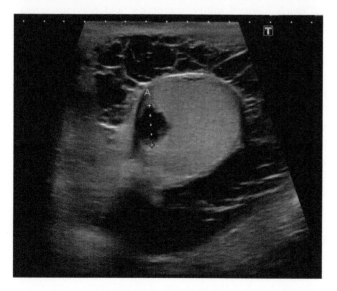

Figure 15.2 Ultrasonography demonstrating a 1-cm intratesticular hematoma. *Source:* courtesy of Davendra Sharma, OBE, FRCS.

Figure 15.3 Axial CT scan demonstrating dislocated right testis lying within inguinal canal. *Source:* courtesy of Davendra Sharma, OBE, FRCS.

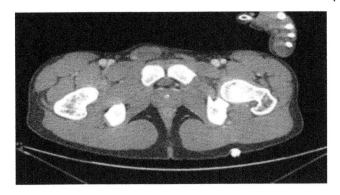

Magnetic resonance imaging (MRI) has been proposed when ultrasonography is inconclusive; however, it does not improve testicular rupture detection [23]. Furthermore, it is time-consuming, logistically difficult, and can potentially delay surgical exploration and repair.

Computed tomography may be useful in suspected testicular dislocation to reveal the position of the displaced testicle (Figure 15.3). Ultrasonography may not always identify the testis; however, if found, color-flow Doppler can assist in evaluating its viability [24].

Management

Acute Management

The majority of scrotal trauma are isolated injuries. Trauma principles should be followed in polytrauma patients, who require a multidisciplinary approach. For penetrating scrotal injuries, prophylactic antibiotics and tetanus prophylaxis are recommended [25].

Scrotal Skin Injuries and Scrotal Reconstruction

Lacerations of the scrotal skin can be closed primarily when there is no suspicion of injury to the scrotal organs. A layered closure of the deep fascia and skin using absorbable interrupted sutures reduces the likelihood of ischemia and allows for drainage between the sutures [6]. If wound contamination is present, extensive washout, and debridement of infected and necrotic scrotal tissue should be undertaken (Figure 15.4). Meticulous hemostasis is important as the low scrotal pressure allows for hematoma development without tamponade. A Penrose drain can be used to limit the amount of hematoma formation [26]. Non-occlusive fine mesh oil emulsion impregnated wound dressings can be applied on the wound, supported by gauze and scrotal support underwear.

The dependent nature of the scrotum allows for extensive mobilization and primary closure of most defects. However, in the presence of scrotal avulsion or when surgical debridement results in significant scrotal skin loss, scrotal reconstruction may be required. The use of vacuum-assisted closure (VAC) systems can be used as temporary coverage for large soft tissue defects requiring multiple surgical debridements and

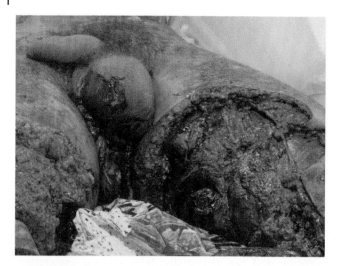

Figure 15.4 Extensive debridement following skin and soft tissue injury including scrotal, perineal, and inner thigh skin loss due to improvised explosive devices (IED)-related injury. *Source:* courtesy of Davendra Sharma, OBE, FRCS.

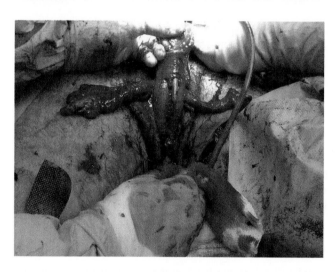

Figure 15.5 Severe IED-related perineal trauma resulting in complete loss of scrotal skin and penoscrotal and most of proximal/mid penile urethra. Note exposed urethral catheter in midurethra. *Source:* courtesy of Davendra Sharma, OBE, FRCS.

reconstructions [27]. Such systems generate a negative topical pressure gradient and increase granulation tissue formation on the wound surface [28]. In the initial management, meticulous wound care with subsequent skin grafting is now the option of choice in most cases (Figure 15.5). Testes and spermatic cords can be buried in a lateral thigh pouch or in a subcutaneous abdominal pouch, but this is rarely necessary. Avulsed skin may occasionally be preserved and prepared for full- or split-thickness skin grafting. In the absence of devastating burns or massive skin injuries, an interval of local care and dressing changes with saline-soaked gauze is favored over immediate grafting [26]. This allows wound decontamination and allows tissue granulation following which split-thickness skin grafts can be used from thigh donor sites [26]. Meshing of the skin graft allows exudate to escape from the interstices, which improves graft take while delivering a good cosmetic result. The spermatic cords and testes may be sewn together before grafting to prevent a bifid neoscrotum.

Thigh flaps can be used for reconstruction when testes have been buried in a thigh pouch [17]. Arrest of spermatogenesis has been shown following scrotal reconstruction with a flap; however, thin-trimming of the reconstruction flap may reverse spermatogenesis arrest [29].

While isolated genital burn injuries are uncommon, they may be present in up to 13% of patients admitted to burns units. Most common causes are flames, hot liquids, and chemical agents. Genital burn management should involve removal of any retained material or clothing followed by cooling down with water. Physiological dressings and topical antibiotics should be applied, while epidermal allografts may enhance epithelialization and reduce hypertrophic scar formation [30]. Urgent debridement is rarely necessary, as structures that appear non-viable may often recover. Conservative approach of even second-degree burns may lead to successful outcome in 61–90% of cases [31]. In third-degree burns or when conservative management of second-degree burns fail, debridement and tissue grafting may be required.

Hematocele

Hematocele is an extratesticular injury in which bleeding is confined within the tunica vaginalis [18]. Small hematoceles may be managed conservatively with elevation, ice packs, non-steroidal anti-inflammatory drugs, bed rest, and close monitoring [32]. Delayed surgical intervention may be necessary in cases of suspected infection or undue pain [25]. Scrotal exploration is indicated when a hematocele is greater than 5 cm or expanding or causes extrinsic compression on surrounding blood vessels and reduced flow on Doppler ultrasonography [18, 33, 34]. Furthermore, ultrasonography may not be able to demonstrate a tunica rupture in the presence of a large hematocele. These cases should be managed operatively with scrotal exploration, evaluation of the blood clot, and meticulous hemostasis, even in the absence of testicular rupture.

Intratesticular Hematoma

Small hematomas confined within the tunica albuginea, with no evidence of rupture, can be managed non-operatively with serial ultrasound examinations until their resolution [21, 33]. Large intratesticular hematomas are best managed by drainage to reduce the risk of pressure necrosis, atrophy, and orchiectomy [2, 18].

Testicular Rupture

The incidence of testicular rupture may be up to 50% in blunt scrotal injuries [2]. Blunt scrotal trauma patients were originally treated conservatively with surgical interventions reserved only when complications arose [35]. In 1969, Gross reported the importance of early exploration and repair. There is no role for conservative management of testicular rupture in contemporary practice [36]. Early surgical intervention may result in testicular preservation in over 90% of cases, while intervention after three days results in orchiectomy rates of 45–50% [2]. Early repair preserves hormonal function and may preserve fertility [37]. Surgical management involves exploration and evacuation of hematoma, excision of any necrotic testicular tubules, and closure of the tunica albuginea, most often with continuous absorbable suture material [25, 35].

Testicular Dislocation and Testicular Torsion

Traumatic dislocation of the testicle rarely happens in victims of motor vehicle collisions. The testis may dislocate subcutaneously with epifascial displacement. The superficial inguinal area is the most common site of dislocation, with perineal, retrovesical, or acetabular regions being less common [18]. Dislocation can occur in blunt abdominal trauma and may often be missed [38]. It occurs rarely and is most common in victims of motorbike accidents as rapid deceleration can cause collision of the scrotum and perineum against the fuel tank resulting in proximal organ displacement [38–43]. Bilateral testicular dislocation has been reported in high impact collisions [43, 44]. Manual repositioning should be attempted with secondary orchidopexy. If this cannot be performed, immediate orchidopexy is indicated [24]. Trauma-induced testicular torsion has also been widely reported in the literature, possibly as a result of forceful contraction of the cremaster muscles [45–47]. Principles of urgent scrotal exploration and orchidopexy apply, as with spontaneous cases.

Extensive destruction of tunica albuginea or excessive testicular swelling may not allow for approximation and closure of the tunica albuginea. In these cases, the parietal lamina of tunica vaginalis can be mobilized as a graft or used as a vascularized flap and sutured to cover the defect.

Penetrating Scrotal Injury

Penetrating injuries to the scrotum generally require surgical exploration with debridement of non-viable tissue. Primary approximation and closure are easily performed in most cases. When complete disruption of the spermatic cord is present, vascular realignment without vaso-vasostomy can be considered when technically feasible [25, 48, 49]. Microsurgical reconstruction of the vas deferens should only be performed in the hemodynamically stable patient or as a secondary surgical procedure.

Testicular salvage in civilian gunshot injuries may be as low as 10%; however, contemporary series show that up to 75% of testes may be successfully reconstructed [6, 50]. When extensive destruction of the tunica albuginea is present, a tunica vaginalis flap can be used. Synthetic grafts should be avoided due to the high infection rate [51]. If there is extensive testicular injury where reconstruction cannot be achieved or the patient is hemodynamically unstable, orchiectomy is indicated [25]. If both testes are not salvageable, acute sperm retrieval should be considered for future assisted reproduction [15, 52]. Consent should be obtained for cryopreservation with clear guidance on future use of the gametes.

Combat-Related Scrotal Injuries

The majority of urological injuries in modern warfare involve the pelvic organs and external genitalia. It is thought that the shift away from torso injuries is due to the use of body armor and the prevalence of ground-level fragmentation devices [11, 13].

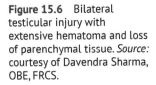

Figure 15.6 Bilateral testicular injury with extensive hematoma and loss of parenchymal tissue. *Source:* courtesy of Davendra Sharma, OBE, FRCS.

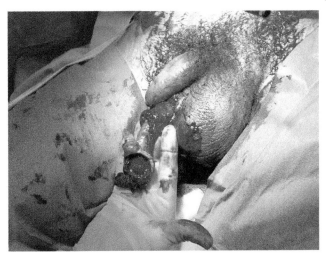

Pelviperineal injuries, primarily due to improvised explosive devices, accounted for 118 (5.4%) of UK military trauma patients with a mortality of 47% [12]. Combined perineal and pelvic fracture injuries have a significantly higher mortality compared to perineal injuries alone (41 vs. 18%) [12]. During the Iraq war, 34% of lower genitourinary trauma cases in a single hospital were scrotal with a high salvage rate of 86%. The leading cause for death in the cohort was associated major blood vessel injury [53]. As a result, modern modified body armors include a detachable flap to protect the genital and medial groin regions [54].

In the setting of traumatic testicular loss in the polytrauma patient, the focus of treatment is damage control by hemostasis, resuscitation, and management of concurrent life-threatening injuries. Multiple reoperations may commonly be required to control infection in combat wounds, which may implicate atypical infections, such as fungal organisms, making management even more challenging [55]. Uncompromising initial debridement, immediate fecal diversion, urinary diversion, and early enteral feeding is recommended in severe pelviperineal trauma (Figure 15.6) [12]. Patterns of survivable injury in warfare have changed in recent years as wounding mechanisms have altered, ballistic protection has improved, and the military chain of trauma care and expertise has evolved [14].

Servicemen that have suffered extensive genital injury highly rate the importance of sexual function as a part of their lives prior to injury. The majority describe their genital injury more important than losing their legs [56]. Close involvement of clinical psychologists is important from the earlier stages. Patients seem to come to terms with their injuries far better if they have fertility preserved or a sperm sample saved. Early aggressive intervention to ensure samples are taken is required. In the United Kingdom, a process for acute sperm retrieval has been developed to meet the injured servicemen's needs, with follow-up to ensure that fertility is preserved through hormonal and surgical interventions [56]. This effort should serve as a model for other countries.

Considerations

Infection

Breach of scrotal skin poses the risk of infection. Antibiotic prophylaxis is therefore recommended for all scrotal penetrating trauma, although data to support this practice is lacking [25]. Animal bites to the scrotum are rare but carry a significant risk of infection. Animal bites are most prevalent in the pediatric population (60–70%) and are mostly from dog attacks (80%) [57, 58]. The relative risk for a dog attack by a German Shepherd or a Doberman may be five times higher than that of a Labrador/retriever or cross-breed [59]. The most common bacterial infection by a dog is *Pasteurella* sp. followed by anaerobic organisms. *Staphylococcus aureus* is the most common aerobic organism occurring in 20–30% of infected dog bite wounds [60]. Other pathogens include *Streptococcus* sp., *Corynebacterium* sp., *Eikenella corrodens,* and *Capnocytaphaga canimorsus* [61]. Surgical exploration with debridement should include thorough irrigation with normal saline followed by daily wound care and further debridement if necessary. Penicillin-based broad-spectrum antibiotic prophylaxis should be administered. Amoxicillin with a beta-lactamase inhibitor (co-amoxiclav) is the first-choice antibiotic [61]. Cephalosporins, erythromycin, or doxycycline may also be considered. There is no consensus on the length of duration; however, 5–7 days of oral treatment for prophylaxis and 7–14 days for treatment of an established infection is recommended [61]. Rabies should be considered for wild as well as for domestic animal bites, especially in endemic rural areas of Africa and Asia. Post-exposure vaccination should be administered in such cases. Tetanus immunization status should be assessed as tetanus immunoglobulin and tetanus toxoid may be required. Human saliva carries a broader range of pathogens than in animals – transmission of viral infections including hepatitis and HIV is possible [26].

Future Fertility

Experimental data in rats suggest that unilateral testicular trauma can significantly reduce fertility to 27% with the contralateral testis showing decreased volume, smaller seminiferous tubular diameters, and various degree of aspermatogenesis due to immunological etiology [62]. A study on pre-pubertal rats showed that even grade I unilateral blunt testicular injury can significantly affect germ cell maturation in both ipsilateral and contralateral testis and alter the sex hormone profile [63]. Another study examined 80 post-pubertal rats subjected to blunt and penetrating unilateral testicular injuries managed by conservative approach, orchiectomy, or repair with sutures or mesh. Fertility rates were significantly lower in all post-injury groups, except the orchiectomy group with histological changes and impaired spermatogenesis in all groups, regardless of treatment group. Contrary to the former studies, contralateral testes showed no evidence of autoimmune injury and showed normal histology [64].

Trauma cases have a notoriously low follow-up rate, therefore analysis of any long-term outcomes is limited. It is estimated that only 22–40% of trauma cases are followed up due to a variety of reasons (resolution of symptoms, socioeconomic factors, incarceration status, or hospitalization for confounding mental illness) [6, 9, 10].

Small case series and case reports suggest that testicular salvage with early testicular repair protects fertility [37, 65]. Testicular atrophy after testicular injury is common and semen analysis may show objective signs of subfertility: oligospermia, asthenospermia, and low sperm motility [37]. Antisperm antibodies can develop; however, levels are unlikely to be clinically significant, therefore subfertility is less likely to be immune-mediated [37]. Sperm density may be reduced but is reported to remain within the normal range following unilateral orchiectomy [65].

Preservation of sperm and testicular tissue has been used for patients with threatened future reproductive function similar to testicular cancer management. This intra-operative practice should be considered in patients with injury to their single testis or patients with bilateral testicular trauma [15, 66, 67]. Acute sperm retrieval can be performed and sperm can be aspirated from the vas deferens, seminal vesicle, or epididymis at the time of surgery [15, 52, 68]. This practice has been observed in severely injured UK soldiers with successful conception achieved in patients with bilateral testicular loss [69]. Testicular replantation can be attempted in selected cases [70]. Sperm retrieval may also be attempted for cryopreservation from semen specimens following surgery [67]. Sperm cryopreservation is also now being offered to British Armed Forces prior to deployment and should be considered in military personnel at high risk of sustaining scrotal injuries to reduce stress in future family planning [71].

As with posthumous sperm extraction, retrieving sperm in an unconscious patient raises several ethical considerations with regards to consent, religion, and the legal rights of the partner and child if this process leads to a live birth [72].

Endocrine

There is conflicting evidence on the effect of testicular trauma on gonadal endocrine function. Kukadia et al. followed eight patients who had normal serum hormonal profiles following operative management [37]. In a seven patient case series, Lin et al. found that baseline follicle stimulating hormone (FSH), luteinizing hormone (LH), and post-stimulation LH were significantly increased in patients that underwent orchiectomy compared to patients that had testicular repair. Serum testosterone, however, was normal, regardless of surgical intervention [65]. Hormone replacement therapy should be considered in hypogonadal patients with bilateral injuries, including bilateral testicular loss [66, 67]. Furthermore, symptomatic swinging temperatures in the patient with significant gonadal loss may be a sign of traumatic andropause and should not be mistaken for sepsis [55]. Secondary hypogonadism should also be considered, especially in patients with chronic pain or those on opiate drugs [73].

Psychological Impact

Genital trauma may cause significant psychological challenges to the patient. Overwhelming emotions and adjusting to injuries may be a long process requiring expert behavioral health input [74]. Following orchiectomy, patients may experience feelings of loss and uneasiness or shame. Testicular prosthesis has been shown to improve the extent of psychological trauma in cancer patients [75].

Testicular amputation may be intentional in certain cases as a result of bizarre autoerotic acts or as an attempt by transgender persons to adjust their body to their gender identity [76]. The majority of genital self-mutilation cases are due to psychosis (65%) and re-attempts are reported in about one-third of patients [77]. Early psychiatric input is therefore important in such cases.

Conclusions

Scrotal and testicular trauma forms a diverse group of injuries, usually affecting the young population. Evaluation should include history and careful examination. Ultrasonography is the diagnostic investigation of choice in blunt trauma. Penetrating scrotal injury, presence of a large or expanding hematocele, or suspicion of testicular rupture should always prompt immediate surgical exploration, debridement, and repair. Orchiectomy should only be considered if reconstruction cannot be achieved. A holistic management approach to scrotal trauma should take into consideration the potential for infection, fertility, hypogonadism, and psychological effects.

References

1 Buckley, J.C. and McAninch, J.W. (2006). Diagnosis and management of testicular ruptures. *Urol. Clin. North Am.* 33: 111–116, vii.

2 Cass, A.S. and Luxenberg, M. (1991). Testicular injuries. *Urology* 37: 528–530.

3 McAninch, J.W., Kahn, R.I., Jeffrey, R.B. et al. (1984). Major traumatic and septic genital injuries. *J. Trauma* 24: 291–298.

4 McGeady, J.B. and Breyer, B.N. (2013). Current epidemiology of genitourinary trauma. *Urol. Clin. North Am.* 40: 323–334.

5 Mulhall, J.P., Gabram, S.G.A., and Jacobs, L.M. (1995). Emergency management of Blunt testicular trauma. *Acad. Emerg. Med.* 2: 639–643.

6 Phonsombat, S., Master, V.A., and McAninch, J.W. (2008). Penetrating external genital trauma: a 30-year single institution experience. *J. Urol.* 180: 192–195; discussion 195–6.

7 Bjurlin, M.A., Kim, D.Y., Zhao, L.C. et al. (2013). Clinical characteristics and surgical outcomes of penetrating external genital injuries. *J. Trauma Acute Care Surg.* 74: 839–844.

8 Simhan, J., Rothman, J., Canter, D. et al. (2012). Gunshot wounds to the scrotum: a large single-institutional 20-year experience. *BJU Int.* 109: 1704–1707.

9 Mohr, A.M., Pham, A.M., Lavery, R.F. et al. (2003). Management of trauma to the male external genitalia: the usefulness of American Association for the Surgery of Trauma organ injury scales. *J. Urol.* 170: 2311–2315.

10 Cline, K.J., Mata, J.A., Venable, D.D., and Eastham, J.A. (1998). Penetrating trauma to the male external genitalia. *J. Trauma* 44: 492–494.

11 Thompson Col, I.M., Flaherty Maj, S.F., and Morey Maj, A.F. (1998). Battlefield urologic injuries: the Gulf War experience11The opinions or assertions contained herein are the private views of the authors and are not to be construed as reflecting the views of the Department of the Army or the Department of Defense. *J. Am. Coll. Surg.* 187: 139–141.

12 Mossadegh, S., Tai, N., Midwinter, M., and Parker, P. (2012). Improvised explosive device related pelvi-perineal trauma: anatomic injuries and surgical management. *J. Trauma Acute Care Surg.* 73: S24–S31.

13 Davendra, M.S., Webster, C.E., Kirkman-Brown, J. et al. (2013). Blast injury to the perineum. *J. R. Army Med. Corps* 159 (Suppl): i1–i3.

14 Sharma, D.M. and Bowley, D.M. (2013). Immediate surgical management of combat-related injury to the external genitalia. *J. R. Army Med. Corps* 159 (Suppl): i18–i20.

15 Gadda, F., Spinelli, M.G., Cozzi, G. et al. (2012). Emergency testicular sperm extraction after scrotal trauma in a patient with a history of contralateral orchiopexy for cryptorchidism: case report and review of the literature. *Fertil. Steril.* 97: 1074–1077.

16 Injury Scoring Scales – The American Association for the Surgery of Trauma. http://www.aast.org/Library/TraumaTools/InjuryScoringScales.aspx#scrotum.

17 Morey, A. and Rozanski, T. (2006). Genital and lower urinary tract trauma. In: *Campbell-Walsh Urology* (eds. A. Wein, L. Kavoussi, A. Novick, et al.), 1274–1292. Saunders: Philadelphia.

18 Nicola, R., Carson, N., and Dogra, V.S. (2014). Imaging of traumatic injuries to the scrotum and penis. *Am. J. Roentgenol.* 202: 512–520.

19 Ugarte, R., Spaedy, M., and Cass, A.S. (1990). Accuracy of ultrasound in diagnosis of rupture after blunt testicular trauma. *Urology* 36: 253–254.

20 Corrales, J.G., Corbel, L., Cipolla, B. et al. (1993). Accuracy of ultrasound diagnosis after blunt testicular trauma. *J. Urol.* 150: 1834–1836.

21 Bhatt, S. and Dogra, V.S. (2008). Role of US in testicular and scrotal trauma. *Radiographics* 28: 1617–1629.

22 Buckley, J.C. and McAninch, J.W. (2006). Use of ultrasonography for the diagnosis of testicular injuries in blunt scrotal trauma. *J. Urol.* 175: 175–178.

23 Muglia, V., Tucci, S., Elias, J. et al. (2002). Magnetic resonance imaging of scrotal diseases: when it makes the difference. *Urology* 59: 419–423.

24 Wu, C.-J., Tsai, W.-F., Tsai, J.-L. et al. (2004). Bilateral traumatic dislocation of testes. *J. Chin. Med. Assoc.* 67: 311–313.

25 Kitrey, N., Djakovic, N., Hallscheidt, P. et al. (2019). *Eur. Urol.* 2019: 47.

26 Wessells, H. and Long, L. (2006). Penile and genital injuries. *Urol. Clin. North Am.* 33: 117–126.

27 Labler, L. and Trentz, O. (2007). The use of vacuum assisted closure (VAC™) in soft tissue injuries after high energy pelvic trauma. *Langenbecks Arch. Surg.* 392: 601–609.

28 Pasquier, P., Malgras, B., Savoie, P.H. et al. (2013). Application of negative-pressure wound therapy for the management of battlefield scrotum trauma. *Injury* 44: 1250–1251.

29 Wang, D., Wei, Z., Sun, G., and Luo, Z. (2009). Thin-trimming of the scrotal reconstruction flap: long-term follow-up shows reversal of spermatogenesis arrest. *J. Plast. Reconstr. Aesthet. Surg.* 62: e455–e456.

30 Michielsen, D.P.J. and Lafaire, C. (2010). Management of genital burns: a review. *Int. J. Urol.* 17: 755–758.

31 Michielsen, D., Van Hee, R., Neetens, C. et al. (1998). Burns to the genitalia and the perineum. *J. Urol.* 159: 418–419.

32 Tiguert, R., Harb, J.F., Hurley, P.M. et al. (2000). Management of shotgun injuries to the pelvis and lower genitourinary system. *Urology* 55: 193–197.

33 Buckley, J.C. and McAninch, J.W. (2006). Use of ultrasonography for the diagnosis of testicular injuries in blunt scrotal trauma. *J. Urol.* 175: 175–178.

34 Buckley, J.C. and McAninch, J.W. (2006). Diagnosis and management of testicular ruptures. *Urol. Clin. North Am.* 33: 111–116.

35 Morey, A.F., Brandes, S., Dugi, D.D. III et al. (2014). Urotrauma: AUA guideline. *J. Urol.* 192 (2): 327–335.

36 Gross, M. (1969). Rupture of the testicle: the importance of early surgical treatment. *J. Urol.* 101: 196–197.

37 Kukadia, A.N., Ercole, C.J., Gleich, P. et al. (1996). Testicular trauma: potential impact on reproductive function. *J. Urol.* 156: 1643–1646.

38 Ko, S.-F., Ng, S.-H., Wan, Y.-L. et al. (2004). Testicular dislocation: an uncommon and easily overlooked complication of blunt abdominal trauma. *Ann. Emerg. Med.* 43: 371–375.

39 Nagarajan, V.P., Pranikoff, K., Imahori, S.C., and Rabinowitz, R. (1983). Traumatic dislocation of testis. *Urology* 22: 521–524.

40 Lee, J.Y., Cass, A.S., and Streitz, J.M. (1992). Traumatic dislocation of testes and bladder rupture. *Urology* 40: 506–508.

41 Shefi, S., Mor, Y., Dotan, Z.A., and Ramon, J. (1999). Traumatic testicular dislocation: a case report and review of published reports. *Urology* 54: 744.

42 Gómez, R.G., Storme, O., Catalán, G. et al. (2014). Traumatic testicular dislocation. *Int. Urol. Nephrol.* 46: 1883–1887.

43 Kochakarn, W., Choonhaklai, V., Hotrapawanond, P., and Muangman, V. (2000). Traumatic testicular dislocation a review of 36 cases. *J. Med. Assoc. Thai.* 83: 208–212.

44 Pollen, J.J. and Funckes, C. (1982). Traumatic dislocation of the testes. *J. Trauma* 22: 247–249.

45 Papatsoris, A.G., Mpadra, F.A., and Karamouzis, M.V. (2003). Post-traumatic testicular torsion. *Ulus. Travma Acil Cerrahi Derg.* 9: 70–71.

46 Elsaharty, S., Pranikoff, K., Magoss, I.V., and Sufrin, G. (1984). Traumatic torsion of the testis. *J. Urol.* 132: 1155–1156.

47 Manson, A.L. (1989). Traumatic testicular torsion: case report. *J. Trauma* 29: 407–408.

48 Altarac, S. (1993). A case of testicle replantation. *J. Urol.* 150: 1507–1508.

49 Chang, A.J. and Brandes, S.B. (2013). Advances in diagnosis and management of genital injuries. *Urol. Clin. North Am.* 40: 427–438.

50 Gomez, R.G., Castanheira, A.C., and McAninch, J.W. (1993). Gunshot wounds to the male external genitalia. *J. Urol.* 150: 1147–1149.

51 Ferguson, G.G. and Brandes, S.B. (2007). Gunshot wound injury of the testis: the use of tunica vaginalis and polytetrafluoroethylene grafts for reconstruction. *J. Urol.* 178: 2462–2465.

52 Baniel, J. and Sella, A. (2001). Sperm extraction at orchiectomy for testis cancer. *Fertil. Steril.* 75: 260–262.

53 Al-Azzawi, I.S. and Koraitim, M.M. (2014). Lower genitourinary trauma in modern warfare: the experience from civil violence in Iraq. *Injury* 45: 885–889.

54 Hudak, S.J., Morey, A.F., Rozanski, T.A., and Fox, C.W. (2005). Battlefield urogenital injuries: changing patterns during the past century. *Urology* 65: 1041–1046.

55 Jones, G.H., Kirkman-Brown, J., Sharma, D.M., and Bowley, D. (2015). Traumatic andropause after combat injury. *BMJ Case Rep.* 2015 https://doi.org/10.1136/bcr-2014-207924.

56 Lucas, P.A., Page, P.R.J., Phillip, R.D., and Bennett, A.N. (2014). The impact of genital trauma on wounded servicemen: qualitative study. *Injury* 45: 825–829.

57 Gomes, C.M., Ribeiro-Filho, L., Giron, A.M. et al. (2001). Genital trauma due to animal bites. *J. Urol.* 165: 80–83.

58 Bothra, R., Bhat, A., Saxena, G. et al. (2011). Dog bite injuries of genitalia in male infant and children. *Urol. Ann.* 3: 167–169.

59 Schalamon, J., Ainoedhofer, H., Singer, G. et al. (2006). Analysis of dog bites in children who are younger than 17 years. *Pediatrics* 117: e374–e379.

60 Goldstein, E.J. (1992). Bite wounds and infection. *Clin. Infect. Dis.* 14: 633–638.

61 Bertozzi, M. and Appignani, A. (2013). The management of dog bite injuries of genitalia in paediatric age. *Afr. J. Paediatr. Surg.* 10: 205–210.

62 Slavis, S.A., Scholz, J.N., Hewitt, C.W. et al. (1990). The effects of testicular trauma on fertility in the Lewis rat and comparisons to isoimmunized recipients of syngeneic sperm. *J. Urol.* 143: 638–641.

63 Srinivas, M., Chandrasekharam, V.V.S.S., Degaonkar, M. et al. (2002). Effects of unilateral grade I testicular injury in rat. *Urology* 60: 548–551.

64 Shaul, D.B., Xie, H.W., Diaz, J.F. et al. (1997). Surgical treatment of testicular trauma: effects on fertility and testicular histology. *J. Pediatr. Surg.* 32: 84–87.

65 Lin, W.W., Kim, E.D., Quesada, E.T. et al. (1998). Unilateral testicular injury from external trauma: evaluation of semen quality and endocrine parameters. *J. Urol.* 159: 841–843.

66 Michael, Ward, A., Burgess, P.L., Williams, D.H., and e.a. (2010). *J. Emerg. Trauma Shock* 3: 199–203.

67 Liguori, G., Pavan, N., d'Aloia, G. et al. Fertility preservation after bilateral severe testicular trauma. *Asian J. Androl.* 16: 650–651.

68 Healy, M.W., Yauger, B.J., James, A.N. et al. (2016). Seminal vesicle sperm aspiration from wounded warriors. *Fertil. Steril.* 0: 2154–2158.

69 Nicol, M. and Gardner, A. (2015). Miracle babies for wounded British soldiers who stepped on Taliban landmines. *Dly Mail.* www.dailymail.co.uk/news/article-3250458/Miracle-babies-wounded-British-soldiers-lost-hope-fatherhood-stepped-Taliban-landmines.html.

70 Starmer, B.Z., Baird, A., and Lucky, M.A. (2018). Considerations in fertility preservation in cases of testicular trauma. *BJU Int.* 121: 466–471.

71 Fertility preservation | Human Fertilisation and Embryology Authority. www.hfea.gov.uk/treatments/fertility-preservation.

72 Strong, C., Gingrich, J., and Kutteh, W. (2000). Ethics of postmortem sperm retrieval: ethics of sperm retrieval after death or persistent vegetative state. *Hum. Reprod.* 15: 739–745.

73 Woods, D.R., Phillip, R., and Quinton, R. (2013). Managing endocrine dysfunction following blast injury to the male external genitalia. *J. R. Army Med. Corps* 159 (Suppl): i45–i48.

74 Frappell-Cooke, W., Wink, P., and Wood, A. (2013). The psychological challenge of genital injury. *J. R. Army Med. Corps* 159 (Suppl): i52–i56.

75 Skoogh, J., Steineck, G., Cavallin-Ståhl, E. et al. (2011). Feelings of loss and uneasiness or shame after removal of a testicle by orchiectomy: a population-based long-term follow-up of testicular cancer survivors. *Int. J. Androl.* 34: 183–192.

76 Van Der Horst, C., Martinez Portillo, F.J., Seif, C. et al. (2004). Male genital injury: diagnostics and treatment. *BJU Int.* 93: 927–930.

77 Aboseif, S., Gomez, R., and McAninch, J.W. (1993). Genital self-mutilation. *J. Urol.* 150: 1143–1146.

16

Testicular Torsion

Alexander J. Skokan[1] and Dana A. Weiss[2]

[1] *Harborview Medical Center, University of Washington School of Medicine, Seattle, WA, USA*
[2] *The Children's Hospital of Philadelphia, Philadelphia, PA, USA*

Introduction

Testicular torsion is a surgical emergency that occurs primarily in childhood and adolescence, but must be suspected in males of all ages. Patients classically present with signs of an *acute scrotum*. Symptoms include scrotal, groin, or abdominal pain, nausea or vomiting, and physical examination findings of scrotal swelling or erythema. Among several potential causes of the acute scrotum, it is critical to distinguish and promptly evaluate patients at risk for acute torsion of the testis and spermatic cord. Testicular torsion remains primarily a clinical diagnosis based upon history and examination, with color Doppler ultrasound (CDUS) used to support clinical suspicion, providing that it will not otherwise delay surgical management. Urologists can offer definitive treatment with urgent or emergent surgical exploration of the scrotum. With timely intervention, organ salvage is feasible in most patients who present within the first several hours after symptom onset. Although long-term follow-up data is limited, many patients may have preserved long-term endocrine and reproductive function, at least in the presence of a grossly normal contralateral testis.

Epidemiology

Torsion of the testis is the most time-sensitive diagnosis to consider in patients presenting with an acute scrotum. Testicular torsion affects up to 1 in 4000 males under age 25 years [1]. Most patients presenting with an acute scrotum will be found to have torsion of the testicular appendage (40–60%), with fewer demonstrating acute testicular torsion (20–30%) or acute epididymitis/epididymo-orchitis (5–15%). Testicular torsion has a bimodal age distribution, affecting boys around the age of puberty and those in the neonatal period. While adults can present with acute testicular torsion, a spontaneous event beyond age 35 years is rare. Patients with torsion of the testicular appendage usually present at a younger age (7–12 years), but they can develop symptoms at any age. Epididymitis can occur in patients of all ages, with noninfectious etiologies predominating in younger children and infectious causes underlying most cases in adolescence and adulthood.

Up to 10% of patients presenting with testicular torsion have an identifiable family history of torsion, suggesting a potential heritable component to patients' risk [2]. In addition, patients with an undescended testis may have up to a ten-fold increased risk of developing a torsion event in their lifetime [3].

Pathophysiology

Torsion of the testis and spermatic cord can occur in one of two anatomical spaces: intravaginal or extravaginal. Intravaginal torsion is the more common event and occurs after the newborn time period. Intravaginal torsion can affect either testis with a slight left-sided predominance (52 vs. 48%), and simultaneous bilateral events can also rarely occur [4]. Most patients who develop intravaginal torsion have an associated anatomical anomaly of the relationship between the tunica vaginalis and the epididymis, known as a *bell clapper deformity* (Figure 16.1). In most males, the potential space between visceral and parietal layers of the tunica vaginalis terminates on the inferior margin of the epididymis. With a bell clapper deformity, the tunica vaginalis and the potential space between its layers extends cranially to cover the posterior surface of the epididymis. This can result in a horizontal lie to the testis as well as free rotation and twisting of the distal-most spermatic cord within the tunica vaginalis. A bell clapper deformity can only be diagnosed at the time of scrotal exploration, where it is identified by direct visual inspection. Patients with a bell clapper deformity seem to be at increased risk for testicular torsion, but not all cases will develop an acute clinical event. Up to 12% of routinely examined testes in one autopsy

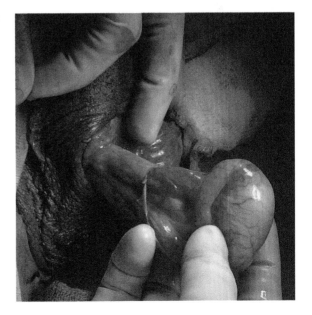

Figure 16.1 Bell clapper deformity with a horizontal testis lie. *Source: courtesy of Dana A. Weiss, MD.*

series had a bell clapper deformity, suggesting that many patients may have this anatomical anomaly but will never have an episode of torsion [5].

Extravaginal torsion is seen in the neonatal period, with most events occurring before birth. Infants with prenatal torsion present with examination findings at birth, while those with a neonatal event have an initial normal scrotal examination followed by new changes within the first one to two months of life. Torsion events occur when the spermatic cord develops a twist before the tunica vaginalis can become fixed to surrounding dartos. The twist in the spermatic cord usually occurs more proximally than with intravaginal torsion, yielding a rotation of all cord structures outside the space of the tunica vaginalis. Children of multiparous mothers and those with large birth weight may be at an increased risk of extravaginal torsion, with up to 60% of cases in one series developing in newborns above the 90th percentile weight at birth [6]. Most perinatal torsion events are extravaginal, but intravaginal torsion can also occur in this period.

Episodes of testicular torsion are treated as surgical emergencies because the torsion event presents a risk of ischemic organ loss. Damage to the Sertoli and germ cells early in an ischemic episode may impact future fertility, and loss of testosterone-producing Leydig cells can affect hormonal function and development. In animal models of torsion/ischemia, there is significant injury to germ cells and Sertoli cells by four hours of complete ischemia, with no evidence of spermatogenesis after six hours [7]. Leydig cell loss also begins at around four hours, with all Leydig cell function in the testis lost by ten hours of ischemia.

There is some evidence that the function of the untwisted contralateral testis is abnormal long-term in patients with a history of acute testicular torsion. This includes borderline or abnormal parameters on hormone assays and semen analyses, although such abnormalities have not consistently borne out to significant differences in overall testosterone production or fertility potential [8, 9]. While some authors hypothesize that either an immunological- or sympathetic-induced ischemic event leads to post-torsion injury of the contralateral testis, the abnormalities seen might actually reflect a preexisting anomaly of the "normal" testis. Testicular torsion may be one manifestation of a congenital testicular dysplasia, which also results in subtle changes in testicular function independent of torsion events [10].

Presentation

The differential diagnosis of the acute scrotum is broad, with the many causes to consider summarized in Table 16.1. Most symptoms and examination findings are nonspecific and can occur with several underlying causes, but the presence of some findings will raise the index of suspicion for an acute torsion event.

Several elements of a patient's history and symptoms will help providers to organize their differential diagnosis. Characterizing the time course and nature of scrotal or abdominal pain is critical during the emergency evaluation. Patients with testicular torsion will classically describe the sudden onset of severe scrotal pain, sometimes waking them up from sleep. This rapid onset of severe pain usually prompts patients to present to a healthcare provider for evaluation early (within 12 hours). In contrast, the gradual onset and worsening of pain over hours or days is more suggestive of acute epididymitis [12]. Torsion can be missed in

Table 16.1 Differential diagnosis of the acute scrotum.

Testicular/spermatic cord torsion

Torsion of the testicular appendage

Acute epididymitis/epididymo-orchitis

Scrotal trauma or hematoma

Incarcerated inguinal hernia

Ureteral calculi

Systemic diseases with scrotal involvement
(Henoch-Schönlein purpura)

Intra-abdominal pathology with scrotal
extension
(Perforated appendicitis or peritonitis) [11]

Varicocele

Testicular tumors

Scrotal cellulitis

Scrotal fat necrosis

Idiopathic

patients who present primarily with abdominal pain and nausea, so it is critical that providers include scrotal examination as a routine component of their evaluation of abdominal pain in males. Providers should suspect torsion of the testis when patients describe associated nausea or vomiting, as these symptoms are uncommon with epididymitis [13]. These symptoms in the setting of testicular torsion may be related to reflex stimulation of the celiac ganglion. Dysuria and fevers are uncommon findings with testicular torsion.

Physical examination findings often help to distinguish torsion from other causes of acute scrotal pain. Tenderness can be localized on examination if a patient is being seen within hours of symptom onset. Tenderness localized to the epididymis suggests epididymitis, while point tenderness at the upper pole of the testis suggests a torsed testicular appendage. Exquisite tenderness throughout the testis will occur early in a torsion event. With delayed presentations, the entire scrotum may be tender, or pain may have even started to subside. During an acute torsion event, the testis may be palpable with an abnormal horizontal lie and may be riding high in the scrotum. Scrotal erythema and edema are nonspecific findings, but these can also occur with delayed presentations of testicular torsion.

Several classic signs have been described in the evaluation of the acute scrotum. Providers may be able to identify the classic *blue dot sign* of a torsed testicular appendage, where a small area of cyanosis is visible through the skin of the scrotum at the anterior upper margin of the testis. However, this finding is apparent in less than one-quarter of patients with a torsed testicular appendage [14]. The *cremasteric reflex* arc involves the major branches of the genitofemoral nerve. Stroking the medial thigh (stimulation of the sensory femoral branch) normally causes contraction of the cremaster muscle and elevation of the ipsilateral testis (activation of the motor genital branch). The cremasteric reflex is absent in most cases of testicular torsion (due to ischemia of the cremaster), although the reflex may be falsely normal in up to 10% of cases [15, 16]. Clinicians should evaluate for the presence or absence of the cremasteric reflex bilaterally, since findings on the unaffected side will help with the interpretation of findings on the side of concern. *Prehn's sign* is also described to distinguish testicular torsion from epididymitis, although its utility in practice is limited. The testis of concern is elevated by the examiner's hand, and the patient is asked to describe changes in the severity of their pain. A positive Prehn's sign occurs when elevating the testis causes increased pain, and is suggestive of testicular torsion; a negative sign indicates improvement in pain with this maneuver, suggesting acute epididymitis.

Perinatal extravaginal torsion usually presents at birth with a firm, swollen, nontender affected testis. Existing findings at birth are thought to suggest a prenatal ischemic event. Synchronous bilateral perinatal torsion can occur in up to 22% of patients, and the affected contralateral testis may appear normal on bedside examination [17]. Metachronous bilateral torsion is a rare event.

Intermittent testicular torsion and torsion-detorsion events deserve unique mention, as it is important for providers to consider these diagnoses in patients with recurrent scrotal pain. This is thought to occur when patients have repeated episodes of acute torsion with spontaneous untwisting of the spermatic cord. Patients will describe several episodes of classic testicular torsion symptoms, with prompt and spontaneous resolution. Torsion-detorsion events can last for three to four hours at a time, and examination may demonstrate evidence of resolving torsion. Such findings may include scrotal swelling, a boggy spermatic cord, or a pseudo-mass palpable within the cord (reflecting a congested epididymis and distal spermatic cord just below the level of cord twisting) [18]. Patients with true torsion-detorsion events may be at increased risk for recurrent twisting or may still have limited partial cord twisting that could progress, so these patients should be taken urgently or electively for scrotal exploration. Intermittent testicular torsion is a diagnosis of exclusion, with episodes often lasting 30–60 minutes usually in the absence of physical findings (since the episodes may be too short for edema or other sequelae of ischemia to develop). The affected testis will usually have a normal vertical lie in the scrotum [19]. Excluding other etiologies of episodic pain is important in these cases. While patients with a history suggesting intermittent testicular torsion do not require emergency surgery, they should be offered timely elective exploration. Observation alone places these patients at risk of an acute torsion event that could compromise the affected testis, while elective intervention may achieve organ preservation and prevent further episodes of distressing symptoms. At the time of surgical exploration, most patients with suspected intermittent torsion will be found to have a bell clapper deformity [19].

Diagnostic Evaluation

In addition to history and physical examination, evaluation of a patient with an acute scrotum should include a urinalysis with reflex urine culture. Pyuria is an uncommon finding with testicular torsion and may suggest an inflammatory or infectious cause for a patient's symptoms. Radiologic studies serve a supportive role in evaluating cases for testicular torsion, with CDUS used most commonly. Ultrasound is useful in cases with low or intermediate suspicion for acute testicular torsion, or in concerning cases where sonographic evaluation can occur rapidly.

Clinical scoring tools may help to risk stratify patients for potential underlying testicular torsion based upon their presenting symptoms and findings on physical examination [16, 20]. This may aid with determining when to order a radiologic study in intermediate-risk patients or those presenting in a delayed manner (>24 hours). The Testicular Workup for Ischemia and Suspected Torsion (TWIST) score is a simple and useful measure that has been validated in children age 3 months to 18 years. A score is calculated by adding points for each of the following findings: a history of nausea/vomiting, scrotal swelling, a high-riding testis, absent cremasteric reflex, and a hard/firm testis. Scores are divided into low, intermediate, and high risk, which can guide providers on when to order an ultrasound or pursue upfront surgical consultation [21]. The use of clinical scoring tools in conjunction with CDUS may avoid a negative surgical exploration in half of patients presenting with an acute scrotum, with no episodes of missed testicular torsion [12, 20].

Ultrasound is a widely available tool in many settings and serves an important role in evaluating patients with an acute scrotum. However, providers should approach testicular torsion as a clinical diagnosis based upon history and examination. CDUS is useful in indeterminate cases or to avoid unnecessary surgical exploration in higher risk cases, but only if it will not delay timely surgical intervention [22]. Ultrasound demonstrates high positive and negative predictive values when evaluating for torsion, and timely use of sonography may help to clarify the diagnosis in indeterminate or intermediate risk cases [23–25]. In addition, ultrasound is a useful aid in the diagnosis of other etiologies of acute scrotal pain, including testis or scrotal tumors, trauma, and epididymo-orchitis. Ultrasound should be performed using a unit capable of color Doppler or power Doppler imaging, using a 4–15 MHz range linear transducer if available [26]. The study should include images of the scrotum on the affected and contralateral sides, as well as dedicated imaging of the inguinal region. Sonographic findings that suggest acute testicular torsion may include diminished or absent Doppler signal or waveforms in an affected testis (Figure 16.2), a thickened spermatic cord, or a *whirlpool sign* [27]. The whirlpool sign is a twist in the spermatic cord that is usually visible at or near the level of the external inguinal ring, and is highly sensitive for testicular torsion. When comparing the Doppler waveform between the affected and contralateral testis, providers may note an increase or decrease in Doppler signal amplitude or reversal of diastolic flow [28]. It is critical for providers to recognize that the presence of any Doppler signal does not indicate normal perfusion, and that they should evaluate for symmetrical arterial waveforms measured from vessels within the parenchyma on the affected and contralateral testes. The testicular parenchyma may appear hypoechoic (early ischemic change) or heterogeneous (late ischemia/delayed presentation, Figure 16.3) relative to the contralateral testis [29, 30]. Heterogeneous parenchyma may indicate a nonviable or severely damaged testis, which could require removal or be at high risk of delayed atrophy with surgical salvage [31, 32]. If available, use of a high-resolution 10–20 MHz probe may significantly improve the ability to identify or rule out testicular torsion on ultrasound [33].

Nuclear scintigraphy was previously utilized, but has mainly a historical role due to the study's inherent radiation exposure and the widespread availability of ultrasound. Magnetic resonance imaging (MRI) with dynamic contrast enhanced and T2 weighted image (T2)

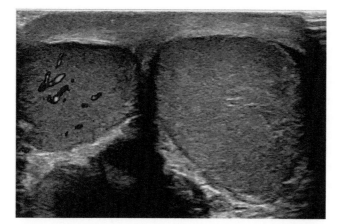

Figure 16.2 Color Doppler ultrasound of a patient with testicular torsion of short duration, showing flow signal in the right testis (RT) with absent signal in the left testis (LT). *Source:* courtesy of Dana A. Weiss, MD.

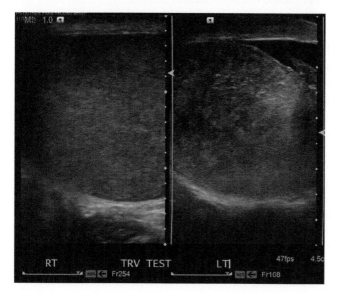

Figure 16.3 Ultrasound of a patient with prolonged torsion, showing heterogeneous parenchyma in the left testis (LT) and normal echotexture within the right testis (RT). *Source:* courtesy of Dana A. Weiss, MD.

sequences may have a limited role in indeterminate cases or to predict nonviable testes, although its use is not standard due to the significant cost and time required [34].

Management

The mainstay of treatment for acute testicular torsion and intermittent testicular torsion remains surgical exploration of the scrotum (Table 16.2). This allows assessment of viability of the affected and contralateral testes, with definitive treatment via detorsion and fixation of a viable testis (an orchidopexy or septopexy) or removal of a grossly unsalvageable organ. In contrast, torsion of a testicular appendage is managed conservatively, with surgical exploration considered if the diagnosis is in question or if patients have prolonged persistent pain [22].

Table 16.2 European Association of Urology summary of evidence and recommendations for the management of acute scrotum in children [22].

Summary of Evidence	Level of Evidence
Diagnosis of testicular torsion is based on presentation and physical exam.	
Doppler ultrasound (US) is an effective imaging tool to evaluate acute scrotum and comparable to scintigraphy and dynamic contrast-enhanced subtraction MRI.	2a
Neonates with acute scrotum should be treated as surgical emergencies.	3

Recommendations	Level of Evidence	Strength Rating
Testicular torsion is a pediatric urological emergency and requires immediate treatment.	3	Strong
In neonates with testicular torsion, perform orchidooexy of the contralateral testicle. In prenatal torsion, the timing of surgery is usually dictated by clinical findings.	3	Weak
Base the clinical decision on physical examination. The use of Doppler ultrasound to evaluate acute scrotum is useful, but this should not delay the intervention.	2a	Strong
Manage torsion of the appendix testis conservatively. Perform surgical exploration in equivocal cases and in patients with persistent pain.	3	Strong
Perform urgent surgical exploration in all cases of testicular torsion within 24 hours of symptom onset. In prenatal torsion, the timing of surgery is usually dictated by clinical findings.	3	Strong

Surgical exploration in an emergent fashion should be offered to all patients with suspicion of testicular torsion presenting within 24 hours of symptom onset [22]. With rare exceptions, children and older patients presenting in a delayed fashion (>24 hours) should also be offered emergent surgical intervention; some patients with prolonged torsion may have had intermittent torsion-detorsion events that transiently restore perfusion and allow salvage of a viable testis, even beyond a 24-hour window. A bilateral scrotal exploration is a rapid and well tolerated intervention with limited morbidity. Surgery is usually performed under general anesthesia, with patients placed in a supine or frog-legged position. Both scrotal compartments can be entered according to surgeon preference, using either bilateral transverse incisions in the anterior scrotum or a longitudinal incision along the midline scrotal raphe. Surgeons should focus on exposing and evaluating the testis of concern first, allowing rapid detorsion and a period of observed reperfusion while the contralateral testis is subsequently delivered (Figure 16.4). Once the affected testis is delivered, its tunica vaginalis is opened sharply and the testis evaluated, noting its color, degree of cord rotation, and the anatomy of the tunica vaginalis, with specific attention to identifying a potential bell clapper deformity. The spermatic cord is untwisted to normal position, then the testis is wrapped in saline-soaked gauze for a period of at least five minutes. The contralateral testis is then exposed, its tunica vaginalis incised, and the testis evaluated in the same

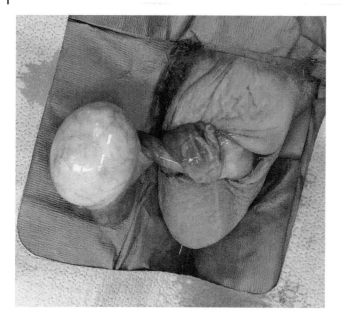

Figure 16.4 A torsed spermatic cord found on early surgical intervention. *Source:* courtesy of Dana A. Weiss, MD.

manner. Once normal position of the contralateral testis is confirmed, a surgical fixation to the scrotum can be performed by placing two or three pexy stitches with a fine nonabsorbable monofilament suture through the tunica albuginea of the testis and adjacent surrounding dartos. This is performed in order to restrict future rotational freedom of the testis and to prevent subsequent torsion events. Attention then returns to the affected testis, and its color is re-evaluated to determine if re-perfusion has demonstrated a return to viable pink parenchyma. If the testis demonstrates improvement in color to suggest viability with restored perfusion, it is pexied in the same manner as the contralateral side. If the testis remains cyanotic or hemorrhagic in appearance, it may be nonviable and orchiectomy may be considered (Figure 16.5).

A small but growing body of literature suggests that some testes may be lost following surgical detorsion due to a testicular compartment syndrome [35]. According to this theory, the fixed volume of the tunica albuginea cannot accommodate parenchymal edema and expansion following a period of prolonged ischemia and re-perfusion, and edema following post-detorsion restoration of flow results in an increased intraparenchymal pressure that impairs further re-perfusion. In cases where a testis remains cyanotic or hemorrhagic intraoperatively, surgeons may consider incising the tunica albuginea to determine whether a compartment release results in signs of re-perfusion with improvement in parenchymal color. If improvement is seen, a segment of tunica vaginalis can be isolated and sutured to the tunica albuginea as a pliable flap that covers the tunical defect, while allowing transient parenchymal expansion at lower pressures. Animal studies have suggested tunica albuginea incision with a tunica vaginalis flap may preserve functional cell groups within the testis, and in clinical cohorts this maneuver has markedly improved testis salvage rates in patients presenting with symptom duration of up to or even beyond 24 hours [36–39].

Testis salvage rates vary widely, with 30–70% being preserved in most studies. The two most important determinants of testis salvage are time from symptom onset to surgery and

Figure 16.5 A cyanotic testis with hemorrhagic change to the epididymis found at surgical exploration after delayed presentation. *Source:* courtesy of Dana A. Weiss, MD.

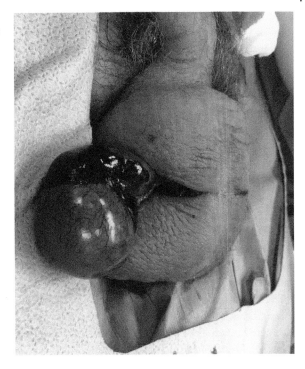

Table 16.3 Relationship between time, testis salvage, and testis atrophy.[a]

Time from Symptom Onset (hours)	Likelihood of Testis Salvage (%)	Risk of Testis Atrophy after Salvage (%)
0–6	95	0–5
7–12	80	5–10
13–18	60	40–45
19–24	45	
25–48	20	80
>48	5–10	

[a] Drawn from Ref. [40].

the degree of cord rotation found at surgery. Among patients who undergo surgical detorsion early (within 12 hours of symptom onset), over 90% will not require orchiectomy (Table 16.3) [32]. In contrast, at least half presenting within 12–24 hours of symptoms may require orchiectomy, and a majority presenting beyond 24 hours will require removal of a nonviable testis. Twisting of the cord beyond 360° can result in severe damage in as little as 4 hours, while patients with incomplete torsion (< 360°) may have a viable testis 12 or more hours after symptom onset. The duration of in-hospital pre-operative care is another critical component of the time from symptom onset, and the "door to OR" time has become a measure of healthcare quality for pediatric centers in the United States [41]. While the measured target from emergency room triage to surgical intervention is less than 240 minutes, it stands to reason that more rapid evaluation and intervention, even within this window, is of significant benefit to patients with concern for testicular torsion.

Pre-operative interventions that may improve the viability of the testis at surgical exploration are also of great interest. Manual detorsion has some evidence to support its use pre-operatively to improve post-operative outcomes, but as with ultrasound, it should not be used in a manner that delays definitive surgical treatment. This is a bedside maneuver that involves externally rotating the affected testis (outward, toward the anterior ipsilateral thigh) as long as there is no resistance to rotation or an acute increase in pain following rotation. This lateral rotation is based upon the predominantly medial twisting of the cord found in cases of acute torsion [4]. The maneuver is performed for one or one-and-a-half full rotations (360–540°), and a successful detorsion is defined by the immediate relief of all symptoms with a normal subsequent scrotal examination. CDUS is a useful tool to confirm the restoration of normal blood flow to the testis with manual detorsion [42]. This maneuver may successfully relieve acute ischemia by untwisting the spermatic cord in 60–95% of cases [4, 43, 44]. Even in cases of successful manual detorsion, the standard of care is to proceed with urgent or emergent scrotal exploration.

There may also be a role for external cooling of the testis and scrotum leading up to surgical exploration. This could limit ischemia–reperfusion injury to the testis itself, improving long-term function. Use of external cooling in an animal model demonstrated improved viability of testicular cell groups after a torsion/ischemia event [45, 46]. Further evaluation of this promising adjunctive treatment is needed in clinical cohorts, but it may be a low-risk option to consider while patients are being prepared for surgery.

Surgical decision-making is approached in a different manner to cases of extravaginal torsion. The rate of testis salvage in patients presenting with evidence of prenatal torsion is low, so surgical intervention is intended to prevent subsequent torsion of the remaining viable testis. This has generated controversy regarding the urgency of surgical management for prenatal torsion events. Although some surgeons advocate delayed surgical exploration to limit the risk of general anesthesia in the neonatal period, most proceed with urgent exploration to protect against the rare but devastating event of a later contralateral torsion. If a neonate has a clear postnatal case (normal newborn examination, subsequent development of abnormal scrotal findings), emergent surgical intervention including contralateral testis exploration and fixation is indicated. Some surgeons advocate an inguinal approach when exploring the affected testis in all cases of extravaginal torsion; this allows adequate exposure of even very proximal twists in the spermatic cord, and ensures the surgeon can manage any unexpected findings such as an inguinal hernia at exploration [47].

Outcomes

While many questions remain, providers can give patients some information on long-term outcomes after fixation or removal of a torsed testis. Historical cohorts suggest that up to 1 in 20 patients may develop a recurrent torsion event in a pexied testis, but the vast majority of recurrences occurred after the use of absorbable suture [48]. Recurrent torsion after use of nonabsorbable pexy sutures is thought to be very rare.

Permanent atrophy of an affected testis after detorsion may occur. While patients who present in a delayed fashion are at high risk of atrophy in salvaged testes, even patients whose testes appeared viable intra-operatively may have long-term atrophy [4, 31, 49]. Atrophy is usually evident in the short- to intermediate term, with most cases identified on follow-up examination by six months post-operatively. Some factors identified at the time of emergency evaluation may predict a patient's risk of long-term atrophy, including a duration of pain greater than 12 hours at presentation, heterogeneous testicular parenchyma on pre-operative ultrasound, and black or hemorrhagic testicular parenchyma on intra-operative evaluation [50]. It is unclear whether patients benefit more from aggressive attempts to preserve a testis at high risk for atrophy or a lower threshold to remove a borderline organ at the time of urgent scrotal exploration.

Although there is some evidence to suggest a potential for impaired fertility after torsion, the studied parameters do not appear to correlate with clinical subfertility or infertility in this patient population [8, 9, 51]. Paternity rates among patients who underwent orchidopexy or required orchiectomy for testicular torsion appear to be comparable to those observed in the general population [52, 53]. While patients may demonstrate abnormal levels of hormonal markers such as luteinizing hormone (LH), total serum testosterone appears to be comparable to the general population, at least into early adulthood [9]. There is little information regarding endocrine and fertility function later in life, and it is possible that preserved function is more fragile with advancing age in patients with a prior torsion event. Data is very limited, but it does not appear that a history of torsion correlates with clinically significant differences in sexual or erectile function long-term [53].

Conclusions and Future Directions

The acute scrotum is approached as an emergency, and current guidelines support prompt surgical exploration in patients whose history and physical examination strongly suggest acute testicular torsion. Ultrasound may identify other causes in some intermediate- or high-risk patients and spare them surgical exploration, but radiologic studies should not be used if clinical suspicion is high and performing such studies would delay surgical management. With early patient presentation (especially within 12 hours of symptom onset) and timely intervention, most testes can be salvaged. Additional investigation focusing on pre-operative and intra-operative maneuvers to improve testis salvage may benefit future patients. Long-term fertility and testosterone production are likely normal or nearly normal at least into early adulthood, but we also do not yet know whether patients with a history of torsion are at a higher risk for hypogonadism or infertility in late adulthood.

References

1 Barada, J.H., Weingarten, J.L., and Cromie, W.J. (1989). Testicular salvage and age-related delay in the presentation of testicular torsion. *J. Urol.* 142 (3): 746–748. https://doi.org/10.1016/s0022-5347(17)38875-4.

2 Shteynshlyuger, A. and Yu, J. (2013). Familial testicular torsion: a meta analysis suggests inheritance. *J. Pediatr. Urol.* 9 (5): 683–690. https://doi.org/10.1016/j.jpurol.2012.08.002.

3 Williamson, R.C. (1976). Torsion of the testis and allied conditions. *Br. J. Surg.* 63 (6): 465–476. https://doi.org/10.1002/bjs.1800630618.

4 Sessions, A.E., Rabinowitz, R., Hulbert, W.C. et al. (2003). Testicular torsion: direction, degree, duration and disinformation. *J. Urol.* 169: 663–665. https://doi.org/10.1097/01.ju.0000047381.36380.0e.

5 Caesar, R.E. and Kaplan, G.W. (1994). Incidence of the bell-clapper deformity in an autopsy series. *Urology* 44 (1): 114–116. https://doi.org/10.1016/s0090-4295(94)80020-0.

6 Brandt, M.T., Sheldon, C.A., Wacksman, J., and Matthews, P. (1992). Prenatal testicular torsion: principles of management. *J. Urol.* 147 (3): 670–672. https://doi.org/10.1016/s0022-5347(17)37342-1.

7 Smith, G.I. (1955). Cellular changes from graded testicular ischemia. *J. Urol.* 73 (2): 355–362. https://doi.org/10.1016/S0022-5347(17)67408-1.

8 Romeo, C., Impellizzeri, P., Arrigo, T. et al. (2010). Late hormonal function after testicular torsion. *J. Pediatr. Surg.* 45: 411–413. https://doi.org/10.1016/j.jpedsurg.2009.10.086.

9 Arap, M.A., Vicentini, F.C., Cocuzza, M. et al. (2007). Late hormonal levels, semen parameters, and presence of antisperm antibodies in patients treated for testicular torsion. *J. Androl.* 28 (4): 528–532. https://doi.org/10.2164/jandrol.106.002097.

10 Anderson, J.B., Cooper, M.J., Thomas, W.E., and Williamson, R.C. (1986). Impaired spermatogenesis in testes at risk of torsion. *Br. J. Surg.* 73 (10): 847–849. https://doi.org/10.1002/bjs.1800731028.

11 Ng, K.H., YFA, C., Wilde, C.C., and Chee, C. (2002). An unusual presentation of acute scrotum after appendicitis. *Singapore Med. J.* 43 (7): 365–366.

12 Boettcher, M., Krebs, T., Bergholz, R. et al. (2013). Clinical and sonographic features predict testicular torsion in children: a prospective study. *BJU Int.* 112 (8): 1201–1206. https://doi.org/10.1111/bju.12229.

13 Nason, G.J., Tareen, F., Mcloughlin, D. et al. (2013). Scrotal exploration for acute scrotal pain: a 10-year experience in two tertiary referral paediatric units. *Scand. J. Urol.* 47 (5): 418–422. https://doi.org/10.3109/00365599.2012.752403.

14 Mäkelä, E., Lahdes-Vasama, T., Rajakorpi, H., and Wikström, S. (2007). A 19-year review of paediatric patients with acute scrotum. *Scand. J. Surg.* 96 (1): 62–66. https://doi.org/10.1177/145749690709600112.

15 Caleb Nelson, B.P., Williams, J.F., and Bloom Ann Arbor, D.A. (2003). The cremasteric reflex: a useful but imperfect sign in testicular torsion. *J. Pediatr. Surg.* 38 (8): 1248–1249. https://doi.org/10.1016/S0022-3468(03)00280-X.

16 Karmazyn, B., Steinberg, R., Kornreich, L. et al. (2005). Clinical and sonographic criteria of acute scrotum in children: a retrospective study of 172 boys. *Pediatr. Radiol.* 35: 302–310. https://doi.org/10.1007/s00247-004-1347-9.

17 Yerkes, E.B., Robertson, F.M., Gitlin, J. et al. (2005). Management of perinatal torsion: today, tomorrow or never? *J. Urol.* 174: 1579–1583. https://doi.org/10.1097/01.ju.0000179542.05953.11.

18 Munden, M.M., Williams, J.L., Zhang, W. et al. (2013). Intermittent testicular torsion in the pediatric patient: sonographic indicators of a difficult diagnosis. *Am. J. Roentgenol.* 201 (4): 912–918. https://doi.org/10.2214/AJR.12.9448.

19 Hayn, M.H., Herz, D.B., Bellinger, M.F., and Schneck, F.X. (2008). Intermittent torsion of the spermatic cord portends an increased risk of acute testicular infarction. *J. Urol.* 180 (4 SUPPL): 1729–1732. https://doi.org/10.1016/j.juro.2008. 03.101.

20 Barbosa, J.A., Tiseo, B.C., Barayan, G.A. et al. (2013). Development and initial validation of a scoring system to diagnose testicular torsion in children. *J. Urol.* 189 (5): 1859–1864. https://doi.org/10.1016/j.juro.2012.10.056.

21 Manohar, C.S., Gupta, A., Keshavamurthy, R. et al. (2018). Evaluation of testicular workup for ischemia and suspected torsion score in patients presenting with acute scrotum. *Urol. Ann.* 10 (1): 20–23. https://doi.org/10.4103/UA.UA_35_17.

22 Radmayr, C., Bogaert, G., Dogan, H. et al. (2019). EAU Guidelines on Paediatric Urology. *Edn Present EAU Annu Congr Barcelona.*

23 Liang, T., Metcalfe, P., Sevcik, W., and Noga, M. (2013). Retrospective review of diagnosis and treatment in children presenting to the pediatric department with acute scrotum. *AJR* 200 (5): W444–W449. https://doi.org/10.2214/AJR.12.10036.

24 Baker, L.A., Sigman, D., Mathews, R.I. et al. (2000). An analysis of clinical outcomes using color Doppler testicular ultrasound for testicular torsion. *Pediatrics* 105 (3): 604–607. https://doi.org/10.1542/peds.105.3.604.

25 Altinkilic, B., Pilatz, A., and Weidner, W. (2013). Detection of normal intratesticular perfusion using color coded duplex sonography obviates need for scrotal exploration in patients with suspected testicular torsion. *J. Urol.* 189 (5): 1853–1858. https:// doi.org/10.1016/j.juro.2012.11.166.

26 Remer, E.M., Casalino, D.D., Arellano, R.S. et al. (2012). ACR appropriateness criteria acute onset of scrotal pain – without trauma, without antecedent mass. *Ultrasound Q.* 28 (1): 47–51. https://doi.org/10.1097/RUQ.0b013e3182493c97.

27 Cassar, S., Bhatt, S., Paltiel, H.J., and Dogra, V.S. (2008). Role of spectral Doppler sonography in the evaluation of partial testicular torsion. *J. Ultrasound Med.* 27 (11): 1629–1638. https://doi.org/10.7863/jum.2008.27.11.1629.

28 Dogra, V.S., Rubens, D.J., Gottlieb, R.H., and Bhatt, S. (2004). Torsion and beyond. *J. Ultrasound Med.* 23 (8): 1077–1085. https://doi.org/10.7863/jum.2004.23.8.1077.

29 Kaye, J.D., Shapiro, E.Y., Levitt, S.B. et al. (2008). Parenchymal echo texture predicts testicular salvage after torsion: potential impact on the need for emergent exploration. *J. Urol.* 180 (4 SUPPL): 1733–1736. https://doi.org/10.1016/j.juro.2008.03.104.

30 Benedetto, G., Nigro, F., Bratti, E., and Tasca, A. (2014). Modifications of echogenicity of the testis during acute torsion may be a predictive factor of organ damage? *Arch. Ital. Urol. Androl.* 86 (4): 371–372. https://doi.org/10.4081/aiua.2014.4.371.

31 Lian, B.S.Y., Ong, C.C.P., Chiang, L.W. et al. (2015). Factors predicting testicular atrophy after testicular salvage following torsion. *Eur. J. Pediatr. Surg.* 26 (1): 17–21. https://doi. org/10.1055/s-0035-1566096.

32 Samson, P., Hartman, C., Palmerola, R. et al. (2017). Ultrasonographic assessment of testicular viability using heterogeneity levels in torsed testicles. *J. Urol.* 197 (3): 925–930. https://doi.org/10.1016/j.juro.2016.09.112.

33 Kalfa, N., Veyrac, C., Lopez, M. et al. (2007). Multicenter assessment of ultrasound of the spermatic cord in children with acute scrotum. *J. Urol.* 177 (1): 297–301. https:// doi.org/10.1016/j.juro.2006.08.128.

34 Watanabe, Y., Nagayama, M., Okumura, A. et al. (2007). MR imaging of testicular torsion: features of testicular hemorrhagic necrosis and clinical outcomes. *J. Magn. Reson. Imaging* 26 (1): 100–108. https://doi.org/10.1002/jmri.20946.

35 Kutikov, A., Casale, P., White, M.A. et al. (2008). Testicular compartment syndrome: a new approach to conceptualizing and managing testicular torsion. *Urology* 72 (4): 786–789. https://doi.org/10.1016/j.urology.2008.03.031.

36 Moghimian, M., Soltani, M., Abtahi, H. et al. (2016). Protective effect of tunica albuginea incision with tunica vaginalis flap coverage on tissue damage and oxidative stress following testicular torsion: role of duration of ischemia. *J. Pediatr. Urol.* 12 (6): 390.e1–390.e6. https://doi.org/10.1016/j.jpurol.2016.06.002.

37 Moritoki, Y., Kojima, Y., Mizuno, K. et al. (2012). Intratesticular pressure after testicular torsion as a predictor of subsequent spermatogenesis: a rat model. *BJU Int.* 109 (3): 466–470. https://doi.org/10.1111/j.1464-410X.2011.10279.x.

38 Figueroa, V., Pippi Salle, J.L., Braga, L.H.P. et al. (2012). Comparative analysis of detorsion alone versus detorsion and tunica albuginea decompression (Fasciotomy) with tunica vaginalis flap coverage in the surgical management of prolonged testicular ischemia. *J. Urol.* 188 (4 SUPPL): 1417–1423. https://doi.org/10.1016/j.juro.2012.02.017.

39 Chu, D.I., Gupta, K., Kawal, T. et al. (2018). Tunica vaginalis flap for salvaging testicular torsion: a matched cohort analysis. *J. Pediatr. Urol.* 14 (4): 329.e1–329.e7. https://doi.org/10.1016/j.jpurol.2018.01.010.

40 Visser, A.J. and Heyns, C.F. (2003). Testicular function after torsion of the spermatic cord. *BJU Int.* 92 (3): 200–203. https://doi.org/10.1046/j.1464-410X.2003.04307.x.

41 Zee, R.S., Bayne, C.E., Gomella, P.T. et al. (2019). Implementation of the accelerated care of torsion pathway: a quality improvement initiative for testicular torsion. *J. Pediatr. Urol.* https://doi.org/10.1016/j.jpurol.2019.07.011.

42 Garel, L., Dubois, J., Azzie, G. et al. (2000). Preoperative manual detorsion of the spermatic cord with Doppler ultrasound monitoring in patients with intravaginal acute testicular torsion. *Pediatr. Radiol.* 30: 41–44.

43 Cornel, E.B. and Karthaus, H.F.M. (1999). Manual derotation of the twisted spermatic cord. *BJU Int.* 83 (6): 672–674. https://doi.org/10.1046/j.1464-410X.1999.00003.x.

44 Dias Filho, A.C., Oliveira Rodrigues, R., Riccetto, C.L.Z., and Oliveira, P.G. (2017). Improving organ salvage in testicular torsion: comparative study of patients undergoing vs not undergoing preoperative manual detorsion. *J. Urol.* 197 (3 Pt 1): 811–817. https://doi.org/10.1016/j.juro.2016.09.087.

45 Power, R.E., Scanlon, R., Kay, E.W. et al. (2003). Long-term protective effects of hypothermia on reperfusion injury post-testicular torsion. *Scand. J. Urol. Nephrol.* 37 (6): 456–460. https://doi.org/10.1080/00365590310014508.

46 Haj, M., Shasha, S.M., Loberant, N., and Farhadian, H. (2007). Effect of external scrotal cooling on the viability of the testis with torsion in rats. *Eur. Surg. Res.* 39 (3): 160–169. https://doi.org/10.1159/000100473.

47 Pinto, K.J., Norman, H., and Jerkins, G.R. (1997). Management of neonatal testicular torsion. *J. Urol.* 158: 1196–1197.

48 Mor, Y., Pinthus, J.H., Nadu, A. et al. (2006). Testicular fixation following torsion of the spermatic cord – does it guarantee prevention of recurrent torsion events? *J. Urol.* 175 (1): 171–173. https://doi.org/10.1016/S0022-5347(05)00060-1.

49 Fisch, H., Laor, E., Reid, R.E. et al. (1988). Gonadal dysfunction after testicular torsion: luteinizing hormone and follicle-stimulating hormone response to gonadotropin releasing hormone. *J. Urol.* 139 (5): 961–964. https://doi.org/10.1016/S0022-5347(17)42731-5.

50 Grimsby, G.M., Schlomer, B.J., Menon, V.S. et al. (2018). Prospective evaluation of predictors of testis atrophy after surgery for testis torsion in children HHS Public Access. *Urology* 116: 150–155. https://doi.org/10.1016/j.urology.2018.03.009.

51 Ozkan, K., Kucukaydin, M., Muhtaroglu, S., and Kontas, O. (2001). Evaluation of contralateral testicular damage after unilateral testicular torsion by serum Inhibin B levels. *J. Pediatr. Surg.* 36 (7): 1050–1053. https://doi.org/10.1053/jpsu.2001.24742.

52 Gielchinsky, I., Suraqui, E., Hidas, G. et al. (2016). Pregnancy rates after testicular torsion. *J. Urol.* 196 (3): 852–855. https://doi.org/10.1016/j.juro.2016.04.066.

53 Mäkelä, E.P., Roine, R.P., and Taskinen, S. (2019). Paternity, erectile function, and health-related quality of life in patients operated for pediatric testicular torsion. *J. Pediatr. Urol.* https://doi.org/10.1016/j.jpurol.2019.10.008.

17

Epididymitis and Orchitis

Norman Zambrano and Juan Fullá

Clinica Las Condes, Las Condes, Chile

Introduction

Epididymitis and orchitis refer to inflammation of the epididymis and testicles, respectively. We can classify these inflammatory processes as acute, subacute, or chronic, based on symptom duration. Acute epididymitis refers to symptoms that have been present for up to five weeks and generally involves scrotal pain and swelling. Chronic epididymitis, in contrast, is generally characterized by pain without notable inflammation, with symptoms persisting for over three months. Differentiation of the acute and chronic phases is critical to appropriate diagnosis, treatment, and resolution of these urological problems.

Anatomy and Physiology

The epididymis is an oblong organ situated above the posterolateral surface of the testis. The internal structure consists of a 3–4-m long tube folded into a tight coil, so that the organ's effective length is 5 cm [1]. The epididymis is covered by the tunica vaginalis, which extends within the interductal spaces to form anatomically and functionally distinct regions commonly referred to as the head, body, and tail.

Histologically, the epididymis is largely composed of two cell types: main cells and basal cells. Main cells have secretory and absorptive functions and vary in height across the length of the epididymis, due to the variable lengths of their stereocilia. Basal cells are derived from macrophages and are found in much lower quantities, dispersed mainly throughout the epithelium [2, 3].

Outside the basal lamina of the epididymal tubes, various contractile cells facilitate sperm transport. The spermatozoa mature as they travel the length of the epididymis and make contact with the fluids and secretions found in the epididymal lumen [4].

The three main functions of the epididymis – maturation, transport, and storage of spermatozoa – are controlled by neurological, hormonal, and thermal factors [5].

A Clinical Guide to Urologic Emergencies, First Edition. Edited by Hunter Wessells, Shigeo Horie, and Reynaldo G. Gómez.

Neurological control regulates the peristaltic progression of spermatozoa through the epididymal lumen. In terms of hormonal regulation, testosterone concentrations within the interstitial compartment of the epididymis are significantly higher than in the serum. Another hormone, dihydrotestosterone (DHT), is responsible for maintaining the structure of the epididymis, as well as functions associated with sperm maturation and storage. As with testosterone, the epididymis shows high DHT levels, attributable to high levels of 5 alpha-reductase expression [6]. Finally, gamete storage and electrolyte transport processes occurring inside the scrotum require a temperature 2–3 °C lower than that of the organism. As a result, increased scrotal temperatures alter epididymal function, potentially compromising the quantity of ejaculated spermatozoa and affecting fertility, as occurs in patients with varicoceles or cryptorchidism [7].

Epidemiology

A variety of inflammatory conditions may affect the epididymis. The most frequent problems include bacterial, viral, and fungal infections, as well as idiopathic and non-infectious diseases. Acute epididymitis is characterized by epididymal inflammation resulting in pain and swelling. The evolution time is short (three to five days), and the condition is typically unilateral. Prevalence is unknown, and the age range for epididymitis episodes is variable.

Epididymitis is the most common urological diagnosis among men aged 18 to 50 years [8]. Approximately 600 000 new epididymitis cases are reported per year in the United States, the majority in men aged 18–35 years [9].

A Canadian study evaluated the prevalence, diagnostic patterns, and typical management of patients with epididymitis seeking outpatient urological treatment from April–July 2004. Participating urologists were selected randomly from the urological associations of Canada and Quebec. Among the 6037 men evaluated, prevalence was 0.9% (n = 57). In 80% of these cases, the inflammation was classified as chronic (duration longer than three months) [10].

A review of 121 epididymitis patients treated on an outpatient basis showed that there was a bimodal distribution, with incidence peaks at 16–30 and 51–70 years of age [11].

Epididymitis is more common than orchitis. Orchitis is an inflammatory reaction of the testis, which usually occurs secondary to an infection. Most cases of orchitis are associated with a viral mumps infection. However, other bacteria and viruses can also cause orchitis. When epididymitis and orchitis coexist, orchitis results from the spread of epididymis inflammation to the adjacent testis [12].

One study reported that orchitis was also found in 58% of men diagnosed with epididymitis [11]. Isolated orchitis is rare and is generally associated with mumps in prepubescent boys.

Pathophysiology

The underlying pathophysiology of epididymitis is not clearly established; however, a leading hypothesis attributes the etiology to retrograde flow of infected urine toward the ejaculatory ducts.

Höppner et al. evaluated the records of 1031 patients with acute epididymitis treated from 1979 to 1989, of which 270 (26%) were managed surgically. Of all surgical interventions, 80% were performed for therapeutic purposes and the remaining 20% for diagnostic purposes, to rule out testicular torsion or tumor. These latter patients would now be diagnosed with ultrasonography. The authors reported that the most common underlying cause of epididymitis among the patients managed surgically was lower urinary tract obstruction [13].

This hypothesis is also supported by results from animal models. Inoculating bacterial pathogens such as *Escherichia coli* or *Chlamydia trachomatis* into the vas deferens produces epididymitis, with a clinical picture, both clinically and microbiologically identical to that found in humans [14, 15].

Tubercular involvement of the genitourinary organs is almost always secondary to pulmonary infection. This subclinical pulmonary infection leads to bacillemia and hematogenous implantation of the tuberculosis bacilli in the kidneys, epididymis, and the prostate [16].

Infectious Epididymitis

Acute infectious epididymitis is generally due to propagation of an infectious agent from the bladder, urethra, or prostate through the ejaculatory ducts and vas deferens into the epididymis. Although about 80% of epididymitis cases are of presumed infectious etiology, the underlying bacterial agent is identified in only 25% of cases [17]. These data come from large epidemiological studies of patients with clinical signs of epididymitis. Patients undergoing urinary tract instrumentation are at elevated risk for epididymitis, supporting the hypothesis that from a physio-pathological point of view, a backflow of infected urine toward the vas deferens is responsible for the infection. Moreover, patients with a urinary tract infection at the time of instrumentation are at even greater risk of epididymitis, and 50% of patients with infectious epididymitis have undergone intermittent catheterization. Among patients younger than 35 years, *C. trachomatis* is thought to be the main agent responsible for infectious epididymitis; however, in about 90% of cases, it is not possible to confirm the presence of the bacteria with PCR [18].

In men older than 35 years, the etiological agents that most typically affect the epididymis are coliform bacteria, of which *E. coli* is the most commonly identified. Other agents have also been implicated in sporadic epididymitis, such as *Ureaplasma urealitycum*, *Corynebacterium* sp., *Mycoplasma* sp., and *Mima polymorpha* [19].

Among children, most epididymitis cases are of viral origin. A study comparing serum viral levels and cultures in patients with and without an epididymitis diagnosis found that antibody titers were significantly higher among those with a history of infection. Infection with mumps has been practically eradicated thanks to the vaccine that was introduced in the United States in 1985 [20].

Chronic epididymal infections are associated with diseases that produce a granulomatous reaction in the parenchyma, the most common of which is infection with *Mycobacterium tuberculosis*. Although there is typically concomitant renal compromise accompanying this epididymal infection, dissemination is thought to occur through the hematogenous route rather than via the urinary tract. Up to 25% of patients have bilateral epididymis, with echographic findings of hyperemic epididymis, involving greater inflammation and multiple cysts and calcifications. Tuberculous epididymitis should be suspected in patients with a history of exposure to tuberculosis, as well as in those whose clinical symptoms do not improve with antibiotics [21].

About 10% of patients with brucellosis develop epididymitis secondary to the presence of this gram-negative coccobacillus. Infection with Brucella occurs via direct contact with infected animals or consumption of unpasteurized milk. In the United States, the states with the highest numbers of cases are California and Texas, due to their proximity to Mexico [22]. The clinical presentation of epididymitis due to Brucella is generally similar to that associated with other infectious agents; however, an ultrasound finding of septated hydrocele is more common with this diagnosis [23]. Diagnosis is based on clinical history and subsequent confirmation with a blood test.

Funiculoepididymitis is a rare cause of epididymitis in the United States, attributable to lymphatic compromise due to filarial infection. About 90% of cases of human lymphatic filariasis are caused by *Wuchereria bancrofti*. The disease typically occurs in patients under 40 years of age. The most common findings are pain, fever, chills, spermatic cord swelling, hydrocele, and leukocytosis with or without eosinophilia. Plain radiographs of patients with filariasis often reveal calcifications [24].

Non-infectious Epididymitis

Unlike infectious epididymitis, thought to be attributable to a backflow of infected urine through the vas deferens, the mechanism behind noninfectious epididymitis (NIE) is less clear.

One hypothesis is that there may be backflow of sterile urine through the vas deferens if the detrusor muscle is contracted when the bladder is completely full. However, less than 10% of patients with NIE have a history of abnormal micturition force, which can produce urinary backflow [17, 18, 25]. Furthermore, NIE symptoms can occur after a vasectomy, in which case sterile urine backflow cannot the principal mechanism of disease. Years after vasectomy, a small number of patients present with epididymal inflammation and intermittent pain in the area. These symptoms are attributable to congestion and inflammation as a result of vas deferens obstruction or epididymal granuloma formation [26].

Sarcoidosis is a granulomatous disease characterized by small accumulations of inflammatory cells in various parts of the body, especially the lungs, lymphatic ganglia, eyes, and skin. It occurs most frequently among African Americans and involves the genitourinary system in 5% of cases. Urological signs may include granulomas in the epididymis, testicles, and vas deferens. Typically, there is a progressive growth of the epididymis, occurring bilaterally in 30% of cases [27]. Echographic findings are variable, generally identifying a heterogeneous growth that may involve multiple nodules. These growths may lead to azoospermia in some cases, and therefore a seminogram should be included in the work-up for patients who plan to have children or who are undergoing surgical exploration [28]. In men with oligospermia, cryopreservation should be offered. The main treatment is corticosteroid therapy, which ameliorates both the pain and the inflammation. In cases for which medical management is not possible, or when response to corticosteroid therapy is poor, surgical management and epididymal extraction may be considered.

Behcet's syndrome is an autoimmune disease of unknown cause affecting the blood vessels (vasculitis). The disease presents with myriad signs and symptoms including mouth and genital sores, uveitis, and epididymitis [29]. In this latter case, patients are prone to concomitant genital ulcers, skin lesions, and arthritis. Treatment is empirical, typically consisting of topical or oral corticosteroids to relieve symptoms.

Chronic use of certain drugs such as amiodarone may cause epididymitis [30]. High concentrations of the drug accumulate in the epididymis, with levels up to 300 times higher than the target serum level, leading to formation of anti-amiodarone antibodies that produce epididymal inflammation and pain. Epididymitis incidence is directly related to dosage, and up to 11% of treated patients with high doses of this medication develop epididymal inflammation. In these cases, the recommendation is to discontinue the drug or reduce the dosage [31].

Schönlein–Henoch purpura is an autoimmune disease of unknown origin. The disease is a type of leukocytoclastic vasculitis characterized by inflammation of small blood vessels, with corresponding skin manifestations. Deposits of immunoglobulin A (IgA) complexes form, potentially leading to acute vasculitic epididymo-orchitis, especially in children aged 2–11 years. Echographic findings include inflammation and increased epididymal volume, increased blood flow, scrotal wall thickening, and sometimes hydrocele. The disease is generally self-limiting and responds well to treatment with corticosteroids [32].

Chronic Epididymitis

Chronic epididymitis is characterized by referred pain in the scrotum, testicles, or epididymis for at least three months. Chronic epididymitis is the reason for 80% of office visits among patients who seek urological treatment for genital pain [10]. Median age at presentation is 49 years, although most patients have had symptoms for at least 5 years prior to diagnosis. Generally, the pain is mild to moderate and does not interfere with activities of daily living. Patients tend to have higher numbers of sexual partners and a greater incidence of erectile dysfunction, musculoskeletal pain, and neurological disorders as compared to healthy controls. In evaluating these patients, it is important to rule out chronic prostatitis and chronic pelvic pain syndrome.

Diagnosis

While most diseases of the epididymis are benign, it is always necessary to take a detailed clinical history and perform a thorough physical exam.

Men with acute epididymitis present with unilateral testicular pain, hydrocele, and significantly increased epididymal volume. In general, the increased volume begins at the tail of the epididymis and then propagates to the rest of the organ, potentially reaching the testicle. The spermatic cord is hypersensitive and in some cases notably thickened. Fever and other symptoms associated with lower urinary tract infections, such as frequent urination, urinary urgency, hematuria, and dysuria, may also be present. It is always important to rule out testicular torsion, which can be accomplished with a testicular Doppler scan.

According to the United States Centers for Disease Control and Prevention (CDC), all patients with suspected acute epididymitis should be assessed for inflammation, evaluating for one of the following findings [33]:

1) Presence of at least two white blood cells in the oil immersion field using gram staining, methyl blue, or gentian violet in a urethral secretion sample
2) Positive leukocyte esterase test in a first-void urine sample
3) Microscopic analysis of urine sediment, demonstrating the presence of 10 or more white blood cells per field.

In children and adolescents who are not sexually active, and in adults over the age of 35 years, a second-void urine sample should be obtained. The urine should be tested using dipstick and microscopy. A urine culture should then be performed for patients with a positive result on either test, as well as for patients at risk for complicated urinary tract infections, such as patients with a recent history of urinary tract instrumentation, urinary catheterization, or anal sex, to rule out the presence of coliform bacteria.

In sexually active men below 35 years of age, the clinician should also rule out *C. trachomatis*. In these cases, testing a urethral exudate sample using gram staining is recommended, in order to assess for urethritis. The definitive diagnosis should be made using nucleic acid amplification (PCR).

Ultrasonography is the first-line imaging modality for evaluating a patient with suspected acute epididymo-orchitis. Over the past decade, ultrasound technology has vastly improved, resulting in increased sensitivity and specificity of scrotal pathology studies. Transducers with a power of 5–10 MHz and color Doppler scans allow for differentiation among a wide variety of conditions that affect scrotal composition.

Ultrasonographic findings which are considered diagnostic of acute epididymitis include an enlarged epididymis with a hypoechoic, hyperechoic, or heterogeneous echotexture and increased blood flow (see Figure 17.1). Also, associated reactive hydrocele and scrotal wall thickening may be present [34].

The main goal of ultrasound is to rule out testicular torsion. However, it is difficult to differentiate a partial torsion from epididymitis, making clinical history crucial.

A finding of decreased flow on Doppler study as compared to the contralateral testicle has a sensitivity of 80–90% and a specificity of nearly 100% for diagnosis of torsion. On the other hand, increased blood flow to the epididymis provides evidence of inflammation.

Magnetic resonance imaging (MRI) allows for detailed evaluation of extra-testicular lesions and can be used when ultrasound alone is incapable of diagnosing an epididymal lesion. On a T1 weighted image (T1) sequence, both testicular and epididymal lesions have an intermediate intensity, while on T2 weighted image T2, they appear hyperintensive, due to elevated water content in the testicle.

Treatment

Treatment for epididymitis includes rest, scrotal suspension, analgesics, and empirical treatment with antibiotics if infection is suspected. Most cases can be treated on an outpatient basis; however, hospital admission is recommended in cases involving intractable

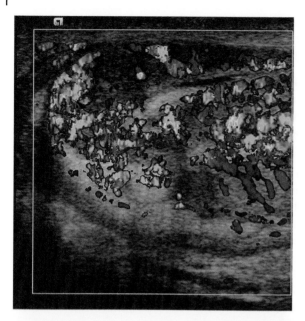

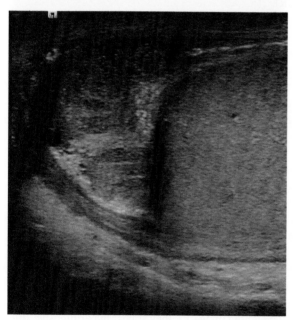

Figure 17.1 Ultrasonographic findings of acute epididymitis showing increased flow on color Doppler (above) and enlarged epididymitis (below) on B-mode. *Source:* courtesy of Andrés O'Brien, MD.

pain, systemic signs (fever or leukocytosis), or other complicating medical conditions, or when a clear diagnosis cannot be otherwise established.

In patients with suspected infectious etiology, empirical treatment with antibiotics should be initiated, even if laboratory tests cannot provide definitive results. The objective of the treatment is to prevent complications and transmission of organisms via sexual contact. Treatment is selected based on the probability of infection with chlamydia, gonorrhea, or enterobacteriaceae.

Recommended Antibiotic Regimens

For acute epididymitis likely due to sexually transmitted chlamydia or gonorrhea:

- Single intramuscular (IM) dose of 250 mg Ceftriaxone +100 mg oral Doxycycline twice daily for 10 days

  For acute epididymitis likely due to chlamydia, gonorrhea, or enteric organisms transmitted via insertive anal sex:

- Single IM dose of 250 mg Ceftriaxone + 500 mg oral Levofloxacin once daily for 10 days, or 300 mg oral Ofloxacin twice daily for 10 days

  For acute epididymitis likely due to enteric organisms:

- 500 mg oral Levofloxacin once daily for 10 days, or 300 mg oral Ofloxacin twice daily for 10 days

Additional Considerations

For patients with confirmed acute epididymitis due to infection with *C. trachomatis* or *Neisseria gonorrhea*, sexual abstinence is recommended for the patient and his partner until both have been treated successfully and the symptoms have disappeared. Screening for other sexually transmitted infections such as HIV is also recommended.

Treatment of Sexual Partners

Evaluation and treatment are recommended for the sexual partners of patients with *C. trachomatis* or *N. gonorrhea* infection, especially if the sexual contact occurred within 60 days prior to symptom onset. If the last sexual contact occurred more than 60 days prior to symptom onset, the most recent sexual partner should be contacted.

Allergies, Intolerance, and Adverse Reactions

In penicillin-allergic patients, there is cross-reactivity with cephalosporins in less than 2.5% of cases. The risk is higher with first-generation cephalosporins and lower with second- and third-generation drugs. There are no studies on the efficacy of alternative regimens; therefore, an infectology consultation is advisable in these cases.

Patients with HIV

For HIV-positive patients with uncomplicated epididymitis, the recommended treatment regimen is identical to that used for immunocompetent patients. It is important to note than in these patients, other etiologic agents should be considered, including cytomegalovirus (CMV), salmonella, toxoplasmosis, ureaplasma, corynebacterium, and Mycoplasma. Infection with fungus and various mycobacteria are also more common among HIV-positive versus HIV-negative patients.

Follow-up

Follow-up is recommended if symptoms do not improve within 72 hours of beginning treatment. If pain or inflammation continues after treatment is completed, a thorough evaluation is recommended to rule out other causes such as tumor, abscess, infarct, tuberculosis, or fungal infection.

Management of Chronic Epididymitis

There are no randomized, placebo-controlled studies evaluating treatments for chronic epididymitis. Most of the available therapies are empirical, and none is effective when used alone. Treatments include local application of heat, nerve blocks, anti-inflammatories, tricyclic antidepressants, and neuroleptics. Successful treatment may involve a combination of various therapies and drug regimens, individualized according to the patient's response.

Staggered management is recommended: for at least the first two weeks, nonsteroidal anti-inflammatories should be used, especially drugs that can be used for long periods, such as naproxen. In addition to pharmacological treatment, rest and testicular suspension are recommended. If symptoms continue, a tricyclic antidepressant or neuroleptic such as Gabapentin may be added to the regimen.

For cases with a poor response, despite several months of treatment, a spermatic cord block with local anesthesia can be considered.

Epididymectomy is reserved for cases with intractable pain. However, this treatment has a failure rate of up to 75% and is therefore not generally recommended.

Complications

Complications are more common in cases attributable to infectious versus uropathogenic processes. Complication rates are higher among older men, patients with bacteriuria, and patients with urological malformations. One study analyzed the evolution of 33 patients with a diagnosis of severe acute epididymitis. Most of the cases were treated on an inpatient basis, with outpatient follow-up to evaluate the incidence of complications. The authors found that in 39% of cases, severe complications developed, including testicular infarct, suppurative necrosis, and testicular atrophy [35].

In patients with delayed antibiotic treatment, 3–8% of patients suffer abscesses during the acute phase, while the rate is less than 3% among those who receive timely treatment [36].

The relationship between acute epididymitis and male subfertility is not clearly established. Inflammation of the testicular parenchyma leads to a deterioration and decrease of spermatogenesis during the acute phase of the disease. However, the incidence of infertility as a result of an epididymitis episode is unknown. Moreover, isolated compromise of an accessory sex gland has been confirmed as the source of subfertility in only 1.6% of infertile men [37].

Conclusion

Acute epididymitis is a common disease in the urological field. Most cases are of presumed infectious etiology. A clinical history and a thorough physical examination help to make a diagnosis and laboratory tests can confirm the etiology in some cases. Ultrasonography of the testes is a useful and quick test to rule out other causes of testicular pain and enlargement, especially acute torsion.

Patients with suspected infectious etiology should be treated with appropriate antibiotics and in cases of suspected sexually transmitted infection (STI), treatment of all sexual partners is required. Acute complications such as abscesses are uncommon and early treatment helps to avoid this complication.

References

1 Lanz, T. and Neuhauser, G. (1964). Morphometrische analyse des menschlichen nebenodens. *Z. Anat. Entwicklungsgesch.* 124: 126–152.

2 Vendrely, E. and Dadoune, J.P. (1988). Quantitative ultrastructural analysis of the principal cells in the human epididymis. *Reprod. Nutr. Dev.* 28 (5): 1225–1235.

3 Robaire, B. and Hinton, B. (2006). *The Epididymis*, 3e, vol. 1. St. Louis: Elsevier, Inc.

4 Holstein, A.F. (1969). Morphologische studien am Nebenhoden des Mensche. *Norm. Pathol. Anat.* 20: 1–91.

5 Sasagawa, M. (1990). Release of leukotrienes (LTC4, D4, E4, B4) from peripheral leukocytes in patients with bronchial asthma. *Arerugi* 39 (12): 1556–1566.

6 Robaire, B. and Henderson, N.A. (2006). Actions of 5alpha-reductase inhibitors on the epididymis. *Mol. Cell. Endocrinol.* 250 (1–2): 190–195.

7 Bedford, J.M. (1991). Effects of elevated temperature on the epididymis and testis: experimental studies. *Adv. Exp. Med. Biol.* 286: 19–32.

8 Collins, M.M., Stafford, R.S., O'Leary, M.P. et al. (1998). How common is prostatitis? A national survey of physician visits. *J. Urol.* 159 (4): 1224–1228.

9 Trojian, T.H., Lishnak, T.S., and Heiman, D. (2009). Epididymitis and orchitis: an overview. *Am. Fam. Physician* 79 (7): 583–587.

10 Nickel, J.C. et al. (2005). Prevalence, diagnosis, characterization, and treatment of prostatitis, interstitial cystitis, and epididymitis in outpatient urological practice: the Canadian PIE study. *Urology* 66 (5): 935–940.

11 Kaver, I., Matzkin, H., and Braf, Z.F. (1990). Epididymo-orchitis: a retrospective study of 121 patients. *J. Fam. Pract.* 30 (5): 548–552.

12 Frungieri, M.B., Calandera, R.S., Bartke, A. et al. (2018). Ageing and inflammation in the male reproductive tract. *Andrologia* 50 (11): e13034.

13 Hoppner, W., Strohmeher, T., Hartmann, M. et al. (1992). Surgical treatment of acute epididymitis and its underlying diseases. *Eur. Urol.* 22 (3): 218–221.

14 Ludwig, M., Johannes, S., Bergmann, M. et al. (2002). Experimental *Escherichia coli* epididymitis in rats: a model to assess the outcome of antibiotic treatment. *BJU Int.* 90 (9): 933–938.

15 Jantos, C., Baumgärtner, W., Durchfield, B. et al. (1992). Experimental epididymitis due to Chlamydia trachomatis in rats. *Infect. Immun.* 60 (6): 2324–2328.

16 Yadav, S., Singh, P., Hemal, A. et al. (2017). Genital tuberculosis: current status of diagnosis and management. *Transl. Androl. Urol.* 6 (2): 222–233.

17 Tracy, C.R., Steers, W.D., and Costabile, R. (2008). Diagnosis and management of epididymitis. *Urol. Clin. North Am.* 35 (1): 101–108; vii.

18 Berger, R.E., Alexander, E.R., Harisch, J.P. et al. (1979). Etiology, manifestations and therapy of acute epididymitis: prospective study of 50 cases. *J. Urol.* 121 (6): 750–754.

19 Tracy, C. (2007). *Anatomy, physiology and diseases of the epididymis.* AUA Update Series. XXVI: lesson 12.

20 Somekh, E., Gorenstein, A., and Serour, F. (2004). Acute epididymitis in boys: evidence of a post-infectious etiology. *J. Urol.* 171 (1): 391–394; discussion 394.

21 Ferrie, B.G. and Rundle, J.S. (1983). Tuberculous epididymo-orchitis. A review of 20 cases. *Br. J. Urol.* 55 (4): 437–439.

22 Pappas, G., Akritidis, N., Bosilkovski, M. et al. (2005). Brucellosis. *N. Engl. J. Med.* 352 (22): 2325–2336.

23 Ozturk, A., Ozturk, E., Zeyrek, F. et al. (2005). Comparison of brucella and non-specific epididymorchitis: gray scale and color Doppler ultrasonographic features. *Eur. J. Radiol.* 56 (2): 256–262.

24 Williams, P.B., Henderson, R.J., Sanusi, I.D. et al. (1996). Ultrasound diagnosis of filarial funiculoepididymitis. *Urology* 48 (4): 644–646.

25 Mittemeyer, B.T., Lennox, K.W., and Borski, A.A. (1966). Epididymitis: a review of 610 cases. *J. Urol.* 95 (3): 390–392.

26 Christiansen, C.G. and Sandlow, J.I. (2003). Testicular pain following vasectomy: a review of postvasectomy pain syndrome. *J. Androl.* 24 (3): 293–298.

27 Ryan, D.M., Lesser, B.A., Crumley, L.A. et al. (1993). Epididymal sarcoidosis. *J. Urol.* 149 (1): 134–136.

28 Rudin, L., Megalli, M., and Mesa-Tejada, R. (1974). Genital sarcoidosis. *Urology* 3 (6): 750–754.

29 Cho, Y.H., Jung, J., Lee, K.H. et al. (2003). Clinical features of patients with Behcet's disease and epididymitis. *J. Urol.* 170 (4 Pt 1): 1231–1233.

30 Greene, H.L., Graham, E.L., Werner, J.A. et al. (1983). Toxic and therapeutic effects of amiodarone in the treatment of cardiac arrhythmias. *J. Am. Coll. Cardiol.* 2 (6): 1114–1128.

31 Ibsen, H.H., Frandsen, F., Brandrup, F. et al. (1989). Epididymitis caused by treatment with amiodarone. *Genitourin. Med.* 65 (4): 257–258.

32 Huang, L.H., Yeung, C.Y., Shyur, S.D. et al. (2004). Diagnosis of Henoch-Schonlein purpura by sonography and radionuclear scanning in a child presenting with bilateral acute scrotum. *J. Microbiol. Immunol. Infect.* 37 (3): 192–195.

33 Workowski, K.A., Bolan, G.A., and Centers for Disease Control and Prevention (2015). Sexually transmitted diseases treatment guidelines, 2015. *MMWR Recomm Rep.* 64 (RR-03): 1–137. Erratum in: MMWR Recomm Rep. 2015, 64(33): 924. PMID: 26042815; PMCID: PMC5885289.

34 Lev, M., Ramon, J., Mor, Y. et al. (2015). Sonographic appearances of torsion of the appendix testis and appendix epididymis in children. *J. Clin. Ultrasound* 43 (8): 485–489.

35 Desai, K.M., Gingell, J.C., and Haworth, J.M. (1986). Fate of the testis following epididymitis: a clinical and ultrasound study. *J. R. Soc. Med.* 79 (9): 515–519.

36 Eickhoff, J.H., Frimodt-Møller, N., Walter, S. et al. (1999). A double-blind, randomized, controlled multicentre study to compare the efficacy of ciprofloxacin with pivampicillin as oral therapy for epididymitis in men over 40 years of age. *BJU Int.* 84 (7): 827–834.

37 Luzzi, G.A. and O'Brien, T.S. (2001). Acute epididymitis. *BJU Int.* 87 (8): 747–755.

Section IV

Pediatric

18

Urologic Neonatal Emergencies

Nicolas Fernandez[1] and Nayib Fakih[2]

[1] Division of Pediatric Urology, Seattle Children's Hospital, University of Washington, Seattle, WA, USA
[2] Division of Urology, Hospital Universitario San Ignacio, Pontificia Universidad Javeriana, Bogota, Colombia

Introduction

Neonatal urological emergencies are uncommon in the general pediatric practice but require highly complex medical infrastructure and a multidisciplinary approach. The aim of this chapter is to describe the most common urological neonatal emergencies that require immediate or early surgical intervention by the pediatric urologist and the multidisciplinary team. The majority of these conditions are detected on routine antenatal ultrasound. Once identified, patients and their mothers should be referred to a specialized center for delivery, as most of these conditions require specific evaluations and treatments, which in the hands of trained multidisciplinary teams improve prognosis and reduce the risk of permanent disability [1].

Posterior Urethral Valves (PUV)

Posterior rethral valves (PUV) is a condition that is usually detected by ultrasound in the prenatal period with a prevalence of 1.4 per 10 000 newborns [2, 3]. It is caused by the abnormal presence of valves at the prostatic urethra that cause bladder outlet obstruction. These membranes are believed to arise from an abnormal development of the urethral crests. By the eighth week of gestation, the prostatic urethra develops and at this point, the mesonephric and paramesonephric ducts fuse with this region of the arising prostatic urethra. When the Wolffian ducts have an abnormal implantation and fusion with the urethra, abnormal urethral membranes develop. According to the original classification described by Hugh H. Young in 1919, there are three different types of PUV, based on 21 cases that were evaluated endoscopically [4]. Type I, which is the most common type accounting for 95% of the cases, presents as a thin membrane that radiates from the distal end of the *verum montanum* to the anterior urethral wall just immediately proximal to the external sphincter. The other two types account for the remaining 5% of the cases. Type II are the least common and were originally described as mucosal folds that start at the *verum montanum* and extend proximally to the bladder neck. Type III, which are the second-most common type, were described as circular membranes that occlude the urethral lumen transversely and are located at the distal to *verum montanum*. Cobb's collar (also called Moormann's ring) has also been considered as a type III PUV [5, 6].

Since Young's classification was proposed, it has been used worldwide; nonetheless, it is important to highlight that some authors have opposing arguments based on the grounds that valves are anatomically disrupted when the urethra is catheterized immediately after birth and before endoscopic evaluation [7]. Also, postmortem evaluations have shown that all cases of PUV are caused by circular diaphragmatic membranes [8]. These findings and arguments suggest a change in the terminology and propose the term "congenital obstructing posterior urethral membranes" (COPUM) [9].

Since the degree of obstruction varies among affected children, there is a spectrum of clinical presentations that vary from oligo/anhydramnios with severe pulmonary dysplasia and high mortality, to late detection of children with voiding dysfunction.

Antenatal Diagnosis and Management

PUV is one of the conditions that can and should be detected during the antenatal period. It is the most common cause of infravesical urinary tract obstruction [10]. Most cases can be detected as early as 12 weeks, but the majority will become clinically and radiologically evident once the kidneys start producing urine around the 16th week of gestation. The best time for urinary tract ultrasonographic screening is at the 20th week of gestation. There are some sonographic findings that suggest the presence of PUV. Bilateral hydroureteronephrosis with a distended bladder or megacystis with thickened walls on a male fetus should always be warning signs to suspect PUV. A classic ultrasonographic finding is the presence of the "keyhole" sign, consisting of the larger lumen of the bladder in continuity with the dilated posterior urethra more caudally (Figure 18.1).

The postnatal positive predictive value, once this classic presentation is seen, is around 48% [11]. Nonetheless, rates of antenatal detection vary among published series. Overall,

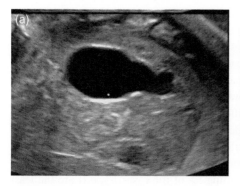 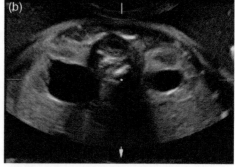

Figure 18.1 Prenatal maternal ultrasound of a fetus with PUV. (a) Bladder projection with classic "keyhole sign." (b) Bilateral hydronephrosis (axial image demonstrating more severe dilation of right kidney). *Source:* courtesy of Nicolas Fernandez, MD, PhD.

Figure 18.2 Neonate with PUV and ascites that extends into the scrotum. *Source:* courtesy of Dr. Jaime F. Perez.

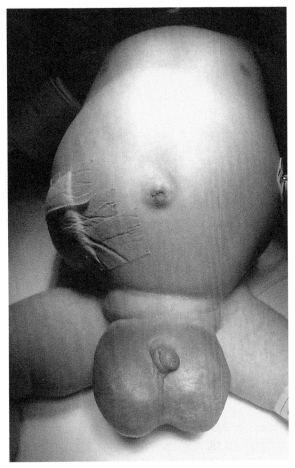

ultrasonographic sensitivity ranges between 90 and 100%. Sequential assessment over time may increase the rate of detection. Other important findings that should be recorded include the echogenicity of the kidneys, which predicts the degree of severity of renal dysfunction. Bladder wall thickness depends on how severely obstructed it is. The presence of oligohydramnios has been reported in around 50% of cases. "Pop-off" mechanisms have been described as protective mechanisms that correlate with better renal function [12, 13]. These pop-off mechanisms are: renal forniceal rupture with perirenal urinoma, bladder diverticuli, and bladder rupture [14]. Severe cases may present with urinary ascites (Figure 18.2).

The incidence of these findings in patients with PUV has been reported to be around 20% [12, 13, 15–17]. Differential diagnosis should include severe vesicoureteral reflux and Eagle Barrett Syndrome (Prune-Belly Syndrome), and urethral atresia.

Antenatal detection allows families to be counseled and referred to tertiary centers for optimal perinatal management. A few centers have advanced antenatal detection for early intervention with the placement of a vesicoamniotic shunt or *in utero* cystoscopy and valve ablation (in those cases with favorable amniotic fluid parameters) [18–20] (Table 18.1).

Table 18.1 Predictive amniotic fluid variables.

Variable	Favorable
Sodium (Na)	Less than 100 mEq/l
Chloride (Cl)	Less than 90 mEql/l
Osmolarity (Osm)	Less than 210 mEq/l
Calcium (Ca)	Less than 2 mmol/l
Beta-2 microglobulin	Less than 2 mg/l

Current evidence fails to support the benefit of early diversion and its impact on long-term outcomes [21]. Nonetheless, the pressure gradient dynamics between the bladder and amniotic fluid, and its impact on appropriate bladder decompression once the shunt has been placed, have never been studied. How much of a role this may play on current outcomes is unknown. It has been identified that amniotic fluid pressures are higher in the first and second trimesters and decrease in the third trimester [22].

The benefit of an early referral enables multidisciplinary planning at the moment of delivery. Therefore, the obstetric and pediatric urology teams can prepare accordingly. It is ideal if the pediatric urologist can participate in any antenatal counseling.

Pre-Operative Management in the Neonatal Unit

At birth, management will be guided based on the severity of pulmonary dysplasia. Early urinary diversion includes the placement of a 5 (1.65 mm) to 6 (1.98 mm) Fr. urethral catheter. Some authors suggest avoiding a Foley, because the balloon irritates the bladder and causes severe spasms and may also occlude ureteral meatus. Nonetheless, based on Penna et al.'s experience with double J stent placement for urinary diversion, we currently use this as the standard method for urinary diversion in all cases (Figure 18.3) [23].

All double J stent placements are performed under ultrasound guidance in order to avoid leaving the proximal coil in the bladder neck or prostatic urethra (Figure 18.3). This initial diversion does not compromise concomitant management required from a pulmonary standpoint and can be left in place until the patient is clinically stable enough to be brought to the operating room for endoscopic valve ablation. Irrespective of the catheter used, all patients should receive antibiotic prophylaxis.

Imaging Diagnosis

Early imaging studies focus on confirming diagnosis. Early postnatal ultrasonography should be performed beyond the first 48 hours to avoid a false negative result secondary to physiological neonatal dehydration.

There is no specific timing for performing a voiding cystourethrogram. Nonetheless, it should be done to confirm diagnosis and establish the presence and severity of vesicoureteral reflux (Figure 18.4). It also helps in the evaluation of bladder capacity and

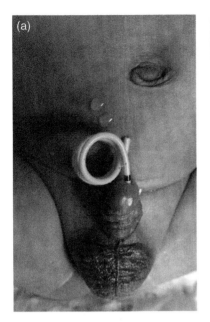
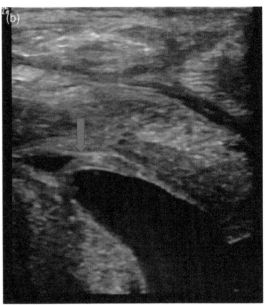

Figure 18.3 (a) Double J stent in place in a patient with PUV with the proximal coil in the bladder. (b) Real-time use of ultrasound to guide double J stent placement. Arrow highlights valves with proximal dilated bladder neck. Courtesy of Dr. Armando Lorenzo.

Figure 18.4 Classic findings of voiding cystourethrogram. Arrow highlights the transition point where valves are present. Note massive vesicoureteral reflux (VUR). *Source:* courtesy of Nicolas Fernandez, MD, PhD.

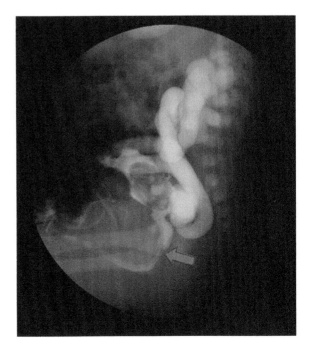

appearance. We have modified our protocol to perform it at the moment of surgery to avoid pain and parents' distress with the study when the patient is awake.

Surgical Management

Current standard of care is endoscopic valve ablation, initially proposed by Young and McKay in 1929 [24]. Most surgeons use cold knife valve ablation, but reports using different cutting or ablating techniques have also been proposed, such as Bugbee or LASER ablation (Figure 18.5) [25]. There is no literature comparing and supporting one or the other. The authors used a neonatal 3Fr. cystoscope for valve ablation with a Holmium LASER fiber.

The Bugbee electrode can be passed through a 5Fr. cystoscope, allowing the possibility of operating on smaller premature babies. Regardless of the type of instrument used for valve ablation, the standard technique suggests incision at 5, 7, and 12 o'clock to accomplish an appropriate ablation. Since the external (striated) sphincter is immediately distal to the location of valve insertion, it is important to avoid injuries that may compromise continence. It is also important to avoid high irrigation pressures as bladder rupture and bacteremia can be possible severe complications. Once valves have been ablated, it is important to confirm a good stream with the patient still intubated. Suboptimal ablation may require re-incision; immediate vesicostomy can also be performed.

There is no evidence supporting the benefit of bladder neck resection when long-term bladder function is assessed. Some surgeons leave an indwelling catheter after ablation. If that is the case, the authors advocate leaving a double J stent in place as described above.

Premature infants may not be immediate candidates for surgical valve ablation due to urethral caliber. Nonetheless, currently available cystoscopes with an 8.5Fr. (2.8 mm) resectoscope allow the possibility of resecting valves on premature babies. A cut-off weight of 2000 g has been suggested to predict the possibility of performing a successful endoscopic valve ablation. Other authors describe a percutaneous antegrade valve ablation for premature children as an alternative to vesicostomy [26]. Although premature low birth weight babies have a higher likelihood of requiring vesicostomy diversion, the long-term renal function outcomes have shown no difference when compared to normal birth weight

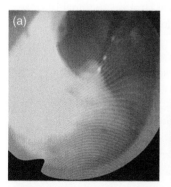 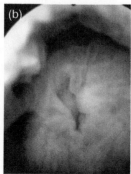 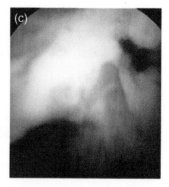

Figure 18.5 (a) Cold knife valve ablation. (b) Verum montanum and utricle orifice with posterior urethral valve extending anteriorly from 9 o'clock of the endoscopic surgical field. (c) Holmium fiber used to perform valve ablation. *Source:* courtesy of Nicolas Fernandez, MD, PhD.

babies [27]. Early intervention should also include circumcision in order to reduce the risks of future urinary tract infections. When endoscopic management is not feasible, or when there are signs of persistent obstruction despite endoscopic management, vesicostomy creation has been shown to be effective. Comparison between endoscopic management and vesicostomy has shown no significant difference in creatinine nadir [28].

Current evidence has proven that vesicostomy is a good method for adequate bladder diversion without compromising future bladder function, as it allows bladder cycling [29]. The most common surgical technique for vesicostomy is the Blocksom technique [30, 31] (see Figure 18.6).

Other types of diversion are the supravesical ureterostomies and pyelostomies (Figure 18.7) [32]. There are multiple types such as distal end ureterostomies, loop, circle, and Y-Sober [33, 34].

In the early 1960s, there were some clinicians who advocated for high urinary diversion with the creation of ureterostomies based on the persistent dilated ureters and clinical signs of poor upper tract drainage and stasis. Subsequent publications reporting the mid- and long-term follow-up of patients with upper urinary tract diversions, showed a detrimental effect on bladder function with no improvement in renal function deterioration [35, 36]. Due to these reports and others, the use of upper tract diversion as a routine practice has slowly been abandoned. Current supporters of high urinary diversion consider its use if no decrease in creatinine is seen after five days after lower diversion, with the belief that a thick bladder may be obstructing ureteral drainage.

Figure 18.6 Blocksom vesicostomy on a neonate with posterior urethral valves. *Source:* courtesy of Nicolas Fernandez, MD, PhD.

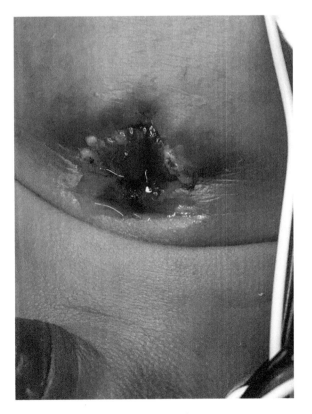

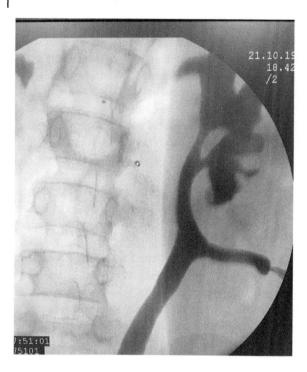

Figure 18.7 Radiologic image of a retrograde pyelogram on a patient with Y-Sober ureterostomy. *Source:* courtesy of Nicolas Fernandez, MD, PhD.

Post-Operative Management and Long-Term Outcomes

After valve ablation or vesicostomy creation, it is very challenging to establish whether persistent hydronephrosis or persistently elevated serum creatinine are due to inadequate diversion or a true nadir. Usually, hydronephrosis tends to take some time to improve after diversion. The concept of persistent obstruction at the ureterovesical junction due to a thick bladder is rare, as this is only present in 4% of the cases [37]. The lack of creatinine improvement may be due to established renal dysplasia that will not improve despite further diversion. Some centers use post-operative voiding cystourethrography (VCUG) to confirm successful ablation. We only consider it if the patient's clinical picture suggests the persistence of obstruction.

A recent debate has focused on the fact that some literature suggests that despite early diversion, there is no impact on reducing long-term development of chronic kidney disease and end-stage renal disease (ESRD). Current literature supports the creatinine nadir as a prognostic indicator for ESRD development [38]. Patients with creatinine higher than 0.8 mg/dl (75 μmol/l) have a higher risk of early ESRD [39].

Irreversible renal damage may occur as an early event *in utero*, explaining why some patients do not benefit from early vesico-amniotic shunt placement. Nonetheless, long-term bladder care (appropriate evacuation with low pressures) might be as important as urinary diversion in preserving renal function.

Management of Valve Bladder Syndrome

Current improvement in antenatal detection and initial aggressive management has improved patient survival. Although most cases will still develop ESRD, the possibility of performing renal transplant on these PUV patients has become more common over the last decades and the key to a better outcome with low rejection rates is an appropriate bladder management.

A number of patients, who suffered from PUV and were ablated as neonates, will still develop persistent renal obstruction due to high bladder pressures and poor emptying [37, 40]. It is not uncommon to see an increase in voiding volumes due to renal dysplasia and poor urine concentration. These high urine volumes may not be efficiently evacuated by the affected rigid "valve bladder." At this point in the natural history of PUV, children will start presenting with urinary incontinence, enuresis, urinary tract infections, and renal function deterioration. Unlike renal function and early valve ablation, bladder function has been preserved with early urinary diversion when compared to late diversion [41].

Epispadias, Bladder and Cloacal Exstrophy

This group of conditions represents one of the most challenging urogenital congenital anomalies, caused by an abnormal migration of mesenchymal cells into the cloacal membrane [42]. The lack of normal migration creates a fragile cloacal membrane that can rupture. The timing of the rupture during morphogenesis creates a spectrum of presentation with the least severe being epispadias and the most severe cloacal exstrophy. The latter is also known as omphalocele, exstrophy of the bladder, imperforate anus, and spinal abnormalities complex (OEIS).

The prevalence of bladder exstrophy has been reported to be 2.07 per 100 000 newborns with a variation between surveillance systems of 0.52–4.63 [43]. For cloacal exstrophy, the estimated prevalence has been reported to be 1 in 200 000 newborns [44].

Antenatal Diagnosis

Exstrophy can be detected with prenatal ultrasound. Suspicion for this diagnosis is made based on the presence of: (i) no bladder cycling during serial ultrasounds (empty bladder); (ii) low implantation of the umbilical cord in the abdomen; (iii) presence of omphalocele; (iv) small genitals; and (v) abnormal pelvic bone structures. A sign that has been described as suggestive of cloacal exstrophy, is the "elephant-trunk-like" sign when the prolapsed terminal ileum is seen [45]. Nonetheless, despite being a major anomaly with significant disability, only one-quarter of the cases are detected with antenatal ultrasound screening [46, 47]. Most reported cases have been identified around the 20th week of gestation. The appearance on physical examination is shown in Figure 18.8.

In cases of high suspicion, a Magnetic Resonance Imaging (MRI) can be performed for a more detailed description of the fetal anatomy.

It is important to note that cloacal anomalies are associated with spinal dysraphism and other severe anomalies such as heart defects [48, 49].

Initial Management in Neonate Unit

The ideal scenario includes antenatal detection and referral to a specialist center. Delivery should be planned, and the multidisciplinary team should be available and ready to take care of the newborn [50, 51]. Obstetricians should be aware that upon cord ligation, they

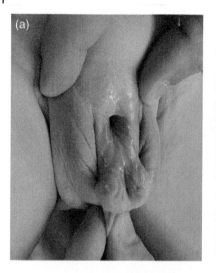
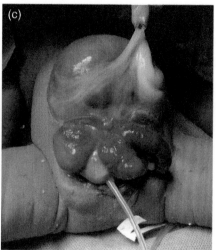
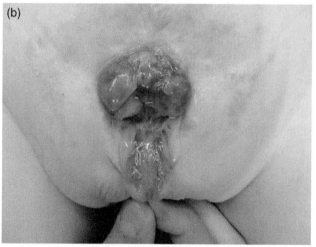

Figure 18.8 (a) Epispadias demonstrating dorsal urethral plate, (b) bladder exstrophy with bladder mucosa visible above epispadiac penis, and (c) cloacal exstrophy with colonic mucosa splayed out below omphalocele. *Source:* courtesy of Nicolas Fernandez, MD, PhD.

should avoid plastic umbilical clamps that may injure the bladder plate. Cord ligation should be done with a 2-0 silk or a rubber band.

The bladder should be covered at all times with a non-adherent plastic film such as Saran Wrap.

Gender assignment in cloacal exstrophy cases is challenging. This is when a multidisciplinary approach is of critical importance [52]. Karyotype will guide the surgical planning and how to counsel families throughout the process. We have found it very useful to use rapid KaryoFISH to more quickly obtain results of the chromosomal sex.

Neurosurgery will proceed with spina bifida repair as soon as the patient is stable enough. Other associated anomalies should be studied and treated accordingly. As important as a good surgical team, a good childcare and family support team is necessary. The process should begin with prenatal counseling. Immediate support after birth is of critical importance, considering that families will be dealing with a lot of information and challenging decisions [53].

General Principles for Surgical Repair

General principles for reconstruction include: (i) abdominal wall closure; (ii) pelvic bone closure; (iii) continence (bladder neck reconstruction with acceptable bladder capacity and compliance); and (iv) genital reconstruction. There are two main surgical trends. One favors a complete primary repair in the neonatal period and the other supports a staged repair [54–56]. Irrespective of technique and although some bladder plates may look small, a successful bladder closure has shown good bladder capacity on follow-up [56]. Continence may be achieved with the help of bladder neck reconstruction. The two most common procedures for bladder neck reconstruction are the Young-Dees-Leadbetter and Pippi-Salle techniques [57, 58]. Continence may also benefit from an appropriate pelvic bone closure [59]. Patients who have had successful primary repairs have a better continence prognosis [60].

Management of epispadias is rarely performed in the neonatal period. Bladder closure aims to allow the bladder to cycle and increase its capacity. Ideally, if needed, bladder neck reconstruction should be performed when patients are mature enough to go through potty training. Some authors have proposed the use of pre-operative testosterone. Recommended protocols use a dose of 2 mg/kg five weeks and then two weeks prior to surgery [61]. The two most common techniques for epispadias repair are the Cantwell-Ransley repair and the Mitchell-Bägli technique [62, 63].

Cloacal exstrophy closure may be more challenging and includes closure of the omphalocele and creation of a colostomy and closure of hemi-bladders [64]. Some groups have attempted a complete repair in a single stage, depending on how stable the patient is during surgery and how feasible it is given patient's anatomy.

Since patients with cloacal exstrophy present with other anomalies like spina bifida, development of neurogenic bladder is possible. Approximately 30% of cases do have spina bifida. This specific association may increase the need for future procedures such as augmentation cystoplasty and possible Mitrofanoff.

Post-Operative Considerations

Immediate post-operative care requires admission to the intensive care unit. All patients should undergo aggressive multimodal post-operative pain control including epidural catheters. Long-term studies have shown that neonates who have been exposed to painful experiences with suboptimal pain control have lower pain tolerance and thresholds when older [65]. Since most of these operations are performed at an early age, narcotics may not be the first line of treatment due to their central respiratory depressive effects. The authors prefer to keep patients intubated, relaxed and sedated during the first 24–48 hours after surgery, with the additional benefit of avoiding increased abdominal pressure when crying. Early feeding should also be an important part of early recovery [66].

Neonatal Testicular Torsion

Torsion that occurs during the perinatal period and until the first 30 days of life [67] (perinatal testicular torsion) has an incidence of 6.1 per 100000 male newborns [68, 69]. It is estimated that about 70% of cases occur *in utero*, with the remaining 30% during the neonatal period [70]. The pathophysiology of neonatal testicular torsion (NTT) is "extravaginal" torsion of the tunica vaginalis including testicle and epididymis. Some reports have presented cases of intravaginal torsion, which is more common during puberty and early adulthood. Vaginal delivery has been identified as a risk factor. It is believed that pressure at the birth canal generates tunica vaginalis torsion due to its loose attachment to the cremasteric muscle. Healthcare providers involved in the immediate neonatal care after delivery should be trained to improve early detection, as this may increase salvage rates [71] (Figure 18.9). Incarcerated inguinal hernia should always be considered as a differential diagnosis.

Since NTT is a rare event, and undiagnosed cases are not included in published series, it is virtually impossible to know the exact prevalence and salvage rates. The literature reports an estimated 5% salvage rate when an early diagnosis is made [72]. The lack of robust evidence creates a debate around whether or not immediate exploration is indicated, and the benefits of performing early surgery. Some authors favor immediate scrotal exploration and contralateral orchiopexy, considering the high risk of asynchronous contralateral torsion and development of anorchia. Opposing positions consider active surveillance as the care of choice, taking into account the risk of general anesthesia plus the unusual

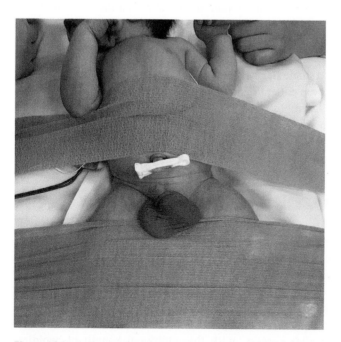

Figure 18.9 Left-side Neonatal testicular torsion. Patient is explored and contralateral orchiopexy is performed with the patient awake under regional caudal anesthesia. *Source:* Nicolas Fernandez, MD, PhD.

possibility of an asynchronic torsion that presents in 4% of cases. We have implemented a protocol of regional/local anesthesia during surgical exploration for the management of NTT with good results while the neonate is awake. This approach avoids the need for general anesthesia and its possible neurotoxicity.

Based on a recent meta-analysis by Monteilh et al., the most common practice is to perform immediate bilateral surgical exploration and contralateral orchiopexy. The decision about orchiectomy varies among surgeons. In general, this approach benefits 12% of the cases, preventing devastating effects of asynchronous torsion [69].

If a decision is made to take the patient to the operating room, several areas have generated debate. Should the affected testicle be explored? If so, depending on viability, should it be left in place or removed? Some authors believe that despite torsion, testicles may maintain endocrine function. For that reason, removal may have adverse effects [73]. The counter-argument supports orchiectomy, considering the future risk of infection or malignancy. More studies will be needed to support these decisions and make specific recommendations.

Disorders of Sex Development

The term "disorders of sex development" (DSD), proposed by consensus in 2006, describes a group of conditions characterized by abnormal genital, chromosomal and gonadal development [74]. It has been estimated that DSD prevalence is 1 per 4500 newborns [75]. Prenatal detection has a high variability that depends on each center's experience and ranges from 24 to 40% of their cases [76]. Prenatally detected cases should be referred to centers with a multidisciplinary team that can start management during the prenatal period. High likelihood cases can be offered fetal circulating DNA testing at 4–5 weeks of gestation, chorionic villus sampling at 10–12 weeks, and amniocentesis at 12–14 weeks to guide diagnosis. Specific conditions, such as congenital adrenal hyperplasia (CAH) in a female fetus, may benefit from dexamethasone treatment during pregnancy in order to reduce virilization [77]. If no genetic diagnosis is made, the chances are that seven out of eight babies are unnecessarily treated. More recently, there is the possibility of genetic diagnosis of *CYP21A2* mutations on fetal cells circulating in the mother's plasma [78].

Patients with CAH detected at birth should be assessed immediately by a multidisciplinary team in order to establish an appropriate management plan [1]. A physical examination should be performed with special attention to describing the anatomy without assignment or conclusions about the gender. An example of notation follows: "Genital tubercle (instead of penis or clitoris), labioscrotal folds, urethral plate, gonads." Other associated anomalies should always be considered and ruled out, because these factor into the discussion about surgical intervention, prognosis, and treatment.

Immediate evaluation is needed to rule out lethal conditions. The most common is salt-wasting adrenal hyperplasia. For that reason, all newborns need a basic metabolic panel, karyotype, and 17β-hydroxyprogesterone. Because the results of a karyotype may take some days, we have implemented the use of karyoFISH, which is quicker and may give initial useful information [79]. This does not replace the high-resolution karyotype. It is very important to highlight that karyotype should be done on at least 50 metaphases, because a mosaicism may not be detected if fewer metaphases are analyzed.

The strategy of early detection is to reduce the risk of lethal hyponatremia. Patients should be started on oral hydrocortisone at 10–15 mg/m^2/day BID. Fludrocortisone should be started at 0.1 mg/day. Early treatment, including prenatal dexamethasone, reduces immediate complications and in one report has shown a positive effect on psychometric intelligence and executive functions in adolescents with CAH [80].

Given the wide range and complexity of conditions included as disorders of sexual development, specific management of each condition is beyond the scope of this chapter.

Female Genital Masses

Inter-labial masses may not always require an emergent consultation for the pediatric urologist. Nonetheless, given the differential diagnosis of possible malignancy or conditions requiring surgical management, it is imperative that these patients are seen as soon as possible. A careful physical examination may be sufficient to make an accurate diagnosis.

Paraurethral Cysts

At birth, an inter-labial mass may present secondary to the obstruction of Skene's glands, usually presenting at the lateral aspect of the meatus between 3 and 9 o'clock. Exact prevalence may be under-reported, as many of these cysts are asymptomatic and elude detection. Depending on how big the cyst is, it can cause displacement of the urethral meatus but rarely obstruction of the lumen. Cysts are usually covered with genital mucosa which may show small vessels with a whitish or yellowish background (Figure 18.10). Theses cysts do not change in size and rarely require drainage [81]. Spontaneous resolution is the usual outcome. Parents need to be counseled and reassured that with time, it will improve on its own.

Ureterocele Prolapse

Ureteroceles close to the bladder neck may prolapse through the urethra and be seen on physical examination (Figure 18.11). The lesion is seen as a bulging mass that can be pink or purple depending on congestion. Size varies but tends to cover the entire introitus, distorting normal anatomy and making it impossible to see the urethral meatus [82]. It is more common in white females during infancy [83]. Although rarely seen in neonates, bladder outlet obstruction is an emergency and requires immediate management with urethral catheter placement. Reduction on physical examination may be challenging and painful. Under general anesthesia, reduction and ureterocele puncture may be sufficient. The majority of cases present with duplex systems and require further studies of the upper tract.

Urethral Prolapse

Neonatal presentation of prolapsed urethral mucosa is uncommon (see Figure 18.12). Its most frequent presentation is at the age of five in black girls [84]. The exact cause is unknown, but constipation may be associated. It is seen as a beefy-red friable tissue with a doughnut shape that bleeds easily to touch (see Figure 18.13).

Figure 18.10 Paraurethral cyst secondary to Skene's glands obstruction. *Source:* courtesy of Dr. Jaime F. Perez.

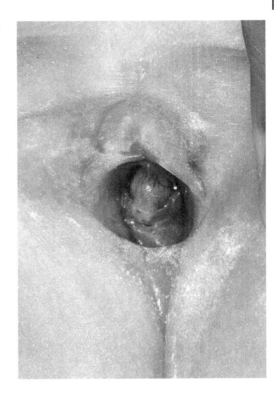

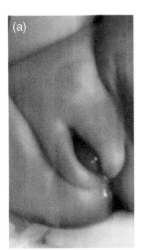

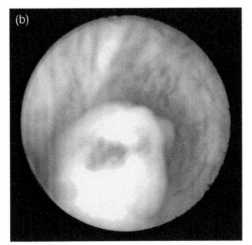

(a)

(b)

Figure 18.11 Prolapsed ureterocele causing urinary retention on a 12-hour neonate with oligohydramnios. Endoscopic image of the ureterocele protruding through bladder neck. *Source:* courtesy of Nicolas Fernandez, MD, PhD.

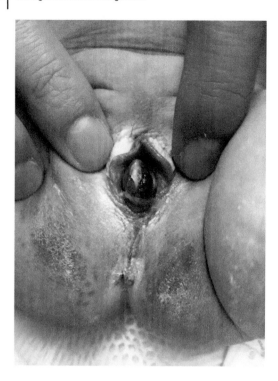

Figure 18.12 Prolapsed ureterocele with some mucosal congestion and urinary retention at birth. *Source:* courtesy of Nicolas Fernandez, MD, PhD.

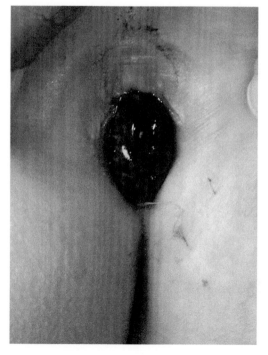

Figure 18.13 Prolapsed urethral mucosa. Beefy-red friable to touch. *Source:* courtesy of Dr. Jaime F Perez.

Most cases can be treated with topical estrogens, and when recurrent, surgical intervention may be required. Some surgeons leave a urethral catheter in place to reduce discomfort, allowing resolution of edema and congestion.

Urethral Polyps

These are very uncommon lesions that arise from the urethra and extend beyond the introitus. They usually have a pedunculated form and may bleed. The majority present as a single lesion (see Figure 18.14), so they should not be confused with other malignant lesions such as sarcomas. Cases that may not be big enough to be visible during physical examination may cause intermittent and recurrent episodes of urinary retention [85].

Sarcoma Botryoides

Malignancy is always part of the differential diagnosis when dealing with genital masses in the newborn female. One of the most important is embryonal rhabdomyosarcoma (ERMS), also known as sarcoma botryoides. Classically described as a "bunch of grapes," it represents a fleshy mass arising from the vagina or urethra. Really uncommon in neonates, it presents most frequently around four to five years of age. This malignancy has an excellent prognosis with early and appropriate management [86].

With new advances in antineoplastic agents and international cooperative groups, aggressive surgery has been replaced by combined organ-sparing and chemotherapeutic approaches [87]. The Intergroup Rhabdomyosarcoma Study Group (IRSG) changed the standard of care establishing the use of vincristine, actinomycin D, with or without cyclophosphamide, as the protocol of choice.

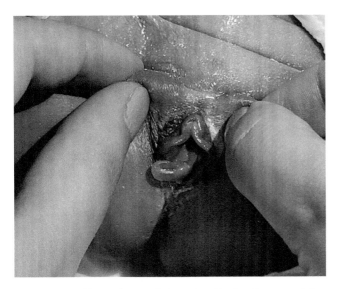

Figure 18.14 Urethral polyp. Pedunculated lesion that extends beyond the introitus. *Source:* courtesy of Dr. Jaime F Perez.

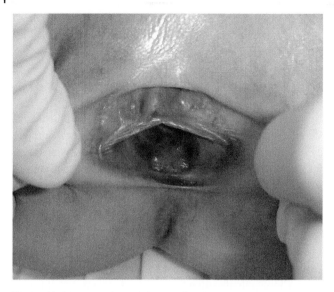

Figure 18.15 Imperforated hymen. Bulging whitish mass with and intact urethral meatus. *Source:* courtesy of Nicolas Fernandez, MD, PhD.

Imperforated Hymen

The presence of a whitish central bulging mass can be seen at birth when an imperforated hymen causes muco-colpos (Figure 18.15). Accumulation can be significant causing anterior displacement of the bladder with some degree of bladder outlet obstruction. Spontaneous rupture and drainage are also possible. Most surgeons favor bedside drainage, while others leave it untreated if not severe [88]. With improvements in prenatal detection, it is not uncommon for it to be detected on ultrasound prior to delivery. If other anomalies are present (postaxial polydactyly and congenital heart defects), the diagnosis of McKusick Kaufman Syndrome needs to be ruled out [89].

Conclusions

Neonatologists, pediatricians, and urologists need to be aware of these conditions, as their appropriate timely diagnosis may significantly improve the patient's prognosis. A decision to operate should always be balanced with the possible risks and outcomes. Nonetheless, aggressive management has been shown to improve patients' conditions in most pathologies, and pediatric urologists need to be involved advocates and team leaders in the care of these patients.

References

1 Fernandez, N., Moreno, O., Rojas, A. et al. (2017). Transdisciplinary management of patients with disorders of sexual development in Colombia. Limiting factors for appropriate management. *Urol. Colomb.* 26: 164–168.

2 Anumba, D., Scott, J., and Plant, N. (2005). Diagnosis and outcome of fetal lower urinary tract obstruction in the northern region of England. *Prenat. Diagn.* 25: 7–13.

3 Thakkar, D., Deshpande, A.V., and Kennedy, S.E. (2014). Epidemiology and demography of recently diagnosed cases of posterior urethral valves. *Pediatr. Res.* 76 (6): 560–563.

4 Young, H., Frontz, W., and Baldwin, J. (1919). Congenital obstruction of the posterior urethra. *J. Urol.* 3: 289.

5 Martins, C.S., Carnevale, J., Vicente, N.C., and Freitas Filho, L.G. (2018). Cobb's collar and chronic renal failure. *Urol. Case Rep.* 18: 75–76.

6 Moormann, J.G. (1973). The problems of the urethral valves according to H.H. Young (author's transl). *Urologe A* 12 (5): 219–226.

7 Parkkulainen, K. (1977). Posterior urethral obstruction: valvular or diaphragmatic? Endoscopic diagnosis and treatment. *Birth Defects* 13 (5): 63–74.

8 Dewan, P., Zappala, S., Ransley, P., and Duffy, P. (1992). Endoscopic reappraisal of the morphology of congenital obstruction of the posterior urethra. *Br. J. Urol.* 70 (4): 439–444.

9 Dewan, P.A., Keenan, R.J., Morris, L.L., and Le Quesne, G.W. (1994). Congenital urethral obstruction: Cobb's collar or prolapsed congenital obstructive posterior urethral membrane (COPUM). *Br. J. Urol.* 73 (1): 91–95.

10 Lundar, L., Aksnes, G., Mørkrid, L., and Emblem, R. (2019). Prenatal extravasation of urine seems to preserve renal function in boys with posterior urethral valves. *J. Pediatr. Urol.* 15 (3): 241.e1–241.e7.

11 Roy, S., Colmant, C., Cordier, A.-G., and Sénat, M.-V. (2016). Apport des signes d'appel échographiques dans le diagnostic anténatal des valves de l'urètre postérieur: expérience de 3ans à la maternité de l'hôpital Bicêtre. *J. Gynecol. Obstet. Biol. Reprod.* 45 (5): 478–483.

12 Rittenberg, M., Hulbert, W., Snyder, H., and Duckett, J. (1988). Protective factors in posterior urethral valves. *J. Urol.* 140 (5): 993–996.

13 Wells, J., Mukerji, S., Chandran, H. et al. (2010). Urinomas protect renal function in posterior urethral valves – a population based study. *J. Pediatr. Sug.* 45 (2): 407–410.

14 Peters, C., Bolkier, M., Bauer, S., and Hendren, W. (1990). The urodynamic consequences of posterior urethral valves. *J. Urol.* 144 (1): 122–126.

15 Heikkila, J., Taskinen, S., and Rintala, R. (2008). Urinomas associated with posterior urethral valves. *J. Urol.* 180: 1476–1478.

16 Bernardes, L., Salomon, R., Aksnes, G. et al. (2011). Ultrasound evaluation of prognosis in fetuses with posterior urethral valves. *J. Pediatr. Surg.* 46: 1412–1418.

17 Yerkes, E., Cain, M., and Padilla, L. (2001). Nutero perinephric urinoma and urinary ascites with posterior urethral valves: a paradoxical pop-off valve? *J. Urol.* 166: 2387–2388.

18 Glick, P., Harrison, M., Golbus, M. et al. (1985). Management of the fetus with congenital hydronephrosis II: prognostic criteria and selection for treatment. *J. Pediatr. Surg.* 20 (4): 376–387.

19 Haeri, S. (2015). Fetal Lower Urinary Tract Obstruction (LUTO): a practical review for providers. *Matern. Heal Neonatol. Perinatol.* 1 (1): 26.

20 Martínez, J.M., Masoller, N., Devlieger, R. et al. (2015). Laser ablation of posterior urethral valves by fetal cystoscopy. *Fetal Diagn. Ther.* 37 (4): 267–273.

21 Morris, R.K., Malin, G.L., Quinlan-Jones, E. et al. (2013). Percutaneous vesicoamniotic shunting versus conservative management for fetal lower urinary tract obstruction (PLUTO): a randomised trial. *Lancet* 382 (9903): 1496–1506.

22 Sideris, I.G. and Nicolaides, K.H. (1990). Amniotic fluid pressure during pregnancy. *Fetal Diagn. Ther.* 5 (2): 104–108.

23 Penna, F.J., Bowlin, P., Alyami, F. et al. (2015). Novel strategy for temporary decompression of the lower urinary tract in neonates using a ureteral stent. *J. Urol.* 194 (4): 1086–1090.

24 Young, H. and McKay, R. (1929). Congenital valvular obstruction of the posterior urethra. *Surg. Gynecol. Obstet.* 48: 509–535.

25 Mandal, S., Goel, A., Kumar, M. et al. (2013). Use of holmium:YAG laser in posterior urethral valves: another method of fulguration. *J. Pediatr. Urol.* 9 (6 Part B): 1093–1097.

26 Zaontz, M.R. and Firlit, C.F. (1985). Percutaneous antegrade ablation of posterior urethral valves in premature or underweight term neonates: an alternative to primary vesicostomy. *J. Urol.* 134: 139–141.

27 Sarhan, O.M. (2017). Posterior urethral valves: impact of low birth weight and preterm delivery on the final renal outcome. *Arab. J. Urol.* 15 (2): 159–165.

28 Seyed, M., Vahid, H., Mohammad, Z. et al. (2015). Comparison of early neonatal valve ablation with vesicostomy in patient with posterior urethral valve. *Afr. J. Paediatr. Surg.* 12 (4): 270–272.

29 Kim, S.J., Jung, J., Lee, C. et al. (2018). Long-term outcomes of kidney and bladder function in patients with a posterior urethral valve. *Medicine (United States)* 97 (23): e11033.

30 Blocksom, B. (1957). Bladder pouch for prolonged tubeless cystostomy. *J. Urol.* 78 (4): 398–401.

31 Duckett, J. (1974). Cutaneous vesicostomy in childhood. The Blocksom technique. *Urol. Clin. North Am.* 1 (3): 485–495.

32 Lusuardi, L., Lodde, M., and Pycha, A. (2005). Surgical Atlas Cutaneous ureterostomy. *BJU Int.* 96: 1149–1159.

33 Kaneti, J. and Sober, I. (1988). Pelvi-uretero-cutaneostomy en-Y as a temporary diversion in children. Soroka experience. *Int. Urol. Nephrol.* 20 (5): 471–474.

34 Williams, D.I. and Cromie, W.J. (1975). Ring ureterostomy. *Br. J. Urol.* 47 (7): 789–792.

35 Hendren, W.H. (1978). Complications of ureterostomy. *J. Urol.* 120: 269–281.

36 Lome, L.G. and Williams, D.I. (1972). Urinary reconstruction following temporary cutaneous ureterostomy diversion in children. *J. Urol.* 108 (1): 162–164.

37 Tietjen, D., Gloor, J., and Husmann, D. (1997). Proximal urinary diversion in the management of posterior urethral valves: is it necessary? *J. Urol.* 158: 1008–1010.

38 DeFoor, W., Clark, C., Jackson, E. et al. (2008). Risk factors for end stage renal disease in children with posterior urethral valves. *J. Urol.* 180 (4 Suppl): 1705–1708.

39 Coleman, R., King, T., Nicoara, C.D. et al. (2015). Nadir creatinine in posterior urethral valves: how high is low enough? *J. Pediatr. Urol.* 11 (6): 356.e1–356.e5.

40 Close, C., Carr, M., Burns, M., and Mitchell, M. (1997). Lower urinary tract changes after early valve ablation in neonates and infants: is early diversion warranted? *J. Urol.* 157 (3): 984–998.

41 Youssif, M., Dawood, W., Shabaan, S. et al. (2009). Early valve ablation can decrease the incidence of bladder dysfunction in boys with posterior urethral valves. *J. Urol.* 182 (4): 1765–1768.

42 Muecke, E.C. (1964). The role of the cloacal membrane in exstrophy: the first successful experimental study. *J. Urol.* 92: 659–667.

43 Siffel, C., Correa, A., Amar, E. et al. (2011). Bladder exstrophy: an epidemiologic study from the international clearinghouse for birth defects survellance and research, and an overview of the literature. *Am. J. Med. Genet. C Semin. Med. Genet.* 15 (4): 321–332.

44 Lee, R.S., Grady, R., Joyner, B. et al. (2006). Can a complete primary repair approach be applied to cloacal exstrophy? *J. Urol.* 176: 2643–2648.

45 Della Monica, M., Nazzaro, A. et al. (2005). Prenatal ultrasound diagnosis of cloacal exstrophy associated with myelocystocele complex by the 'elephant trunk-like' image and review of the literature. *Prenat. Diagn.* 25 (5): 394–397.

46 Zarante, I., Franco, L., López, C., and Fernández, N. (2010). Frequencies of congenital malformations: assessment and prognosis of 52,744 births in three cities of Colombia. *Biomedica* 30 (1): 65–71.

47 Goyal, A., Fishwick, J., Hurrell, R. et al. (2012). Antenatal diagnosis of bladder/cloacal exstrophy: challenges and possible solutions. *J. Pediatr. Urol.* 8 (2): 140–144. https://doi.org/10.1016/j.jpurol.2011.05.003.

48 Ben-Neriah, Z., Withers, S., Thomas, M. et al. (2007). OEIS complex: prenatal ultrasound and autopsy findings. *Ultrasound Obstet. Gynecol.* 29 (2): 170–177.

49 Austin, P.F., Homsy, Y.L., Gearhart, J.P. et al. (1998). The prenatal diagnosis of cloacal exstrophy. *J. Urol.* 160 (3 Pt 2): 1179–1181.

50 Massanyi, E.Z., Gearhart, J.P., and Kost-Byerly, S. (2013). Perioperative management of classic bladder exstrophy. *Res. Rep. Urol.* 5: 67–75.

51 Joshi, R.S., Shrivastava, D., Grady, R. et al. (2018). A model for sustained collaboration to address the unmet global burden of bladder exstrophy-epispadias complex and penopubic epispadias the international bladder exstrophy consortium. *JAMA Surg.* 153 (7): 618–624.

52 Gordetsky, J. and Joseph, D.B. (2015). Cloacal exstrophy: a history of gender reassignment. *Urology* 86 (6): 1087–1089. https://doi.org/10.1016/j.urology.2015.06.056.

53 Mednick, L., Gargollo, P., Oliva, M. et al. (2009). Stress and coping of parents of young children diagnosed with bladder exstrophy. *J. Urol.* 181 (3): 1312–1317.

54 Grady, R.W. and Mitchell, M.E. (1999). Complete primary repair of exstrophy. *J. Urol.* 162 (4): 1415–1420.

55 Jeffs, R. (1977). Functional closure of bladder exstrophy. *Birth Defects Orig. Artic. Ser.* 13 (5): 171–173.

56 Stec, A.A., Baradaran, N., Schaeffer, A. et al. (2012). The modern staged repair of classic bladder exstrophy: a detailed postoperative management strategy for primary bladder closure. *J. Pediatr. Urol.* 8: 549–555.

57 Purves, T., Novak, T., King, J., and Gearhart, J.P. (2009). Modified young-dees-leadbetter bladder neck reconstruction after exstrophy repair. *J. Urol.* 182 (4 Suppl): 1813–1817. https://doi.org/10.1016/j.juro.2009.03.017.

58 Pippi Salle, J.L., McLorie, G.A., Bägli, D.J., and Khoury, A.E. (1997). Urethral lengthening with anterior bladder wall flap (Pippi Salle procedure): modifications and extended indications of the technique. *J. Urol.* 158: 585–590.

59 Wild, A.T., Sponseller, P.D., Stec, A.A. et al. (2011). *Semin. Pediatr. Surg.* 20 (2): 71–78.

60 Husmann, D.A. (2018). Lessons learned from the management of adults who have undergone augmentation for spina bifida and bladder exstrophy: incidence and management of the non-lethal complications of bladder augmentation. *Int. J. Urol.* 25 (2): 94–101.

61 Gearhart, J.P. and Jeffs, R.D. (1987). The use of parenteral testosterone therapy in genital reconstructive surgery. *J. Urol.* 138 (4): 1077–1078.

62 Gearhart, J.P., Sciortino, C., Ben-Chaim, J. et al. (1995). The Cantwell-Ransley epispadias repair in exstrophy and epispadias: lessons learned. *Urology* 46: 92–95.

63 Mitchell, M.E. and Bägli, D.J. (1996). Complete penile disassembly for epispadias repair: the Mitchell technique. *J. Urol.* 155 (1): 300–304.

64 Soffer, S.Z., Rosen, N.G., Hong, A.R. et al. (2000). Cloacal exstrophy: a unified management plan. *J. Pediatr. Surg.* 35 (6): 932–937.

65 Roth, E., Goetz, J., Kryger, J., and Groth, T. (2017). Post-operative immobilization and pain management after repair of bladder exstrophy. *Curr. Urol. Rep.* 18 (3): 19.

66 Okonkwo, I., Bendon, A.A., Cervellione, R.M., and Vashisht, R. (2019). Continuous caudal epidural analgesia and early feeding in delayed bladder exstrophy repair: a nine-year experience. *J. Pediatr. Urol.* 15 (1): 76.e1–76.e8.

67 Callewaert, P.R.H. and Van Kerrebroeck, P. (2010). New insights into perinatal testicular torsion. *Eur. J. Pediatr.* 169 (6): 705–712.

68 Mathews, J.C., Kooner, G., and Mathew, D. (2008). Neonatal testicular torsion – a lost cause? *Acta Paediatr.* 97: 502–504.

69 Monteilh, C., Calixte, R., and Burjonrappa, S. (2019). Controversies in the management of neonatal testicular torsion: a meta-analysis. *J. Pediatr. Surg.* 54 (4): 815–819. https://doi.org/10.1016/j.jpedsurg.2018.07.006.

70 Das, S. and Singer, A. (1990). Controversies of perinatal torsion of the spermatic cord: a review, survey and recommendations. *J. Urol.* 143: 231–233.

71 Mano, R., Livne, P., and Nevo, A. (2013). Testicular torsion in the first year of life characteristics and treatment outcome. *Urology* 82: 1132–1137.

72 Yerkes, E., Robetson, F., Gitlin, J. et al. (2005). Management of perinatal torsion: today, tomorrow, or never? *J. Urol.* 174: 1579–1583.

73 Arena, F., Nictotina, N., and Romeo, C. (2006). Prenatal testicular torsion: ultrasonographic features, management and histopathological findings. *J. Urol.* 13: 135–141.

74 Hughes, I.A., Houk, C., Ahmed, S.F., and Lee, P.A. (2006). Consensus statement on management of intersex disorders management of intersex disorders. *Arch. Dis. Child.* 9 (7): 554–563.

75 Lee, P.A., Nordenström, A., Houk, C.P. et al. (2016). Global disorders of sex development update since 2006: perceptions, approach and care. *Horm. Res. Paediatr.* 85 (3): 158–180. https://doi.org/10.1159/000442975.

76 Finney, E.L., Finlayson, C., Rosoklija, I. et al. (2019). Prenatal detection and evaluation of differences of sex development. *J. Pediatr. Urol.* 16 (1): 89–96.

77 Mouriquanda, P., Gorduzaa, D.B., Gaya, C.-L. et al. (2016). Surgery in disorders of sex development (DSD) with a gender issue: if (why), when, and how? *J. Pediatr. Urol.* 12 (3): 139–149.

78 New, M.I., Tong, Y.K., Yuen, T. et al. (2014). Noninvasive prenatal diagnosis of congenital adrenal hyperplasia using cell-free fetal DNA in maternal plasma. *J. Clin. Endocrinol. Metab.* 99 (6): E1022–E1030.

79 García, M., Moreno, O., Suárez, F. et al. (2019). Disorders of sex development: genetic characterization of a patient cohort. *Mol. Med. Rep.* 21 (1): 97–106.

80 Messina, V., Karlsson, L., Hirvikoski, T. et al. (2020). Cognitive function of children and adolescents with congenital adrenal hyperplasia: importance of early diagnosis. *J. Clin. Endocrinol. Metab.* 105 (3): e683–e691.

81 Fujimoto, T., Suwa, T., Ishii, N., and Kabe, K. (2007). Paraurethral cyst in female newborn: is surgery always advocated? *J. Pediatr. Surg.* 42 (2): 400–403.

82 Fletcher, S.G. and Lemack, G.E. (2008). Benign masses of the female periurethral tissues and anterior vaginal wall. *Curr. Urol. Rep.* 9 (5): 389–396.

83 Caldamone, A.A. (1985). Duplication anomalies of the upper tract in infants and children. *Urol. Clin. North Am.* 12 (1): 75–91.

84 Ninomiya, T. and Koga, H. Clinical characteristics of urethral prolapse in Japanese children. *Pediatr. Int.* 59 (5): 578–582.

85 Akbarzadeh, A., Khorramirouz, R., and Kajbafzadeh, A.-M. (2014). Congenital urethral polyps in children: report of 18 patients and review of literature. *J. Pediatr. Surg.* 49 (5): 835–839.

86 Hays, D.M., Newton, W., Crist, W.M. et al. (1984). Clinical staging and treatment results in rhabdomyosarcoma of the female genital tract among children and adolescents. 61 (9): 1893–1903.

87 Raney, R.B., Maurer, H.M., Anderson, J.R. et al. (2001). The Intergroup Rhabdomyosarcoma Study Group (IRSG): major lessons from the IRS-I through IRS-IV studies as background for the current IRS-V treatment protocols. *Sarcoma* 5 (1): 9–15.

88 Khanna, K., Sharma, S., and Gupta, D.K. (2018). Hydrometrocolpos etiology and management: past beckons the present. *Pediatr. Surg. Int.* 34 (3): 249–261.

89 Slavotinek, A.M. (2002). McKusick-Kaufman syndrome. In: GeneReviews® (eds. M.P. Adam, H.H. Ardinger and R.A. Pagon). Seattle, WA: University of Washington, Seattle.

Section V

COVID-19

19

Urologic Emergency Care in the COVID-19 Pandemic Era

Rishi R. Sekar, Sarah K. Holt, Joseph Meno, Rachel McKenzie, and Hunter Wessells

Department of Urology, University of Washington School of Medicine, Seattle, WA, USA

The COVID-19 pandemic has placed unprecedented strain on health care systems throughout the world, requiring a delicate balance of providing appropriate and necessary health care while emphasizing public health preventative measures to minimize virus transmission. Though the global medical community quickly enacted protocols to escalate care for the critically ill with healthcare workforce and resource mobilization, access to healthcare for other acute, chronic, and emergent conditions may have been strained as part of this restructuring. Further, local and national public health measures, such as stay-at-home orders as well as patient hesitation to seek medical care during a pandemic, likely contributed to lapses in standard of care management of chronic conditions and delays in presentation of acute and emergent conditions. As the COVID-19 pandemic continues to evolve, the impact on the presentation and management of urologic conditions is becoming evident and may have long-term implications for our patients. In this brief chapter we review the initial response of urologists from a variety of settings, the impact on care delivery at several academic settings, as well as predications on the long-range impact of care deferral on population health.

Immediate Responses of Urology Departments

Faced with the rapid upswing in COVID-19 cases during the month of March 2020 (see Figure 19.1 for Washington State), health systems in the United States, in parallel with those in Europe, began planning for a dramatic change in work dictated by resource constraints, restrictions on elective surgical cases, and protection of their workforces. Incident Command Centers were established at all major hospitals to implement the enormous numbers of changes to day-to-day operations. Each hospital and practice was forced to assess stocks of personal protective equipment (PPE) and redeploy healthcare workers to Emergency Departments, Intensive Care Units, and other "front line" responsibilities. Enunciating ethical rationale for redeployment, based on a "duty to care" allowed our

A Clinical Guide to Urologic Emergencies, First Edition. Edited by Hunter Wessells, Shigeo Horie, and Reynaldo G. Gómez.

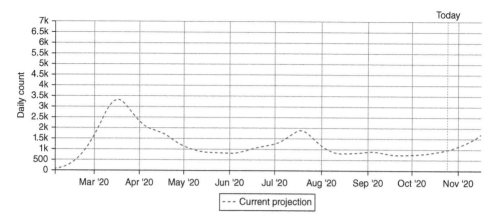

Figure 19.1 COVID-19 case rates in Washington State, March–October 2020. Institute for Health Metrics and Evaluation, accessed October 24, 2020 at https://covid19.healthdata.org/united-states-of-america/washington?view=total-deaths&tab=trend

institution and many others to create lists of attending and housestaff physicians and advanced practice providers willing and able to redeploy [1]. The numbers of individuals deployed, and responsibilites assigned, varied dramatically based on rates of COVID-19 transmission, ED and ICU occupancy, and population demographics.

Urology Departments around the world developed systems to protect the workforce and patients from high risk and COVID-19 positive patients. The Society of Academic Urologists hosted Roundtable webinars to disseminate information and share best practices on the administrative and educational challenges of the pandemic [2]. These ranged from establishing chains of command and decision-making to protection of workforce, protection of learners and the learning environment, and patient triage systems. Because of the high numbers of potential COVID-19 patients presenting to Emergency Departments, specialty services like urology devised strategies to expedite specialist consultation, as well as physical separation of these lower acuity patients from the COVID-19 section. One in particular, the Kaiser Permanente LA Medical Center, physically restructured speciality consultation to one area of the ED, and designated urologists to perform primary assessments of acute urologic emergencies under conditions of high COVID census (see Figure 19.2).

Surgical Triage

In March 2020, surgical services across the western United States rapidly ceased elective surgery in response to PPE shortages and state Executive Orders, as well as recommendations from professional organizations. The American College of Surgeons called for a cessation of elective surgery as early at March 13, and on March 17 issued triage guidance for non-emergent surgical care [3]. These recommendations had substantial impact of surgical volumes, which varied by speciality. Within our own department, the delivery of

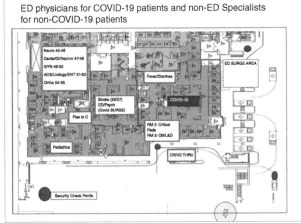

ED physicians for COVID-19 patients and non-ED Specialists for non-COVID-19 patients

Phase 1 (up to 120 patients per day):

• Normal operations

Phase 2 (up to 145 patients per day):

• Add physician pool Orthopedics, Pediatrics, and Anesthesia airway team to ED

Phase 3 (165+ patients per day):

• Physician specialty pool to cover all non-COVID 19 patients, including Neurology, Acute Care Surgery, Urology, HNS, Cardiology, Gastroenterology, Nephrology, and OB/GYN

Figure 19.2 Diagram of physical layout and criteria for specialty consultation prepared by Kaiser LA Medical Center leadership. Note "Red Zones" for COVID-19 related symptom triage and separate "Green Zones" designated for non-COVID-19 patients along with guidance for initiating direct urologic consultation. *Source:* courtesy of Polina Reyblat, MD, Crisis Command Center, Kaiser Permanente, Los Angeles with permission.

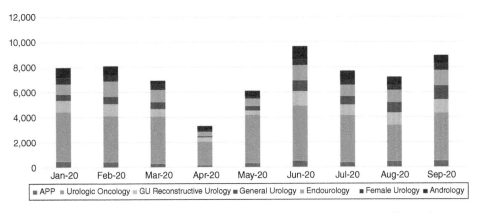

Figure 19.3 Clinical activity including outpatient and surgical cases as measured by work relative value units (wRVU) and subspecialty within UW Medicine Department of Urology. Note the total reduction in volumes (y-axis, wRVU) by month with a nadir in April 2020 and a rebound in June 2020 reflecting a backlog of untreated surgical cases, and return to baseline levels of clinical activity. All subspecialties experienced reduced volumes, with the degree of reduction and time to recovery varying substantially. APP: advanced practice provider.

emergency surgery for trauma, infection (e.g. necrotizing soft tissue infection, complicated UTI), and urinary obstruction required continuous deployment of on-call teams. Most elective surgery was canceled, with the exception of selected patients with active urinary stone disease and those with high risk malignancies (e.g. aggressive bladder, kidney, and other cancers) [4]. The variation in the amount of clinical care (in particular surgery) delivered by each urologic subspecialty also reflects variation in hospital policies and access to PPE (see Figure 19.3).

Telemedicine

Telemedicine evolved as an important means to sustain essential patient care during the pandemic, with additional benefits of protecting patients and healthcare providers and their staff from potential exposure. The rapid adoption in the US, abetted by liberalized state licensing decisions and Medicare payments, will permanently change care delivery and accelerate the digitalization of healthcare [5]. The trends in outpatient encounters (see Figure 19.4) for the Department of Urology at UW Medicine reflect events in many surgical practices. The near complete cessation of in-person office visits in March and April of 2020, with a commensurate rise in telemedicine and telephone visits, allowed continued access to care for approximately 50% of normal outpatient visit volumes. The eventual drop off in telephone encounters reflects implementation of video teleconferencing as well as the lower reimbursement compared to telemedicine consults. The ability to rapidly convert in-person visits to telemedicine visits will be key to managing successive waves of COVID-19 infection, when rising rates of transmission may require stay-at-home orders, as well as when members of the healtcare team must quarantine as a result of workplace or social exposure to the coronavirus.

Consequences of COVID-19 on Urologic Care

Deferred care as a result of COVID-19 will impact every specialty of medicine and surgery, and these may be far reaching. Delays in care for urologic emergencies such as acute urinary tract obstruction, hematuria, nephrolithiasis, urologic trauma, and other conditions covered in this book can have severe sequelae including compromised renal function,

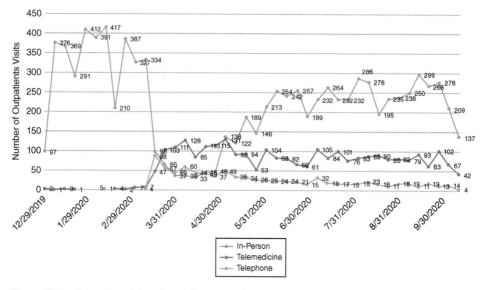

Figure 19.4 Outpatient visit volumes by type within UW Medicine Department of Urology. Note previous nominal use of telehealth prior to March 2020.

Table 19.1 Urgent and emergent urological patients, mean (standard deviation), ANOCA.

	Reference week	COVID-19 week 1	COVID-19 week 2	COVID-19 week 3	*p* value
Emergent/urgent cases, total	35.4 (24.3)	20.3 (15.3)	17.8 (14.2)	10.8 (11.8)	**<0.001**
Emergent/urgent cases in surgery, total	8.7 (7.4)	4.4 (4.1)	3.6 (3.3)	3.4 (3.8)	**<0.001**
Cases by type					
Haematuria	7.1 (5.7)	4.3 (3.5)	3.4 (2.8)	2.2 (2.3)	**<0.001**
Urinary retention	6.3 (5.7)	3.8 (3.6)	3.3 (3.2)	1.9 (2.4)	**<0.001**
Urinary tract infection	4.4 (3.5)	2.2 (2.3)	2.2 (2.4)	1.1 (1.7)	**<0.001**
Scrotal pain	3.7 (4.0)	2.1 (2.3)	1.6 (1.8)	0.9 (1.2)	**<0.001**
Renal colic	10.9 (6.9)	7.1 (6.2)	6.3 (5.4)	3.9 (4.8)	**<0.001**
Trauma	0.7 (0.8)	0.4 (0.8)	0.4 (0.6)	0.2 (0.6)	0.158
Emergency operating facilities					
Endourology (URS, ureteral stenting)	5.0 (4.2)	2.9 (2.4)	2.2 (1.9)	2.2 (2.4)	**0.002**
Transurethral resection of bladder tumor	2.3 (3.0)	0.9 (1.9)	0.9 (1.6)	0.8 (1.3)	**0.023**
Urethrotomy	0.5 (0.8)	0.3 (0.6)	0.1 (0.5)	0.1 (0.4)	0.081
Testicular detorsion	0.8 (0.8)	0.4 (0.8)	0.2 (0.5)	0.2 (0.4)	**0.006**

Bold indicates statistical significance (*p* < 0.05). COVID-19, coronavirus disease 2019; URS, ureteroscopy. Drawn from Reference 6, with permission.

life-threatening infection, and lifelong disability in voiding and sexual function. As such, several institutions, particularly in Europe, have sought to investigate changes in emergent presentations and procedures in the setting of the COVID-19 pandemic. The AGILE group, a large multicenter collaborative in Italy, reported a significant decrease in cases of hematuria, urinary retention, urinary tract infection, scrotal pain, and renal colic during the first several weeks of the COVID-19 pandemic compared to the prior year (see Table 19.1). They similarly showed a significant decrease in emergent urologic procedures performed during this timeframe [6]. Further, a retrospective study comparing urologic consultations in the ED at Padua University Hospital (Italy) in February and March of 2020 to the same months in 2019 demonstrated an approximate 60% reduction in total and daily average consultations, as well as a significant reduction in the number of invasive procedures performed [7]. In terms of the impact of the pandemic on management of nephrolithiasis, multiple studies have demonstrated a higher complexity of patient presentations with higher rates of positive urine cultures, antibiotic requirement, need for percutaneous nephrostomy tube placement over ureteral stent placement, and length of hospital stay [8–10]. Though these data focus on changes in care observed during the height of the pandemic, likely when the most stringent virus containment strategies were in effect, it is evident that the COVID-19 pandemic has contributed to significant variation in the presentation of emergent urologic conditions; however, the short- and long-term implications remain to be investigated.

In addition to the total burden of deferred urologic care, the pandemic also has uncovered disparities in impact of the disease by race, ethnicity, and other factors [11]. We assessed rates of ED access and overall urologic healthcare visits during the period before and during the COVID-19 pandemic. Preliminary analysis demonstates a reduction in frequency of urologic care-seeking early in the pandemic, with a slight rebound as time went on (unpublished data.) This finding parallel's results shown in Figures 19.3 and 19.4. Notably, the concurrent increase in telemedicine use during the pandemic also may create health disparities related to access to technology. Future analyses will focus on detailed trends with care access and utilization by demographic groups and urologic subspeciality.

Conclusions

The COVID-19 pandemic affects every aspect of healthcare and will have a lasting impact on many facets of urologic patient care. The reduction in access to outpatient consultation and elective surgery will translate into more complex management due to deferred care; delays in cancer screening; a reduction in routine and emergency diagnostic studies that detect serious urologic conditions; lower case numbers for trainees; and challenges for clinical trials and basic research. The collaboration and innovation required to meet patient needs and protect healthcare workers will yield important advances including digitalization of the outpatient and inpatient environments, remote care delivery, and new clinical trials approaches. Further research is needed on vulnerable populations that may have experienced greater impact from COVID-19 illness, access to telemedicine, as well as a larger burden of deferred care of non-emergent urologic conditions.

References

1 Dudzinski, D.M., Hoisington, B.Y., and Brown, C.E. (2020). Ethics lessons from Seattle's early experience with COVID-19. *Am. J. Bioeth.* 20 (7): 67–74.

2 Society of Academic Urologists. SAU Chairs' Roundtable Webinar: Sharing Experiences to Cope With The COVID-19 Pandemic. https://sauweb.org/resources/covid-19-resources.aspx accessed October 25, 2020.

3 American College of Surgeons. COVID-19: Guidance for Triage of Non-Emergent Surgical Procedures. https://www.facs.org/covid-19/clinical-guidance/triage accessed October 25, 2020.

4 Metzler, I.S., Sorensen, M.D., Sweet, R.M., and Harper, J.D. (2020). Stone Care Triage During COVID-19 at the University of Washington. *J. Endourol.* 34 (5): 539–540. https://doi.org/10.1089/end.2020.29080.ism. Epub April 17, 2020. PMID: 32302502.

5 Industries in 2021. The Economist Intelligence Unit. https://www.eiu.com/n/campaigns/industries-in-2021/ accessed October 25, 2020.

6 Porreca, A., Colicchia, M., D'Agostino, D. et al. (2020). Urology in the time of Coronavirus: reduced access to urgent and emergent urological care during the Coronavirus disease 2019 outbreak in Italy. *Urol. Int.* 104 (7–8): 631636. https://doi.org/10.1159/000508512.

7 Motterle, G., Morlacco, A., Iafrate, M. et al. (2020). The impact of COVID-19 pandemic on urological emergencies: a single-center experience. *World J. Urol.* Published online May 23. doi:https://doi.org/10.1007/s00345-020-03264-2.

8 Gul, M., Kaynar, M., Yildiz, M. et al. (2020). The increased risk of complicated ureteral stones in the era of COVID-19 pandemic. *J. Endourol.* 34 (8): 882–886. https://doi.org/10.1089/end.2020.0658.

9 Tefik, T., Guven, S., Villa, L. et al. (2020). Urolithiasis practice patterns following the COVID-19 pandemic: overview from the EULIS Collaborative Research Working Group. *Eur. Urol.* 78 (1): e21–e24. https://doi.org/10.1016/j.eururo.2020.04.057.

10 Proietti, S., Gaboardi, F., and Giusti, G. (2020). Endourological stone management in the era of the COVID-19. *Eur. Urol.* 78 (2): 131–133. https://doi.org/10.1016/j.eururo.2020.03.042.

11 Price-Haywood, E.G., Burton, J., Fort, D., and Seoane, L. (2020). Hospitalization and mortality among black patients and white patients with Covid-19. *N. Engl. J. Med.* 382 (26): 2534–2543.

Index

a

AAST. see American Association for the Surgery of Trauma (AAST)
abdominal plain films/"x-rays" 71
abrasions penile 185
acute epididymitis 232
acute kidney stone management. see kidney stone management
acute prostatitis 158
acute pyelonephritis
  clinical presentation 41
  epidemiology 41
  imaging 43–44
  laboratory findings 42
  microbiology and pathophysiology 42–43
  treatment 44–45
acute renal colic 64
acute scrotum 216
adrenal gland swelling 86
adrenal hemorrhage. see traumatic adrenal hemorrhage
Age Adjusted Charlson Comorbidity Index 170
Al-Ghorab shunt 195–197
alpha-1 adrenergic receptor blockers 72
American Association for the Surgery of Trauma (AAST) 6, 7, 9, 11, 27, 28, 85, 92, 93, 100, 119–120, 132, 180, 202, 203
amputation penile
  initial evaluation 183
  penetrating penile injury 181
  penile injury management 184–185
anaerobic bacteria 167
anorectal abscess 167
anterior urethra injury 131
antibiotic prophylaxis 210
augmented anastomotic buccal ureteroplasty 100
auto-transplantation 114
avulsion. see blunt penile injury

b

Behcet's syndrome 236
bell clapper deformity 217
bilateral adrenal injury 83
bilateral XGP 49
bites
  animal 210
  avulsion 181
  human 181
  penile injury management 185–186
bladder distension 120
bladder exstrophy
  antenatal diagnosis 255
  general principles for surgical repair 257
  initial management in neonate unit 255–257
  post-operative considerations 257
bladder injuries 122–123
  clinical symptoms and imaging diagnoses 121–122
  complications 123
  etiology 119–121
  long-term consequences 123
  treatment 122–123
blast injury 26
Blocksom vesicostomy 253
blue dot sign 219
blunt penile injury 179–180
blunt renal injuries
  complications and follow-up 14–15
    chronic pyelonephritis 18
    fistulae 18
    flank pain 18
    hypertension 17
    mortality 18
    post-trauma hydronephrosis 18
    renal insufficiency 16–17
    secondary hemorrhage 15–16
    stone formation 18

A Clinical Guide to Urologic Emergencies, First Edition. Edited by Hunter Wessells, Shigeo Horie, and Reynaldo G. Gómez.
© 2021 John Wiley & Sons Ltd. Published 2021 by John Wiley & Sons Ltd.
Companion website: www.wiley.com/go/wessells/urologic

urinary extravasation and perinephric
  abscess 16
diagnosis
  radiographic evaluation 6–9
  workup 5–6
epidemiology 3–4
etiology 3–4
management
  in children 12
  indications for intervention 10–11
  issues in operative technique 14
  non-operative management 9–10
  non-operative *vs.* operative management
    11–12
  operative technique 12–14
  predictors of failure of non-operative
    management 12
pathophysiology 3–5
blunt trauma 84–85, 132
boari flap procedure 113
bony pelvis anatomy 134
Buck's fascia 168
bulbar urethra 131
burns 181
  genital burn management 207
  penile injury management 181, 186

c
children, renal trauma management 12
Chlamydia trachomatis 234
chronic epididymitis 232, 236
chronic kidney disease (CKD) 159
chronic pyelonephritis 18
  clinical presentation 51
  management 52
  radiologic findings 52
civilian *vs.* military trauma 25–26
cloacal exstrophy
  antenatal diagnosis 255
  general principles for surgical repair 257
  initial management in neonate unit 255–257
  post-operative considerations 257
Cobb's collar 248
cocaine 191
cold knife valve ablation 252
Colles fascia 168
color Doppler ultrasound 216
color duplex ultrasonography 193
combat-related scrotal injuries 208–209
complete IVU 94
complete ureteral loss 113–114
computed tomography (CT) 6, 28, 30, 50,
    56, 70, 161
  acute pyelonephritis 43–44
  cystography 121–122
  gas in scrotal wall 171
  lower urinary tract injury 127

modality of choice 47
non-contrast 68
post-operative 106
renal infection protocol 43–44
traumatic adrenal injury 86, 87
ultra-low dose 78
XGP 51
concomitant injuries 92–93
congenital adrenal hyperplasia
    (CAH) 259
congenital obstructing posterior urethral
    membranes (COPUM) 248
contained hilar vascular injuries 6
contrast enhanced computed tomography
    (CT) 43, 107–108
contrast extravasation 94
corpora cavernosa 193
Corynebacterium sp. 234
costovertebral angle tenderness 67
COVID-19 pandemic
  consequences on urologic care 276–278
  immediate responses of urology
    departments 273–275
  surgical triage 274–275
  telemedicine 276
cremasteric reflex 219
CT cystography 122
cyanotic testis 225
cystography 121

d
Dartos fascia 168
deferred urethroplasty 138
delayed hemorrhage 15
delayed renal bleeding 35
deoxygenated hemoglobin S (HbS) 192
diagnostic endoscopy 96–97
diffuse hemorrhage 86
diffuse irregular hemorrhage obliterating the
    gland 86
dihydrotestosterone (DHT) 233
direct uretero-neocystostomy 112
direct vision internal urethrotomy (DVIU)/
    dilation 149
disorders of sex development (DSD)
    259–260
doxycycline 210

e
Eagle Barrett Syndrome 249
empagliflozin 169
emphysematous pyelonephritis (EPN) 45
  clinical presentation 47
  diagnosis 47–48
  pathogens and pathogenesis 46–47
  treatment 48–49

end-stage renal disease (ESRD)   254
enteric gram-negative rods   169
epididymitis   216–217
    and orchitis
        anatomy and physiology   232–233
        chronic epididymitis   236
        complications   240
        diagnosis   236–238
        epidemiology   233
        infectious epididymitis   234–235
        non-infectious epididymitis
            235–236
        pathophysiology   233–234
        treatment   237–240
epispadias exstrophy
    antenatal diagnosis   255
    general principles for surgical repair   257
    initial management in neonate unit
        255–257
    post-operative considerations   257
erectile dysfunction (ED)   190
erythromycin   210
Escherichia coli   234
excision and primary anastomosis (EPA)   150–151
external ureteral trauma   119
    anatomical considerations   91–92
    complications   101–102
    concomitant injuries   92–93
    diagnosis
        delayed diagnosis   96–97
        diagnostic endoscopy and urography   96–97
        diagnostic imaging   93–95
        intra-operative diagnosis   95–96
    management   97–98
        damage control surgery   100–101
        delayed management of injuries   101
        surgical principles   98–100
        ureteral contusions   98
    mechanisms of injury   92
external wounds   167
extravaginal torsion   218

f
"false" penile fracture   180
female genital masses
    imperforated hymen   264
    paraurethral cysts   260–261
    sarcoma botryoides   263
    ureterocele prolapse   260–261
    urethral polyps   263
    urethral prolapse   260, 262–263
female urethra   132
fistulae   18
flank pain   18
focal adrenal hematoma   86
follicle stimulating hormone (FSH)   211
fossa naviculares   131
Fournier's gangrene (FG)

bacteriology   169
clinical symptoms and imaging   170–172
epidemiology   167–168
etiology   168–169
treatment   171–175
Fournier's Gangrene Severity Index (FGSI)   170, 172

g
Gelfoam   33–34
gram-positive cocci   169
gross hematuria   121
GSW. see gunshot wounds (GSW)
gunshot wounds (GSW)   26, 92
    abdominal   92
    low-velocity   29
    management   184
    penetrating penile injury   180–181
    renal   30
    and stab wounds   184
    ureteral injuries   92

h
hematocele   207
hemorrhoids   167
heparin   191
heterogeneous parenchyma   221
Holmium fiber   252
human immunodeficiency virus (HIV)   159
hypertension   17

i
iatrogenic bladder injuries   121
iatrogenic ureteral injury
    etiology   105–106
    management   106–108
    outcomes and complications   114–115
    surgical technique
        boari flap procedure   113
        complete ureteral loss   113–114
        direct uretero-neocystostomy   112
        psoas hitch procedure   112–113
        trans-uretero-ureterostomy   113
        uretero-calicostomy   109–112
        uretero-pyelostomy   109–110
        uretero-ureterostomy   109–110
    timing of repair   109
iatrogenic urethral strictures   144
idiopathic strictures   144
imperforated hymen   264
infectious epididymitis   234–235
intentional injuries   25
intermittent testicular torsion   220
internal trauma   133
intratesticular hematoma   207
intravaginal torsion   217

intravenous pyelogram (IVP) 9
intravenous urography (IVU) 93
ipsilateral delayed pyelogram/hydronephrosis
      94–95
ischemic priapism 190–192

k

kidney stone management
   acute procedural intervention
      indications 74–75
      stone treatment 77
      upper urinary tract decompression 75–77
   history and physical 64–66
      additional relevant history 66
      diagnostic evaluation 67–71
      physical exam 66–67
   management of symptoms 71–72
      trial of stone passage/medical expulsion
         therapy 72–73
   medical dissolution therapy 73–74
   prognosis 77–78
   special considerations
      pediatric patients 79
      pregnant patients 78–79

l

lacerations penile 185
lichen sclerosus (LS) 144
luteinizing hormone (LH) 211

m

magnetic resonance imaging (MRI) 44, 52, 78, 106,
      147–148, 161, 181, 205, 221, 237, 255
male urethra
   anatomy of 130–131
   anterior urethra 131
   bulbar urethra 131
   innervation 130
   membranous urethra 131
   navicularis fossa 131
   penile urethra 131
   posterior urethra 131
   pre-prostatic urethra 131
   prostatic urethra 131
   sphincter complex 130
   urethral meatus 131
   vascularization 130
malignant priapism 192
medical dissolution therapy 73–74
membranous urethra 131
metachronous bilateral torsion 220
military trauma, civilian *vs.* 25–26
Mima polymorpha 234
Moormann's ring 248
mortality 18
Mycobacterium tuberculosis 234
Mycoplasma sp. 234

n

necrotizing soft tissue infection (NSTI) 175
negative-pressure wound therapy 173
neonatal testicular torsion 258–259
neonatal urological emergencies
   antenatal diagnosis and management 248–250
   disorders of sex development 259–260
   epispadias, bladder and cloacal exstrophy
      antenatal diagnosis 255
      general principles for surgical repair 257
      initial management in neonate unit 255–257
      post-operative considerations 257
   female genital masses
      imperforated hymen 264
      paraurethral cysts 260–261
      sarcoma botryoides 263
      ureterocele prolapse 260–261
      urethral polyps 263
      urethral prolapse 260, 262–263
   imaging diagnosis 250–252
   management of valve bladder syndrome 254–255
   neonatal testicular torsion 258–259
   posterior urethral valves 247–248
   post-operative management and long-term
      outcomes 254
   pre-operative management 250–251
   surgical management 252–254
non-infectious epididymitis 235–236
non-ischemic priapism 192
nonsteroidal anti-inflammatories (NSAIDs) 71–72
norepinephrine re-uptake inhibitor 191
nuclear scintigraphy 221

o

omphalocele, exstrophy of the bladder, imperforate
      anus, and spinal abnormalities complex
      (OEIS) 255
open primary realignment urethral 137
opioids 71–72
orchitis, epididymitis and
   anatomy and physiology 232–233
   chronic epididymitis 236
   complications 240
   diagnosis 236–238
   epidemiology 233
   infectious epididymitis 234–235
   non-infectious epididymitis 235–236
   pathophysiology 233–234
   treatment 237–240

p

paraurethral cysts 260–261
parenchymal renal lacerations 6
partial/complete lesions 140
pediatric patients, acute kidney stone
      management 79
pelvic fracture urethral injury (PFUI) 145

pelviperineal injuries   209
penetrating adrenal trauma   85
penetrating penile injury
   gunshot wounds   180–181
   stab wounds/amputation   181
penetrating renal trauma
   anatomy   26–27
   civilian *vs.* military trauma   25–26
   evaluation   28–29
   management
      complications   35
      non-operative   29–32
      operative   31–35
   pathophysiology   26
penetrating scrotal injury   208
penetrating ureteral trauma   92, 133
penile arteriography   193–194
penile blood gas testing   193
penile fracture. *see also* blunt penile injury
   initial evaluation   181–182
   management   183–184
penile injury
   avulsion   181
   bites   181
   burns   181
   penetrating. *see* penetrating penile injury
penile ultrasonography   193–194
percutaneous cavernosal spongiosal shunts   195, 196
periadrenal fat stranding   86
perinatal extravaginal torsion   220
perirenal hematomas   6
permanent atrophy testicular   227
persistent urinary extravasation   35
plain film cystography   120–122
posterior urethral valves (PUV)   247–248
post-stimulation LH   211
post-trauma hydronephrosis   18
post traumatic renal insufficiency   16–17
predictive amniotic fluid variables   249–250
Prehn's sign   220
priapism
   definition   189
   effects on erectile function   198
   epidemiology   189–190
   evaluation and diagnostic workup
      192–194
   ischemic   190–192
   non-ischemic   192
   stuttering   192
   treatment   194–199
primary adrenal insufficiency   86
primary blast injury, renal   26
primary endoscopic realignment   136–137
primary urethral realignment   136
prostatic abscess   161–163
prostatic urethra   131
prostatitis
   classification   158
   diagnostic imaging   161–162

   management   159–161
   presentation   158–159
   prostatic abscess   161–163
Prune-Belly Syndrome   249
pseudoaneurysm (renal)   15
psoas hitch procedure   112–113

q
quaternary blast injury   26

r
renal abscess
   clinical presentation   53
   epidemiology   52–53
   imaging   53–54
   laboratory diagnosis   53
   management   54–55
   microbiology   53
renal colic pain   64
renal contusions   6
renal hilar avulsion injuries   6
renal infections
   acute pyelonephritis
      clinical presentation   41
      epidemiology   41
      imaging   43–44
      laboratory findings   42
      microbiology and pathophysiology
         42–43
      treatment   44–45
   chronic pyelonephritis
      clinical presentation   51
      management   52
      radiologic findings   52
   emphysematous pyelonephritis   45
      clinical presentation   47
      diagnosis   47–48
      pathogens and pathogenesis   46–47
      treatment   48–49
   renal abscess
      clinical presentation   53
      epidemiology   52–53
      imaging   53–54
      laboratory diagnosis   53
      management   54–55
      microbiology   53
   tuberculosis of the kidney
      clinical presentation   55–56
      imaging   56
      laboratory findings   56
      treatment   56
   xanthogranulomatous pyelonephritis   49
      clinical presentation   50
      diagnosis and treatment   51
      imaging   50
renal injuries
   grade I injuries   6
   grade II injuries   6
   grade III injuries   6

grade IV injuries   6
grade V injuries   6
renal ultrasound (US)   70
renin-mediated hypertension   35
renorrhaphy   33
renovascular hypertension   17
retrograde pyelogram   253–254
retrograde urethrogram (RUG)   127
retrograde urethrography   127–128
ruptured arteriovenous fistulas (AVFs)   15

s
Saran Wrap   256
sarcoidosis   235
sarcoma botryoides   263
Scarpa's fascia   168
Schönlein–Henoch purpura   236
"Scout Film" Kidney, Ureter, Bladder
      (KUB) static radiograph
      120–122
scrotal skin injuries and scrotal
      reconstruction   205–207
scrotal ultrasonography   204
secondary blast injury   26
secondary hemorrhage   15–16
segmental arterial bleeding   15
segmental vessel injury   6
serotonin re-uptake inhibitor   191
SGLT2 inhibitors   169
"shattered" kidneys   6
sickle cell disease (SCD)   189–190
silent hydronephrosis   78
simple urethral catheterization   136
stab wounds, penetrating penile injury   181
stone passage/medical expulsion therapy   72–73
stone treatment   77
stuttering priapism   192
subcapsular hematoma   6
substitution ureteroplasty, using bowel segments   114
substitution urethroplasty   151–152
suprapubic cystostomy   138, 159
Surgicel   33–34
synchronous bilateral perinatal torsion   220

t
telemedicine   276
tertiary blast injury   26
testicular dislocation and testicular torsion   208
testicular rupture   207–208
testicular torsion   216
   diagnostic evaluation   220–222
   epidemiology   216–217
   management   222–226
   outcomes   226–227
   pathophysiology   217–218
   presentation   218–220
Testicular Workup for Ischemia and Suspected
      Torsion (TWIST) score   221

tile A fractures   135
tile B fractures   135
tile C fractures   135–136
torsed spermatic cord   224
trans-uretero-ureterostomy   113
transurethral procedures, for strictures   149–150
trauma during sexual activity   133
traumatic adrenal hemorrhage
   complications   89
   etiology
      blunt trauma   84–85
      penetrating trauma   85
   imaging   86–88
   management   88
   presentation   86
   relevant anatomy   83–84
   staging   85–86
traumatic anterior urethral strictures   144
traumatic penile injuries
   American Association for the Surgery of
      Trauma   179–180
   blunt penile injury   179–180
   initial evaluation
      amputation   183
      penetrating injury   182–183
      penile fracture   181–182
   lacerations   185
   management
      abrasions   185
      amputation   184–185
      avulsion   185
      bites   185–186
      burns   186
      gunshot wounds   184
      lacerations   185
      penile fracture   183–184
   penetrating penile injury   180–181
traumatic renal injuries   25
traumatic scrotal and testicular injuries
   AAST scrotal injury scale   202–203
   AAST testicular injury scale   202–203
   combat-related scrotal injuries   208–209
   considerations
      endocrine   211
      future fertility   210–211
      infection   210
      psychological impact   211–212
   general evaluation   203
   imaging   203–205
   management
      acute management   205
      hematocele   207
      intratesticular hematoma   207
      penetrating scrotal injury   208
      scrotal skin injuries and scrotal
         reconstruction   205–207
      testicular dislocation and testicular
         torsion   208
      testicular rupture   207–208

traumatic ureteral injuries   91
traumatic urethral injuries
   delayed management   140–141
   initial management   126–130
   management in the acute phase   140
   urethral trauma
      anterior urethra   139–140
      classification   132–133
      posterior urethra   133–139
      urethral anatomy   130–132
trazodone   191
tricyclic antidepressants   191
tuberculosis of the kidney
   clinical presentation   55–56
   imaging   56
   laboratory findings   56
   treatment   56
tube ureterostomy   100

u
ultrasound urethrography   147
Uludag Fournier's Gangrene Severity Index   170
unintentional injury   25, 91
upper urinary tract decompression   75–77
Ureaplasma urealitycum   234
ureteral contusions   98
uretero-calicostomy   109–112
ureterocele prolapse   260–261
uretero-pyelostomy   109–110
uretero-ureterostomy   109–110
urethral atresia   249
urethral contusion   140
urethral meatus   131
urethral polyps   263
urethral prolapse   260, 262–263
urethral rest   146
urethral stent   150
urethral stricture
   elective management
      transurethral procedures   149–150
      urethroplasty   150–152
   emergency management   148
   etiology   144–145
   evaluation   145–146
      magnetic resonance imaging
        147–148
      ultrasound urethrography   147
      urethro-cystoscopy   147
      urethrography   146–147
      voiding symptoms and uroflowmetry   146
   patient history and physical examination   145
   post transurethral procedures   153
   post urethroplasty   153
urethral trauma
   anterior urethra   139–140
   classification   132–133
   posterior urethra   133–139
   urethral anatomy   130–132
urethro-cystoscopy   147

urethrography   146–147
urethroplasty   150–152
uric acid stones   73
urinary extravasation and perinephric abscess   16
urinary tract infections (UTI). *see* renal infections
urine culture and sensitivity testing   160
uroflowmetry   146
urography   96–97
urologic emergency care, COVID-19 pandemic
      era   273–278
urologic neonatal emergencies
   antenatal diagnosis and management   248–250
   disorders of sex development   259–260
   epispadias, bladder and cloacal exstrophy
      antenatal diagnosis   255
      general principles for surgical
        repair   257
      initial management in neonate unit   255–257
      post-operative considerations   257
   female genital masses
      imperforated hymen   264
      paraurethral cysts   260–261
      sarcoma botryoides   263
      ureterocele prolapse   260–261
      urethral polyps   263
      urethral prolapse   260, 262–263
   imaging diagnosis   250–252
   management of valve bladder syndrome   254–255
   neonatal testicular torsion   258–259
   posterior urethral valves   247–248
   post-operative management and long-term
      outcomes   254
   pre-operative management   250–251
   surgical management   252–254

v
vacuum-assisted closure (VAC) therapy   174
valve bladder syndrome   254–255
veru montanum and utricle orifice   252
vesicoureteral reflux   249
voiding cystourethrography (VCUG)   254

w
warfarin   191
whirlpool sign   221
wound care   174
Wuchereria bancrofti   235

x
xanthogranulomatous pyelonephritis (XGP)   49
   clinical presentation   50
   diagnosis and treatment   51
   imaging   50

y
Yang-Monti tube   114
Y-Sober ureterostomy   253–254

Printed and bound by CPI Group (UK) Ltd, Croydon, CR0 4YY